WITNESSES FROM THE GRAVE

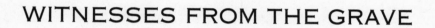

ALSO BY ERIC STOVER

The Breaking of Bodies and Minds
(*coeditor with Elena O. Nightingale*)

WITNESSES FROM THE GRAVE

THE STORIES BONES TELL

Christopher Joyce
and Eric Stover

Little, Brown and Company

Boston   Toronto   London

FIRST EDITION

The authors are grateful for permission to include the following previously copyrighted material:

Federico García Lorca, "The Ballad of the Civil Guard," from *Selected Poems*. Copyright 1952 by New Directions Publishing Corporation. Reprinted by permission of New Directions.

Excerpts from *Preludes* by Conrad Aiken. Copyright © 1966 by Conrad Aiken. Reprinted by permission of Oxford University Press, Inc.

"Last Will and Testament" by Ariel Dorfman, from *Missing — Poems by Ariel Dorfman*, published by Amnesty International, British Section, London.

LIBRARY OF CONGRESS CATALOGING-IN-PUBLICATION DATA

Joyce, Christopher, 1950–
    Witnesses from the grave: the stories bones tell / Christopher
Joyce and Eric Stover.
      p.   cm.
    Includes index.
    ISBN 0-316-47399-5
    1. Forensic anthropology. 2. Human skeleton. 3. Snow, Clyde C.
I. Stover, Eric. II. Title.
GN69.8.J69 1991
614'.1 — dc20   90-44068

10 9 8 7 6 5 4 3 2 1

MV PA

Published simultaneously in Canada by Little, Brown & Company (Canada) Limited

Printed in the United States of America

For the disappeared

"Death has two faces. One is nonbeing; the other is the terrifying material being that is the corpse."

MILAN KUNDERA
The Book of Laughter and Forgetting

And finally
when
the day
comes when they ask you
to identify the body
and you see me
and a voice says
we killed him
the poor bastard died
he's dead,
when they tell you
that I am
completely absolutely definitely
dead
don't believe them,
don't believe them,
don't believe them.

ARIEL DORFMAN, "Last Will and Testament,"
from *Missing — Poems by Ariel Dorfman*

CONTENTS

ACKNOWLEDGMENTS

Foremost among those who helped us write this book was Nancy Heneson, who shepherded our prose with acumen and compassion and kept it from wandering into uncharted territory. Jerry Snow's insights helped illuminate our main character, as did the assistance of Marguerite King at the Ralls Historical Museum. We would like to thank several friends and colleagues who reviewed earlier drafts of the book: Joyce Kornblatt, Richard P. Claude, Juan Méndez, Tom Gergely, Gerald Posner, Pamela Blotner, Martin Anderson, and Richard Joyce.

The American Association for the Advancement of Science, and its former executive officer, William D. Carey, enabled the work in Argentina described herein to take place, and Cristian Orrego of the University of California at Berkeley also lent knowledgeable assistance. Many in Argentina aided the project, especially Coche Pereyra and the Abuelas de Plaza de Mayo, the staff of the Movimiento Ecumenico de Derechos Humanos, María Julia Bihurriet, Mauricio Cohen, and Brian Thomsen. We would like to note Susana Méndez's bravery in driving us through the streets of Buenos Aires. We were also assisted by a research grant from the European Human Rights Foundation in the Netherlands.

David Marwell of the U.S. Justice Department, Ralph Blumenthal of the *New York Times*, and writer Richard White provided valuable information about the pursuit of Josef Mengele. Patricia Feeney of Amnesty International did likewise for the Bolivian episode. Of course, everyone who endured being interviewed for this book de-

ACKNOWLEDGMENTS

serves a thank you. So does Steve Rubin, computer wizard, for explaining how to route the words through the machinery. Kristine Dahl, our agent, and Karen Dane, our editor at Little, Brown, got us, respectively, into and out of this project, and William Phillips of Little, Brown fortunately decided it was worth doing.

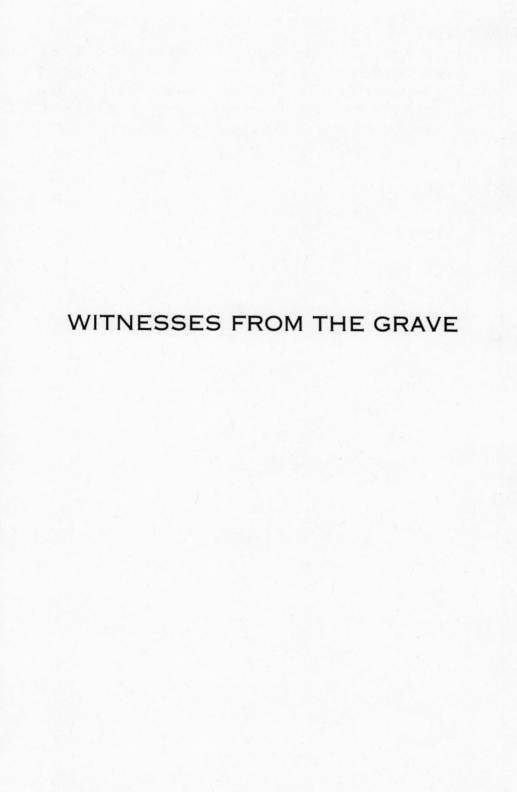

WITNESSES FROM THE GRAVE

PROLOGUE

ON a warm October morning in 1989, Clyde Collins Snow, his straw cowboy hat pulled low over his forehead, stood on a bluff overlooking the valley of Granja de Espejos in central Bolivia. Parrots flashed through the undergrowth near the escarpment. He could hear troops of monkeys chattering in noisy confrontation somewhere on the ridge behind him. Gazing down at the valley, he imagined this place, with its silver-braided streams and semitropical forests, as a kind of Eden. But as he had learned over the past few days, for the eighty or so men who lived in the whitewashed longhouses below it was more like Hell.

Snow had arrived in the nearby town of Santa Cruz a week before. He came as a scientist, but no ordinary one. He had no interest in curing the sick, discovering a rare plant or animal, or even publishing his findings in a professional journal. He was a forensic anthropologist, an expert who applied his knowledge of human skeletal variation to civil and criminal investigations. Few people practiced Snow's profession. Fewer still, no more than a handful, had ever used their skills as he had to expose atrocities committed by governments. And only Snow, the scientific detective, could offer the special kind of expertise demanded by the bloody events that had taken place in this valley amid Bolivia's cocaine country.

The American had come here to investigate the Granja de Espejos, a work camp — a prison without walls. Since 1967, Bolivian police had swept hundreds of boys and young men from the streets of their cities and dumped them in camps like the Granja. Some were the chaff from Bolivia's huge coca operation — addicts who, unlike the traffickers, inhale cocaine instead of selling it for export. Many others, however, were street kids, petty thieves, or what the law labeled as

3

"vagrants and miscreants." Older inmates at the Granja called them *palomillos*, or little pigeons. Many of them were addicted to *pitillos*, cigarettes rolled with coca paste, which they smoked to blunt their hunger and despair. Even if a palomillo had a family, they might never learn of their son's fate, or be able to challenge his imprisonment. Or even care.

Those brought to the Granja were never formally charged, never tried, never sentenced. They were sent there for rehabilitation, to learn self-discipline by working the fields and orchards and by tending the farm animals. They stayed a year or so, until they straightened out and kicked their habit. Unless they died first.

Snow arrived in Santa Cruz, a humid boomtown in Bolivia's heartland, on Thursday, October 12. He was met at his hotel near the city's main plaza by three young Argentine men, all members of the Buenos Aires–based *Equipo Argentino de Antropología Forense*, or Argentine Forensic Anthropology Team, the only group of its kind in the world. Thickset, over six feet tall in his Luchesse cowboy boots, Snow towered over the Argentines. Gravity was winning a battle with the contours of his face, abetted by the man's love of hard liquor and late nights. His accented Spanish bespoke a Texas upbringing. Deliberate in speech and gait, he moved like a timeworn battleship, the Argentines darting around him like tugs leading him to safe harbor.

Over the previous five years, in the graveyards and morgues of Argentina, Snow had passed on to this young team many of his skills, along with a few gems of west Texas wisdom. Now they had established themselves in a specialty of his making and had called on him to help in their latest investigation. The group repaired to a café near the hotel. Snow folded himself into a comfortable cane chair, lit his first cigarette of the day's second pack, and turned his gray gaze to Morris Tidball Binz. Tidball, a wiry, athletic man with the fair complexion and blue eyes of his English ancestors, described the course of the investigation so far. His colleague, Alejandro Inchaurregui, an intense, bearded man in his mid-thirties, ordered a round of coffee and a scotch for Snow. The third Argentine, Luis Fondebrider, an anthropologist and, not yet thirty, the youngest of the three, let his friends do most of the talking.

The Argentines had first come to Santa Cruz in early September.

Their host was a Bolivian human rights lawyer named Alejandro Colanzi. Since 1984, Colanzi had sought to reform Bolivia's one-hundred-year-old law that empowered the police to send most anyone they pleased off to the Granja, forty-four kilometers southwest of Santa Cruz, or to one of its sister camps near the cities of Cochabamba and La Paz. To bolster his case, he had interviewed dozens of former Granja inmates in his office at the *Centro de Estudios Legales y Sociales*, or Center for Social and Legal Studies, in Santa Cruz. They had told him of camp guards grown sadistic from boredom, of beatings for unexplained transgressions, and of executions and burials on a hillside cemetery they called the Plantanales.

Cruzeros, as the inhabitants of Santa Cruz are known, paid little attention to the Granja de Espejos until May 1987. That month a local newspaper reported that a young university student named Hernan Callau Flores had been shot while trying to escape from the camp. Months later, when the deceased's widow asked for the body to be returned for burial, the camp's superintendent, Luis Camacho, told her it had already been interred. Moving it, he said, would be an incovenience.

A year later, another inmate died at the Granja. He, too, had been shot while trying to flee. That, at least, was the official story. Former Granja prisoners, however, told Colanzi a different story. Edwin "Bubby" Parada Vaca, though a pitillo addict, was hardly the typical Granja inmate. He was a gifted university student, a poet, and, in the eyes of the guards, a troublemaker. He taunted the guards, calling them peons. He even organized his fellow inmates to demand better food and less work. Then one day he escaped.

Later that evening a guard named José Soliz took out after him. An unwritten rule at the camp held that when an inmate escaped, the guard on duty was responsible for capturing him — dead or alive. At noon the next day, Soliz returned with Bubby. Soliz marched the men to the camp football field where they watched as he beat the young poet with a rubber strap. When the boy collapsed to the ground, Soliz drew a pistol and fired into his twisted and bleeding body.

Bubby's murder, involving as it did a middle-class boy, drew more outrage than others that had been reported at the Granja. University students demonstrated, distributing leaflets demanding justice for their fellow classmate. Seizing the moment, Colanzi pressured the governor's office to investigate the camp. The guard Soliz, as it turned out, was eventually taken into custody and, in mid-1989, Colanzi was given permission to inspect the Granja and the cemetery mentioned in the testimonies of former inmates. In a matter of days, he had contacted Amnesty International in London, which, in turn, had referred him to the Argentine team.

In September Colanzi and the Argentines made the three-hour journey over dirt tracks and rain-swollen rivers to the Granja. At the camp's entrance, the group was met by Luis Camacho, a beefy and imposing man clad in a green, epauleted uniform and knee-high commando boots.

Camacho carefully inspected the delegation's papers and then led them on a tour of the camp. At times beaming unctuously under his bush hat, at others brusque and defensive, he showed them the living quarters, the open-air kitchens, the livestock pens, the duck pond, and the lemon groves. He even called the inmates to drill. Rousted from their cells, they stood at attention in ragged formation, their brown uniforms unwashed and torn. Camacho commanded them to run in single file to the outdoor mess, each clutching his own colored plastic bowl to his chest, for a helping of gelatinous green soup ladled out of a fifty-gallon drum.

Camacho denied that any prisoner had ever been beaten unnecessarily during his ten years at the camp. It was true that the law gave his guards the power to shoot escapees, and some had. But, he insisted, such incidents were rare.

When Colanzi asked Camacho if the delegation could visit the cemetery, he reluctantly led the group to the crest of a hill overlooking the camp. The Argentines walked down the row of graves, pushing aside small shrubs. Between some of the markers the earth had collapsed, forming shallow depressions. In all, they counted over sixty graves.

Two days later, the group returned to the Granja with the governor's legal-affairs director. This time they brought a new order, instructing Camacho to allow the Argentines to exhume graves at the cemetery. He took one look at it and ordered them out of the camp.

Back in Santa Cruz, the group, more determined than ever to nail Camacho, debated how to proceed. Colanzi, it was decided, would obtain a judicial order, something Camacho could not so easily dismiss. The Argentines, meanwhile, would return to Buenos Aires and enlist Snow, whose international reputation might give them more clout.

On October 10 — two days before Snow's arrival — the Argentines, along with Judge Hernan Cortez of the First Criminal Court of Santa Cruz and a troupe of journalists, returned to the Granja. Camacho, both outranked and seemingly outnumbered, conceded to the exhumations.

Under the noonday sun the Argentines marked out the boundaries of a grave. Its wooden cross bore the name Hernan Callau Flores. Starting at the foot of the grave, they dug down until they located the feet, giving them an idea of the body's depth below the surface. Within hours, they had scraped away the soil to reveal a skeleton. The grave's occupant, a male, had been buried facedown on a crude stretcher of wood and palm leaves. From the soil and vegetation in the grave, the team calculated that the burial had taken place one or possibly two years earlier.

The following day, the Argentines unearthed another skeleton, this one in an unmarked grave. He, too, had been buried facedown. He became, for the record, SC2. A third grave proved empty, but a fourth, which they designated SC4, contained another young man. A nearly illegible inscription on the cross read, "Escobar."

The team completed five exhumations and recovered four skeletons. With the assistance of several inmates, they packed the remains in wooden crates, carried them down the hill, and transported them by jeep to Santa Cruz. The lawyer Colanzi, Tidball explained to Snow, was now waiting for them to begin the laboratory work at a hospital morgue on the other side of the city.

For the next three days, Snow inspected and measured the Granja bones to determine each skeleton's sex, race, and age at death. He consulted mathematical tables for calculating stature from the arm and leg bones, and X-rayed each bone for signs of fractures and other abnormalities. For tools, he used only a hand-held magnifying glass, a pair of calipers, a pencil and paper, and a small calculator. Mindful that murder in a third-world country far from home was at issue, he carefully dictated a description of each step of the process into a microcassette recorder.

One of the skeletons, he determined, belonged to a boy of about fifteen. Another skeleton was of a twenty-four-year-old. His was the skeleton raised from the grave marked "Escobar." Turning over the left forearm and the finger bones of the left hand, he found several hairline fractures. Taken together, these were typical in cases where a person defends himself from a beating with a baton or club. He also saw similar fractures on the lower ribs on both sides of the skeleton. All were perimortem — wounds received at about the time of death.

On the skeleton taken from the grave marked Hernan Callau Flores, Snow found that a .22-caliber bullet — the guards at the Granja carried .22-caliber rifles — had blasted through a rib on the left side of the body and exited through another rib on the right side, leaving metal particles behind as a calling card.

The last skeleton told the most detailed story. Snow, a smoldering Havana cigar in one hand and his tape recorder in the other, held up the skull to the onlookers in the morgue and, as he described it, "parsed" its features. A small-caliber bullet, he explained, had entered the back of the head, a couple of inches behind the left ear. Traveling upward and to the right, it would have exited just above the right eye had it not spent its energy and lodged inside the skull. Tilting the skull downward, Snow let the bullet fall with a clatter to the floor. "What we have here," he said, "is a case of acute lead poisoning."

Picking up the left thighbone, Snow pointed to another bullet wound at the end where the bone forms part of the knee. "It looks as if he was kneecapped here and then finished off," he said. Indeed, inmates had told the Argentines that the man had been beaten and then shot in the leg. The guards had carried him up to the cemetery, dumped him facedown into an open grave, and shot him in the head.

Things happened fast after Snow's examination at the morgue. Judge Cortez ordered the arrest of Camacho and three of his guards. He also closed down the Granja, releasing the minors first. The remaining guards at the camp collected the other inmates, led them to the road to Santa Cruz and, giving each a few coins for bus fare, abandoned them. Meanwhile, a government official from the capital of La Paz flew to Santa Cruz and announced at a press conference that his government would reassess the system of agricultural labor camps and the police law that permitted detention without trial. Ca-

macho and several of his henchmen were jailed. As for the four inmates exhumed from the Granja cemetery, they were later identified
and returned to their families.

Curious to see the scene of the crimes, Snow spent his last day in
Bolivia on a visit to the Granja with Colanzi. The two climbed the
bluff above the camp where the cemetery lay and stood for a few quiet
moments looking down at the abandoned buildings. Reaching into
his jacket pocket, Snow pulled out a cigar, about as big around as a
shotgun barrel, and handed it to the lawyer. "You know," Snow said,
cupping his hand around a match, "back in 1979, I was pulled into
a case where I had to identify a bunch of boys killed by a psychopath
in Chicago. I never imagined that ten years later I'd be down here
doing pretty much the same thing." He paused, searching for the
right words that would sum up a lifetime of calling witnesses back
from the grave. "But there's a big difference in this case," he finally
said. "Camacho and his men murdered those kids with the power of
the state behind them. Now, for me, that's the worst crime of all."

PART

I

1

LESSONS IN THE
BONE TRADE

B Y the time he was six years old, Sonny Snow had shared a bed with most of the kids in Crosby County. An only child of a country doctor in the 1930s, he was nonetheless on roughhousing terms with most of the boys in this Texas county, and he knew the names of the girls' dolls and their pets and which kids got switched or not. He knew more than the local telephone operator about what went on in the townfolks' parlors and kitchens, about their joys and squabbles and their dust-bowl misfortunes.

Sonny's father, W.C. (for Wister Clyde) Snow, would call him down from his room, or if the boy was asleep, he would quietly bundle him up and carry him down to the car. His mother, Sarah Isabel Snow, would pack the linen, the medical instruments, some fried chicken and biscuits. The three of them would drive out into the plains of the Texas panhandle, a land as flat as sheet metal where the summer air rises in ripples and the "blue northers" of winter can deliver a deadly front of frozen air like a flash flood over a salt flat. The back seat of the black Chevy sedan was Sonny's domain. When they traveled by day, he read books on Indians or the adventures of Davy Crockett or the battle of the Alamo. Tiring of that, Sonny would watch for jackrabbits, roadrunners, and prairie dogs or count the silhouettes of the windmills.

Sometimes they'd drive for hours among the fields, their car disappearing into an ocean of frothy cotton plants, visiting one farmhouse or tenant shack after another. W.C. would pull the car up to a house and Sonny would climb out and stretch and pet whatever dog offered itself while his father talked quietly with the farmer or his wife. With W.C. carrying his medical bag and Isabel bringing whatever else was necessary for the job at hand, the couple would enter the sickroom — the bedroom in winter, or, if the weather was hot, perhaps the cool shade of a screened front porch. As often as not, "Dr. Snow" or "Doc," as the country folk called him, knew the patient by his or her Christian name, and he knew that a touch on the shoulder and small talk about the good cotton crop or last month's rodeo was as powerful as most store-bought medicine. Sonny, meanwhile, would poke around the house, meet the kids, or just play with the dog. If it was late, he'd be tucked into bed with the kids.

The Texas panhandle was a dusty place in the 1930s, so dry, people would say, that the bushes followed the dogs around to get a little moisture. Most people who lived off the land had no choice but to live simply. W. C. Snow was one of two doctors in the town of Ralls back then. He delivered a couple of thousand babies during his sixteen years in the panhandle, charging twenty-five dollars total for delivery and pre- and postnatal care. There were plenty of broken bones to set as well. And with so much dust in the air, pneumonia carried off a lot of folks. With pneumonia, before the advent of sulfa drugs or antibiotics, there wasn't much one could do but just sit with the family and make small talk until the fever broke or death came. Sonny Snow saw a lot of new life come into the world, and quite a lot of tired life take leave of it.

Highway 82 linked Ralls with Lubbock, twenty-seven miles to the west and the nearest big town. The railroad kept Ralls's thirteen hundred or so inhabitants supplied with goods and news from towns like Fort Worth and Dallas to the east. Rodeos, football games, church suppers, and the Crystal Theater, the town's only picture show, provided about the only entertainment available. Once in a while, a carnival or medicine show would roll in. For the men, there was a combination domino and pool parlor, and on Saturday afternoons in the summer they played softball in the dusty park across from the town square. Crosby County was "dry," but liquor was easy to find since bootleggers were so thick they had to make signals to keep from selling it to each other. During the Depression most people hunted jackrabbits to eat without thinking much about sport.

The Snows lived in town above the "Clinic," which besides the doctor was attended by his wife. Isabel had come to Texas from Wisconsin to work beside her husband. She was a Yankee from a devout Irish Catholic family who married one of two doctors in a Texas way station of a town full of cowboys, cotton farmers, and Baptists. But Isabel, an outspoken, hardworking woman, made the rounds, tended the wounds, and helped bring forth the babies. In the hardest years of the Depression, W.C. would work for nothing but an IOU. Isabel and Sonny would spend days driving from farm to farm, walking the rows of cotton plants to find the farmer, asking if maybe he could manage five dollars or so for the services Dr. Snow had rendered to his kin.

Often, W.C.'s payments came in the form of barnyard animals, either dressed or on the hoof. Word around Crosby County also had it that the Snows would raise any critter as a pet. So Sonny acquired something of a menagerie. He had a lamb called "Eleanor," whose teeth were as big and white as her namesake, Eleanor Roosevelt. During hunting season farmers stopped by the two-story brick house on the town square to leave wounded wildlife — a sparrow hawk, a golden eagle, a prairie dog that Sonny named Oscar and carried around in his jacket pocket, a raccoon, an opossum, and a steady flow of wild ducks. On hot summer afternoons, if someone remembered to turn on the sprinklers in the town park, the Snows' mixed flock of shot-crippled mallards, redheads, and pintails would cross the street in a leisurely file for a shower.

The Snows were bookish by Ralls standards, and Sonny regarded a trip to the bookstore in Lubbock as a treat. But if the boy was clever in school, he also had earned a reputation for doing what he damn well pleased. And his father indulged him, sharing with Sonny his knowledge of medicine and his love of the spare land. Riding in the car, W.C. would point out the dry gullies and copses where he hunted dove and quail, and name the mesquite, scrub cedar, and the sharp-bladed yucca.

As for the local inhabitants, the desolation of the place seemed to breed extravagant personalities, as if, like the yellow blossoms on the prickly pear cactus, they were compensation for the land's topographical plainness. Boys in the panhandle were raised on tales of Texas royalty, the oil and cattle barons who out-owned and outspent the richest Yankees, people like the Irishman P. H. "Pat" Landergin, who followed the cattle trail to Texas to found the one hundred-thousand-acre XIT ranch in Oldham and Deaf Smith Counties. The house that Landergin built, over twenty rooms in brick under a green glazed terra-cotta roof in neoclassical and Georgian splendor, was surely the finest home in Amarillo.

Perhaps no one captured Sonny's world better than Bob Wills. Texas loved Wills, though then only a princeling of western swing. Folks in Ralls, doing their wash or weekend chores, regularly tuned their radios to Wills and his Light Crust Doughboys, who were broadcast from Saginaw, near Fort Worth. The band was sponsored by the Cargill Burrus Mill, whose flour inspired the band's name. The Doughboys toured Texas and the southwest in a custom-built bus and hit most towns, large and small. Ralls occasionally stood in their path, and the band would set themselves up atop a flatbed truck and make a one-night stand of it. Sonny never missed a show.

In the autumn, W.C. and Sonny spent a lot of time hunting. Around Ralls there were birds to shoot — ducks on the lakes that dotted the panhandle, doves around the ponds, and in the rugged canyons, fat bobwhite and blue quail. In November, Sonny and his father made an annual trek to New Mexico to hunt the big mule deer amid the pine and juniper in the mountains west of the Pecos River.

It was on such an autumn trip, near Silver City in New Mexico, that Sonny saw his first skeleton.

Sonny was only twelve years old in 1940 but already had experienced more of death than most kids; his friends even called him "Little Doc." He knew the quiet way an old rancher passed in the night when his father's medicines offered no cure. He had felt the pall of grief settle over a home when a baby was stillborn. Standing silently in the background, he had seen that absolute stillness of a body that meant life had flown.

A group of hunters came to the lodge in New Mexico where Sonny and his father were staying and asked to see the doctor. The men said they had found something up in the next canyon. It must have been something strange, Sonny thought, because men at hunting lodges didn't normally talk so quietly. Then his father walked over to him. "Looks like they've found a skeleton up in the woods," he told his son. "Let's go have a look."

The local deputy sheriff joined the group, and they hiked over to the other side of the mountain, about a half hour's brisk walk through pine forests and over granite bluffs. The hunters said they figured the bones were human. But they had seen other bones in with them that maybe weren't human. It was pretty hard to tell exactly what they were, they said. Finally, the hunters led them down an embankment to a thicket near a clearing and pointed at something in among the roots and dessicated leaves.

Sonny's father squatted over the heap, freeing one bone after another from a netting of rotted clothing. The bones looked like brown tree branches to Sonny, who wondered why they weren't white, like the skeletons in comic books and movies. Apparently these hadn't been exposed long enough to the elements to have been bleached. The hunters peered over his father's shoulders, keeping a respectful silence as the expert performed his examination. The doctor said nothing, letting his eyes do the work. He stood up finally and turned to them.

"Yeah, they're human enough. And these here, mingled in with them, are deer, a good-sized buck judging from the size of the antlers. This guy probably shot it somewhere in there," he said pointing away from the road toward the dense undergrowth, "and tried to haul it out by himself. Probably had a coronary."

They went through what was left of the pockets in the body's clothing looking for something that might identify it. All they found was a set of keys. The deputy sheriff had a hunch, though, that the body might belong to a fellow who lived in Silver City, a regular hunter, who had disappeared a couple of years before. Dr. Snow and Sonny went with the deputy sheriff into town. They drove straight to the hunter's house. The deputy sheriff walked up to the front door and knocked. No one answered, so he tried one of the keys they'd found. It fit the lock perfectly.

It is a story that Sonny has told many times during his life, especially when asked about his first experience in forensic anthropology. He always remembered how straightforward it seemed. You just had to know what kind of bones belong to what kind of body. Essentially, you needed to know the basics before taking the first step in solving a mystery. After that, things sort of fell into place.

An educated man, Sonny's father had to practice more than just medicine. Folks believed Dr. Snow, as someone who had graduated college and medical school, to be a deep thinker, a man whose intellect gave him insight into cause and effect in a world that so often made little sense. In Sonny's view, his father was actually like a detective called in by the citizenry not just to set a fracture or to calm a fever, but to put an explanation on what was cockamamy, cussed, or mysterious.

Murder was something that required such an expert's hand. About the same time that Sonny saw his first forensic case solved, someone murdered a man in Lorenzo, another apostrophe of a town just west of Ralls. Lorenzo stretched all of two blocks. Its most notable building, the bank, sat on a corner of Main Street. After the bank's bookkeeper, twenty-two-year-old Irvin Bownds, was found one afternoon in the vault with his throat cut, Dr. Snow was called to examine the body and Sonny tagged along. They found poor Bownds laid out in the funeral home, located on the second floor of the furniture store (the two businesses shared a common need for wood and carpentry and were often joint enterprises in those days). Establishing death and its cause took little more than a glance. Figuring out how and when it was done, and by whom, however, proved beyond the skills of Dr. Snow and everyone else who worked on the case.

The bank closed every noon. Bownds regularly left the bank and walked home for lunch and to listen to the 12:30 news on KFYO, the local radio station. He was always the first one back to work, entering through the side door. He would bring the cash out of the vault for the afternoon's transactions, then unlock the front door at one o'clock with the punctuality that banks normally look for in their accountants.

When Woodrow Watts, the bank's accountant, walked through the front door at one o'clock on the fateful day, the place was empty. It being a small bank, Watts shortly discovered Bownds in the vault. His throat was slit in three places and blood was splattered everywhere. One thousand four hundred and eighty-seven dollars was missing.[1]

The general store was located directly across the street from the bank, and its front porch provided a daylong meeting place for local loafers who in the town vernacular were known as the "Spit and Whittle Club." No, they hadn't seen anyone come or go during the lunch hour, they told Dr. Snow. The bank and the vault held no clues, and nobody looked guilty. The doctor was as mystified as everybody else. The FBI eventually sent someone in to nose around town, but the crime was never solved.

Ralls didn't usually offer such tantalizing mysteries. But at least there was chess. Sonny learned the game from Dave Schein, thought to be the only Jew in Ralls at the time and one of its leading eccentrics. Schein had escaped Russia through Turkey and eventually got a job as a newspaperman in New York City. He drank jubilantly, which kept him on the move until he ended up working on the newspaper in Ralls. He lived in a back room at the newspaper's office and painted signs to supplement his income. Schein taught chess to Sonny, whom he regarded as bright and aggressive enough to make a good player. Sonny didn't disappoint him, and soon was winning games, although not without some risk; Schein had a habit of knocking the board over "accidentally" if he fell behind too quickly.

Dr. Snow gave his son a long leash, and Sonny used every inch of it. Once, just before Christmas, he took his wrapped gifts from their hiding place and X-rayed them in his father's clinic to see what was inside. Even his father was fair game for tricks. "One of the things I would do," Snow remembers from his childhood, "would be to wait until he was delivering a baby. He'd added a wing to the house, putting in about five or six beds so that women would come to have their babies there and we wouldn't have to be up all night all over the county. He'd have his hands all gloved up, so I could walk in while he was delivering, and I'd stick my hand down his pocket and get a quarter or two. And there wasn't a damn thing he could do about it."

Eventually, one of Sonny's pranks ended his days in Ralls. As a sophomore in high school, he and his best friend, Charlie Dial, made special preparations for a school visit by the superintendent of schools for the state of Texas, a mighty man in the estimation of most folks in Ralls, whose impending visit caused much ado at the high school. Minutes before the superintendent's arrival, Sonny and Charlie hid two dozen firecrackers in several lockers and inserted each fuse into

19

the butt end of a burning cigarette. The prank succeeded beyond their expectations when multiple explosions and chaos ensued. Justice was swift: Sonny and Charlie were given the choice of corporal punishment or expulsion. They chose the latter.

Life changed abruptly. Packed off by W.C. to the New Mexico Military Institute in Roswell, Sonny left Ralls, his family, and even his nicknames behind. He became Clyde Snow and the lowest of creatures in a world of spit and polish. He had no idea what to make of himself, although he did learn to ride, since the institute was among the last military institutions in the 1940s to still maintain that men on horseback made the best soldiers. For two years, Snow, a gangly six-footer with jug ears and a quick wit, turned in a most lackluster academic performance. Then he met Abe Cornell, who transformed Clyde the country boy into a scholar.

Cornell, from Albuquerque, was everything Snow wasn't — an excellent athlete, an outstanding scholar, and a shrewd, albeit somewhat unorthodox, entrepreneur. Snow drew Cornell as a roommate, and his recollection of the man remains sharp:

> Everybody was always short of money. Our allowance was two dollars a week. Abe lent money at some exorbitant rate. He was a big guy, very tough, and established his reputation pretty fast. When he came to collect, he also carried a blackjack.
>
> One of the big things in military school in those days was the annual "GI inspection" by a team of officers sent down from Washington, D.C., to rate military schools all over the country. Getting ready for it was incredible. We would start a week before. We had to scrub our rooms, shine brass, clean rifles. We were up until three or four o'clock in the morning. Everything, you see, had to be perfect.
>
> One of the big things was to have the floors just gleaming. A troop would put in their money and go down and rent waxers and sanders, because during the year we were throwing cigarettes on the floor, and you'd get these black marks on those nice oak floors. They'd send somebody down to two or three places in Roswell and rent the sanders and waxers. But one year, I think it was '44 or '45, everything was the same all over town. These sanders and waxers were reserved. Who were they

reserved for? "Well," they'd say, "a cadet named Abe Cornell came in here about a month ago, you see . . ." It turned out Abe had every sander and waxer in Roswell tied up. And he was charging something outrageous per hour or minute or something. It didn't make him very popular.

Cornell took Snow into his confidence. In addition to being a businessman, Cornell led his class academically. So he taught Snow how to study. He showed the kid from Ralls how to keep notes on three-by-five cards, indexing the important points and condensing them so that three cards eventually became two, and two shrank to one. They spent evenings drilling each other from the cards.

"At first, it was sheer drudgery, rote memorization," explains Snow. "Sometimes he would keep me up until two or three o'clock in the morning, quizzing me with those goddamn three-by-five cards. If I got sleepy or rebellious, there was always that damn blackjack!" But when the mid-semester grades came out, Snow astounded his instructors and himself with straight A's.

Snow stuck to the Institute for four years, which put him through the equivalent of his second year of college. He'd become a pretty good rider, although a horse once fell on him, leaving a trace of gimpiness in his walk. At least it kept him off the polo team, which was always getting whipped by a bunch of local Mexican ranch hands. "Those Mexicans were just a pickup team," Snow remembers with some fondness. "They worked for a local rancher, and they beat everybody. No uniforms, just mangy-looking guys on ranch horses." In their starched uniforms astride their high-strung ponies, the boys from NMMI found these defeats particularly humiliating.

Snow had done well enough in class to overcome an abysmal high-school record, and he took the entrance examinations for Harvard, which accepted him. He had a commission to fulfill, however, and he spent that summer at Fort Hood, Texas. Meanwhile, Charlie Dial, his fellow incendiary from Ralls High School, was partying hard at Southern Methodist University in Dallas, where Snow spent his weekends. Harvard was far away, Snow thought, and Texas was swinging. Snow decided to enroll at SMU.

Far from Cornell's blackjack, Snow lapsed into his old ways. He spent more of his time in Dial's yellow Cadillac convertible at Sybil's, a Dallas drive-in with roller-skating waitresses in shorts, than he did in classes. By the end of his second semester, he had tallied about eighteen hours of F's. Thence began an odyssey through college campuses in the southwest. Snow squeaked into the only college that would have him, Eastern New Mexico State, a campus in the middle of nowhere that offered few temptations. He earned a bachelor's degree in 1951 and moved on to Texas Tech in Lubbock, shooting for a master's degree in zoology. Before he finished, he decided to switch to medical school at Baylor in Houston. Medical studies failed to interest him, however, and two years later he quit and went back to Texas Tech. He passed up an offer to transfer to Iowa State to study physiology — a fortuitous decision, he remembers, as he heard later from some of the students there that they spent much of their time making bulls ejaculate. He got his master's in zoology in 1955.

Snow's college ramble might have continued indefinitely had the draft board not intervened. In 1954 his number came up at the board's Roswell office. Alarmed, he reported to the board, but after a few minutes contemplating life as a grunt in green fatigues, he walked next door to an air force recruiting office. There he found that his zoology degree qualified him to become a clinical laboratory officer. He signed up on the spot.

His orders were to appear for swearing in at 8:00 A.M., April 1, 1955, just over five months from then, in Montgomery, Alabama. But the army wanted him now. He walked back to the draft board to explain his predicament. They were unsympathetic. Come November 15, he was going to be a G.I., he was told.

Doubting the army's power to do such a thing, Snow returned to Lubbock and called Congressman George Mahon, then head of the House Appropriations Committee and the congressman for Snow's district. Mahon said he'd put in a word in the right places. Some very long hours passed, during which Snow compiled a long mental list of things he hated about governments. Then he got a call from an air force colonel at the Pentagon.

"Don't quote me on this," the colonel warned, "but we don't give a damn what you do between now and the first of April. If you walk into Montgomery at eight o'clock on April 1, you're going to be sworn in as a second lieutenant in the Air Force. So get lost."

Over five months to go, Snow thought. The army seemed determined to have him, and surely would track him down. Where could he "get lost"? Where better than in the rugged wilderness where he and his father had spent so many summers, up in his family's cabin in Ruidoso. Snow packed up his Chevy with bourbon, canned food, and long underwear and vanished into the Sacramento Mountains of southern New Mexico. He had never wintered there before and half froze to death, keeping warm most of the day by chopping wood to burn through the night. Even then, a glass of water left out by his bedside grew a cloudy crust of ice on its surface by morning. When he wasn't chopping, he buried himself in blankets and books, the latter a hodgepodge of detective stories, a complete John Donne, a portable Faulkner, some Dickens, and of course tales of the chapped and frozen land that lay outside his window and the desperados who had, like him, disappeared now and then into its crenellated valleys and scarps.

Snow stayed undiscovered, and on March 31, 1955, he thawed out the car and roared nonstop to Montgomery. The air force took him in, and he spent three years as a clinical laboratory officer. It may have been uneventful, but at least he didn't have to march around with a rifle. Toward the end of his commission, he wrangled an early discharge by promising to go back to college.

As a graduate student in archaeology at the University of Arizona, Snow spent a good part of his time roaming the countryside digging in the dirt. But southwestern archaeology consisted primarily of collecting and examining bucketfuls of potsherds. As much as he enjoyed fooling around in the dirt, working under someone else could get exasperating. He had learned a few lessons during his time at Texas Tech from a man named William Holden. Holden, as Snow describes him, was a "cowpoke" with an archaeology degree who enforced a strict code on his digs. For example, students could use only number-two pencils; if Holden found any other writing utensil, he usually broke it. Students proved themselves by how much dirt they could move, carefully. On Snow's first outing, he was quickly challenged.

We had found a cistern, which the Indians had dug, maybe about 1,000 A.D., to store rainwater. It must have been about fifteen feet deep and about six feet square. The Indians dug them out and plastered them and diverted water into them. Old man Holden got the idea that he wanted to dig out one of these things. Well, they were filled with sand. You'd get down in there, with no breeze, and you'd have a shovel, and maybe a handful of sand would make it out from each shovelful. You see, if you screwed up on the site, that's where you'd get sent.

Eventually, we got it cleaned out. Holden got up on the edge, took a picture down inside there, then turned to me and said, "Okay, fill 'er up." He told us that if we didn't fill it in again, the ranchers would lose a steer down there and there'd be hell to pay.

Holden's unadorned professionalism stuck with Snow the rest of his life, as did his habit of putting his students' devotion to the test, although Snow was never quite as harsh in his demands. Archaeology did not stick, however. Snow was still dabbling. By now, switching academic tracks was second nature to him, so he moved into anthropology, something more akin to his training in zoology. The university sent him to Puerto Rico for a year to study rhesus monkeys, a species of primate he learned to dislike heartily, he remembers, because of its unrelenting, noisy obnoxiousness. The pace of life in Puerto Rico agreed with him, however.

Snow knew well enough that physical anthropology, the study of evolutionary changes in the human skeleton, rewards very few of its disciples with wealth or fame. Except for fossil-hunters such as the Leakey family and Donald Johanson, who through genius, cunning, and good fortune have pried several of humanity's ancestors from the African earth, most anthropologists labor quietly in classrooms. Snow most likely would have followed that path, for he tended to drift from one course to another, directed by circumstances, and remaining happy as long as his curiosity could be satisfied. Had anyone told him that someday his name would be synonymous with a scientific discipline which in that day barely existed, or that he would fly to faraway cities to track down Nazis and help put dictators in jail, he would have scoffed.

Proud of the breadth of his interests, Snow was still a Ralls boy at heart, just intent on having a good time. He rode like a cavalry man, chased skirts, and could do major damage to a fifth of Jack Daniels.

If the devil came to take names, beside his name would go not "Ph.D" but "Texan."

So things stood when Jerry Snyder, an old classmate of Snow's, called him in Puerto Rico one day in 1960. Snyder had done his graduate work in anthropology at Arizona with Snow and was now employed by the Federal Aviation Administration. He had racked up a distinguished combat record as a P-51 pilot in Korea, then decided to return to academic life in physical anthropology. Snyder asked his former classmate if he remembered the midair collision of the TWA Super Constellation and United Airlines DC-7 over the Grand Canyon in June 1956. Sure, Snow replied. Snyder said it had prompted the government to lay aside some serious money for aviation safety research. There was a job for Snow in Oklahoma City, Snyder said, at his new laboratory in anthropology at the FAA's newly built Civil Aeromedical Institute (CAMI). Snyder was running the physical anthropology lab and needed someone who understood the human body and could help redesign airplanes and anything else that humans used in the business of flying airplanes. Snow could finish his dissertation (on the growth and physical development of the savannah baboon) while at the FAA.

Snow had had enough of monkeys and black beans. He took the job, saying good-bye forever, or so he thought, to the Spanish language that he never had quite been able to wrap his Texas tongue around.

During the 1960s, the FAA was generous to the institute, and the scientists at CAMI got just about whatever they wanted. Their mission was to translate aviation medicine into standards for the airlines. The anthropologists built and brutalized dummies in simulated crashes in order to better the design of passenger and pilot seats, or they helped engineers construct consoles around air-traffic controllers. They also did more traditional anthropological work, taking batteries of physical measurements on pilots and others in the aviation trade to provide engineers with data.

The work had its light moments; Snow once spent months measuring stewardesses. The idea seemed reasonable to him. CAMI was supposed to help the FAA set standards for the design of the interiors of planes. They had to make seats that fit right, cabinets at the correct

25

height, and emergency equipment that young women could manage. Working stewardesses had been complaining of frequent injuries in aircraft accidents. Many of the injuries could be traced to the shoddily designed protection and survival equipment allocated to them, well below the standards of equipment enjoyed by the male pilots. Deadly sideways-facing jumpseats and poorly anchored restraint harnesses topped the list. In low-impact accidents, passengers were being overcome with deadly fumes and fire, and Snow reasoned that wherever one found dead stewardesses, one would find a lot of dead passengers.

Snow threw himself into the work, compiling over a hundred body measurements for each of 423 stewardesses during the spring of 1971. For his work with the tape measure and calipers, the project earned the uncoveted distinction of being one of the first to win the Golden Fleece award, an honor given on an irregular basis by Senator William Proxmire to scientific projects paid for by the taxpayer that Proxmire deemed a waste of money.[2]

Some of Snow's duties were grim, however. It was part of CAMI's job to study air crashes, and it was an anthropologist's expertise that the institute needed to determine what happened to a plane's passengers after it fell out of the sky.

Few events provoke as much public shock as an air crash. The perpetual tabulation of deaths by auto, accident, or crime accumulates victims comparatively slowly, and the victims aren't all in one place at one time. The image of a downed plane, however, captured in newspaper photos and flashed repeatedly across the country's television screens, tends to rivet people to the event and unhinge the imagination of anyone who has ever flown. Who cannot have wondered what it must be like during those last horrible seconds? Moreover, big crashes happen too infrequently to grow boring the way floods in India or slayings in urban America do. And unlike some of the victims of crime or auto crashes, who may have contributed to their own undoing, casualties of plane crashes are presumably just decent, ordinary people sitting in the wrong place at the wrong time.

Like archaeologists re-creating the past from rubble, the experts at CAMI sifted through the wreckage of broken planes and bodies to extract fact from tragedy. Depressing work, it also intrigued them, like a puzzle whose pieces, when finally arranged through careful deduction, spell out messages in code. These messages could then be hammered into hardware or procedures that could save lives the next time.

The work fascinated Snow. Scientifically, methodically, he reconstructed momentous events from tiny clues, using his knowledge of human form and behavior. In fact, these re-creations exercised the same skills that constitute the backbone of forensic science. Most people associate forensic science with the investigation of crimes. Crash investigations by teams of specialists from CAMI did not involve a "crime" as such, unless sabotage was involved, but technically they were legal matters in that the law requires determination of the cause of each accident.

CAMI's investigators operated much the same as police scientists. They worked in teams, not only identifying the cause of crashes but sometimes the victims and their cause of death. Pathologists might determine whether most passengers in a fatal crash died of trauma, fire, or smoke inhalation. Meanwhile, a toxicologist might burn materials found in the passenger cabin to determine what kind of gases could have been produced by fire. Engineers would search the wreckage for signs of structural or engine failure.

When fire or the sheer violence of a crash either burned bodies beyond recognition or dismembered them, it fell to the anthropologists and odontologists, the savants of bone and teeth, to try to identify the victims. True, airlines keep records of who buys tickets and boards their aircraft. But for legal purposes, such as settling an estate or an insurance claim, identities should be confirmed by a medical examiner or coroner. These authorities are usually hesitant to sign a death certificate without a body. Besides, as Snow and the other investigators learned, the person named on an airline ticket isn't always the same person who boards the aircraft. An injured athlete might turn over his or her ticket to a teammate; business people charging their companies for trips with spouses fly instead with secretaries or lovers.

For Snow, part of the excitement of accident investigations was getting there. Jerry Snyder had bought a World War II–surplus P-51 Mustang and had converted it into a two-seater. Snyder and Snow would fly "Phoebe," named after Snyder's wife, all over the country, Snow crammed into a back seat so tight there wasn't enough room for him to wear a parachute. Snyder explained that a chute wouldn't do any good anyway because there wasn't space to squeeze around the front seat and out of the cockpit should he feel the need to bail out. "He'd just grin and say, 'Trust me, Clyde,' " Snow remembers. "I went ahead and trusted him, but I always wondered why *he* wore a chute."

Snow spent much of his time during crash investigations interviewing survivors and piecing together a picture of the inside of the plane during a given crash. For example, did seat belts adequately protect the average passenger in a "survivable" accident such as a forced landing? What, in fact, was the shape of the "average" passenger? How would a seatbelt fit over a pregnant woman? Would it hold the unusually corpulent, say, someone whose weight put him above the ninety-fifth percentile of the population, that is, among the fattest 5 percent?

One survivable crash, of a United Airlines 727 in 1965 at Salt Lake City, provided the CAMI group with an idea for saving lives that has yet to receive a full hearing among aviation experts. On November 11, the plane pancaked and skated off the runway. It quickly caught fire and forty-three of the ninety-one people aboard died. Few people suffered injuries on impact; as is often the case in such crashes, most who died succumbed to smoke inhalation. Ernie McFaddin, a respiratory physiologist at CAMI, and Snow, sitting in a motel room near the airport, got to kicking around the idea that, as Snow describes it, "if you just had a sack over your head you'd have a few minutes to breathe and get out of the plane."

CAMI let the two scientists pursue the idea. McFaddin rigged up a treadmill and had people put plastic bags over their heads to see how long they could breathe comfortably. He and Snow also searched for a material that wouldn't burn, settling for a while on Mylar, a tough synthetic made by DuPont that resists flame. They fiddled with various designs and materials, testing one after the other on their long-suffering volunteers on the treadmills. Snow eventually moved on to other projects. The airlines were never very thrilled about the idea anyway. But McFaddin stuck with it for years, eventually creating a "smoke hood" with drawstrings that theoretically would give a passenger precious seconds of air to make an escape from a burning plane. The airlines balked, arguing that reaching under the seat for

28

the bag and putting it on would slow passengers down. The smoke hood never got off the ground.

The first accident that Snow investigated involved a United DC-8 that crashed at Stapleton Airport in Denver on July 11, 1961. It was a survivable landing, but eighteen passengers died. Back at CAMI, McFaddin put together a mock-up of the fuselage and ran volunteers through it to see how fast people could get out. Snow watched this little drama for a while and decided to apply a little scientific methodology to the question of why some people survive such accidents and others don't. It was the sort of problem he had begun to enjoy, worthy of lengthy thought and analysis in the classical inductive manner of drawing conclusions dispassionately from the facts.

Snow drew on the methodology of fellow scientists in another discipline, toxicology, for a rough model of how to examine fatalities in air crashes. Those who examine the effects of substances on organisms apply a measure called the LD50 to the poisons they study. To measure accurately the toxicity of a chemical, one must administer it to a large group of organisms, usually laboratory mice, rather than just a few, because each organism may respond differently. A commonly used measure of a chemical's toxicity is the dose at which it kills half of the animals. That dosage earns the name LD50, "LD" meaning lethal dose, "50" representing the percentage killed at that dose. Chemical toxicity can be characterized by LD25 and LD75 as well. Although toxicologists now attempt to substitute tissue or even computer models, testing on live animals was usually the only method available in the 1960s.

Snow and colleagues Jack Carroll from the National Transportation Safety Board and Mackie Allgood at CAMI applied the LD50 concept — retrospectively, of course — to the crash environment.[3] They carefully monitored the number of survivors from three air disasters: the Denver and Salt Lake City crashes, and another in Rome on November 23, 1964, a TWA flight, in which forty-eight of seventy-three occupants died. "All three of the accidents had this in common: that impact injuries were nonexistent or minimal," Snow explains. "So it was a pure problem of getting from your seat to your exit." In each, fire erupted in the passenger cabin. The crash in Denver represented a "thermotoxic environment" that could be labeled

29

an LD25 — it killed fewer than 25 percent of the passengers. The passengers' environment in Salt Lake City represented an LD50, while in Rome it was closer to an LD75.

In those days CAMI had plenty of money, and when one of their scientists got excited about a new project, he or she had free rein to follow it to its conclusion. Snow dogged his project for about two years. Using the ticket lists, which included diagrams kept by flight attendants of who sat where (now replaced by computer lists), he plotted where everyone had been sitting in relation to exits. He recorded the passengers' ages, sex, and whatever else he could find out about them. He studied the survivors' official statements and interviewed some as well.

Some of what he discovered didn't surprise him. People who sit nearest the exits, all other things being equal, had a better chance of getting out. Other findings required more sophisticated statistical analysis. Looking at the range of ages and sizes of the passengers on each flight, for example, Snow wondered if there might be something unexpected that would indicate that some had an advantage over others.

What he determined, and presented in a scientific paper for a meeting of the Aerospace Medical Association in St. Louis in 1973, unsettled his superiors at the FAA and, in Snow's words, landed him in "deep shit."

"Males get out," Snow concluded. "Businessmen who fly a lot, they get out. The odds are roughly two to one in favor of adult males. There's a lot of physical stuff going on in there and they certainly do not behave like gentlemen. Another thing is traveling companions. That is significant in that if you are traveling in a group, family groups tend to do a little better. Blood relatives are more likely to help each other. Age-wise, it amounts to the fact that if you are under twelve years old, forget about it, only about 10 percent of them get out, at least in the 1960s. And if you are male over fifty-five, you survive about the same as females do. As the toxic environment becomes more extreme, as in the Rome crash, age, sex, and experience become less important for survival."

The FAA's administrators were horrified. Children don't survive? The public would blanch at this cold portrayal of jungle law aboard the nation's air carriers. Characteristically, Snow hadn't pulled any punches, and although the FAA couldn't find fault with his statistics, they demanded that he soft-pedal the paper's conclusions. They were particularly indignant at the literary grace note in Snow's preface, something that perhaps as bureaucrats they neither appreciated nor fathomed.

"I used a quotation," Snow says, "a little piddling thing, the old Hippocratic aphorism, 'Life is short and Art long, the occasion instant, decision difficult, experiment perilous.' " It fit his conclusions, Snow thought, because the crashes present the passenger with just such an instantaneous occasion and difficult decision. Moreover, the paper referred to the crashes as "natural experiments" for the scientist. It was an observation not without regret over the loss of lives; nonetheless, the nuance was lost on the FAA, who said it suggested that commercial-aviation accidents were an "experiment." Snow would have to withdraw the paper. He refused. In the end, Snow missed the conference, although he eventually published the paper.

Snow spent the next decade locked in a love-hate relationship with the FAA. The big budgets continued long enough and Snow's professional reputation grew strong enough to allow him to be indulged, to follow paths of his choosing often enough to keep his disdain for governmental rules under control. A believer in the adage, Don't get mad, get even, Snow attacked through his wit. He was quick with the civil servant's sidearm, the memo, and a stream of them flowed from his office, a practice he called "hustlin' the monkey." Their combination of dry sarcasm and blunt force, a blend one might expect from a scientific mind formed from the clay of northwest Texas, made them collector's items among the appreciative civil servants whose lives had been circumscribed within margins drawn in red ink.

One memo to a senior official at CAMI is representative. Dated August 14, 1970, over Snow's signature, it reads (with the victims' names deleted for obvious reasons):

I have been informed that, during the recent meeting in Washington, a great deal of time was consumed in an argument between you and Dr. ———— concerning whether sharks are attracted to their victims by smell or by taste.

After pondering the question, it occurred to me that it could be easily and economically settled by a simple experiment. This would entail placing you and Dr. —— in the CAMI survival tank, introducing a large shark to the tank, and observing its behavior.

If the shark attacks Dr. ——, it will be evidence that it cannot smell; if it goes for you, it will be equally obvious that it has poor taste. In either event, the experiment would answer an important scientific question with very little expense to the government.

If you concur, I will be happy to prepare a form 1750 for this project.

In addition to his job at CAMI, Snow lectured on physical anthropology at the University of Oklahoma, which further strenghthened his reputation in the field, at least locally. Had he worked in a city in the East, he might never have polished his bone craft to the point where he could point the science in new directions. In urban centers such as New York or San Francisco, as Snow has observed, sophisticated citizens may be inclined to tolerate or ignore many forms of bizarre behavior, but they are apt to draw the line at decomposition.[4] Thus a body in such environs rarely gets the chance to reach a state that would interest an expert in skeletons. But Oklahomans spread themselves like pollen across the dry plains. When someone disappeared over the horizon, he sometimes wasn't found until the body had gone the way of all flesh, leaving nothing behind except an image in the memories of friends and relatives and a bagful of bones. Also, under the Oklahoma sod lay Indian burial grounds, occasionally unearthed when earthmovers prepared the land for another road or shopping mall. At such times, it required the expertise of someone who knew that a pair of shovel-shaped incisors or a skull's prominent cheekbones suggested a long-dead Indian and not Uncle Bobby who went out for smokes three years before and never returned.

Before long, the staff of the medical examiner's office in Oklahoma City took notice of this anthropologist, and Snow started spending more of his time with the M.E.'s staff. The Charons of central and western Oklahoma ushered those who died violently or suspiciously into the afterlife through the portals of a rundown one-story building in a desolate part of town. Like most morgues, it was purposely nondescript, though unmistakably official in its foursquare stolidness, as if the corpses somehow had to be reassured that their exit from the world would be handled through official channels. When the police dropped by with a box of mysterious bones, the authorities would flip through their file cards to find the number for Clyde Snow, that tieless, unmade bed of a man in boots who always arrived late and usually brought along a dog. Snow himself jumped at the chance to escape the strictures of the FAA now and then, and he slipped easily into the role of cowboy professor and expert-on-call.

In 1967, the Oklahoma medical examiner, Dr. James Luke, brought Snow into an investigation that had stumped the M.E.'s office.[5] As in Snow's first experience with a skeleton as a boy in New Mexico, it was hunters who first alerted the authorities to something suspicious in the woods.

Hunters occupy a special place in police investigations. Apart from those who accidently kill themselves, other hunters, innocent passersby, or surprised livestock, hunters occasionally call in the police when they stumble across the remains of people who breathed their last in the woods. These hunters did exactly that. On November 19, hoping to bag dinner for Thanksgiving, they had been stalking quail near an abandoned farmhouse on the southeastern outskirts of Oklahoma City when they stumbled across a skull and some other bones in the brush. Curious, they took the bones home to compare them with illustrations of human skulls in an encyclopedia. Realizing the importance of their discovery, they called the police the next day and led them to the site.

There, the police found more bones, mostly fragments of ribs and vertebrae, and a child's dress, all located about 150 feet south of the vacant farmhouse. In the sandy soil at the center of a thicket lay a shallow depression. It was a makeshift grave, dug only about eighteen inches deep, and it yielded more bones, a mass of tangled hair, and a badly deteriorated piece of a child's underwear. The investigators returned the next day and performed a meticulous search over about a hundred acres, dividing the area into rectangular plots measuring two hundred by one thousand feet. Some fifty volunteers, equipped with probes and rakes, combed every plot. Search parties examined nearby ditches, culverts, and wells, while a small grader skimmed the surface vegetation from a forty-by-forty-yard area around the shallow grave. They even searched badger holes and coyote dens within a mile or two of the grave.

The field, located on Reno Road, was thickly overgrown with weeds. A truckload of bones could be lying unseen and they'd never find them, thought Bill Forney, a police investigator on the case. He called Snow at the FAA for advice.

"I was thinking," he asked the professor, "would it hurt anything if we burned those weeds? Would it hurt the bones?"

Snow reasoned that the kind of heat generated by that kind of fire probably wouldn't destroy any osteological evidence. It was a calculated risk, for a fire might burn other evidence, but they had already found what the person most likely had been wearing. He told Forney to go ahead. But Forney couldn't get the fire department to agree to it. So he and his team spent the next two days on their hands and knees picking through the underbrush.

The authorities probably would not have mounted this Herculean effort had the city not already been agitated over a tragedy that had occurred a little over four months before. A child of five, known in court documents only as Anna, had disappeared on July 6. She had last been seen playing near her home late in the afternoon. Exactly four weeks later, another child, a six-year-old named Brenda White from a suburb several miles south of Oklahoma City, also disappeared. Her bicycle had been found in an alley behind a neighborhood grocery. Later, one of her playmates said she had seen Brenda in a car with a young man with light blond hair, although she could not describe the make or model of the car. Neither Brenda nor Anna had been found on that day when the hunters excitedly called the police.

The massive search garnered bags full of bones, ranging from delicate shards from field mice to a piece of a horse's skeleton the size of a baseball bat. Snow was given the job of sifting through this brittle detritus for more clues. He knew that skeletal identification of a child posed one of the most difficult challenges to an anthropologist. Underneath the skin and tissue, young children are remarkably alike. Certainly the size of the skull suggested a child. But getting the sex right on a child's skeleton can be especially trying. Most of the classic markers of gender, such as the shape of the pelvic opening or the features of the skull, are "secondary" sexual characteristics, that is, they don't usually develop fully until puberty.

At his lab at the FAA, on an aluminum examining table under the harsh fluorescent light of the tiled examination room, Snow laid out the bones. They made up about one third of a human skeleton. Most important so far was the skull, although the mandible, or lower jaw, had not turned up. Also important were two ribs; a left fibula, one of the two bones of the lower leg; and the right femur, the long bone of the thigh. The femur was a bonus, being the best bone to use to calculate a person's height. Snow carefully placed each in the position it would have occupied in the living person. Down the middle of the table he arranged several cervical vertebrae, the part of the spine that forms the neck. Below these he placed several thoracic vertebrae, those that articulate with the ribs. As the police brought in more bones, Snow added more pieces to the skeleton, like an archaeologist reassembling pieces of broken pottery. Two gently curved clavicles, like slender boomerangs, formed what had been the child's shoulders. The ribs, almost all recovered, filled out what had been the thorax. Snow also had the two humeri, the bones of the upper arm, and at least one of the two bones, the radius and ulna, of both lower arms. Unfortunately, the pelvic bones were missing, along with the smaller bones of the hands and feet.

Presumably, the bones belonged to Brenda, whose mother had recognized the hair and the dress found at the site as her daughter's. If a suspect were ever found, however, refuting this tenuous identification would hardly tax the skills of an experienced defense attorney. Luke needed a clear indication, one way or another, of whether this was either Brenda or Anna, or bones from both girls. It was even within the realm of possibility that they were from yet another girl whose disappearance, for one reason or another, had not been reported.

The thoroughness of the search assured Snow that this was all he was going to get. Bearing in mind the forensic scientist's axiom that the first case you blow is likely to be your last, he set to work.

Without pelvic bones, the long hair and dress found at the make-shift grave had to suffice as evidence that the victim was female. The hair was slightly wavy and the strands were thin and lightly pigmented, the best evidence Snow had that the body belonged to a Caucasian. Snow also was reasonably certain that these were not Indian bones, for an incisor tooth that had not yet erupted from the maxilla, the upper jaw, lacked the shovel shape that occurs in at least 80 percent of Indians.

Snow picked up the skull, inverted it, and peered into the cavity. Packed in with some sandy dirt were cobwebs and some dead insects. He made a mental note of this as he mounted the skull on a craniostat, an aluminum stand made specifically for such work, and took a long look at the visage. The relatively large brain case but small face were those of a child, an opinion he confirmed with his calipers by taking twenty measurements at different points on the skull. Holding the skull close and squinting through his horn-rimmed, hand-held magnifying glass, he slowly scanned the sutures, where the separate bones of the cranium join. When viewed under a magnifying glass, or even by the naked eye, the sutures traverse the cranium in tight, looping switchbacks, the way a river meanders back and forth across a delta. The clues to age don't lie in the undulations, however, but in the degree to which the sutures have closed.

The cranium of a newborn child is like an egg whose shell has been broken into several pieces, then glued back together so that the joints show. Bone being a living tissue, however, the cranial pieces slowly, but on a regular schedule, expand and close the joints. Like a camera, death forever freezes this dynamic process in a snapshot from which the anthropologist gleans details of that instant. Snow could see clearly that the occipital bone at the back of the skull, which at birth is in four pieces, had completely fused, an event that normally doesn't take place until a person reaches four or five years of age.

Snow had also read the work of T. Dale Stewart of the Smithsonian Institution, among the living masters of forensic anthropology in the 1960s, and other experts who had listed other parts of the body where such snapshots of growth and change could be found. Among these are the shafts, or diaphyses, of the arm and leg bones. None of the shafts that Snow held up to the light had yet fused completely with the knobby ends, or epiphyses. That suggested that the victim had to be younger than about fifteen. Similar assessments of fusion in parts of the vertebrae narrowed the age to between five and twelve years.

With some help from an odontologist, Snow then mapped which teeth had erupted. Even though many of the teeth had not been found, X rays of the sockets revealed whether permanent teeth still lay embedded in the jaw, a code that could reveal the child's age. Tooth and bone agreed: this was indeed a child, who died somewhere between five and a half and eight years of age.

As for height, Snow consulted standardized tables that equate the lengths of long bones to a person's overall stature. The femur and humerus on the examining table brought the examination one step closer to its bitter conclusion: they belonged to a child of about four feet in height — 49.5 to 52.5 inches, to be exact.

By now, Snow had spent almost two weeks piecing together the skeleton. He had dragged his textbooks down to the morgue and, except for consultations with doctors, dentists, and teachers who had known the two missing girls, had spent most of his waking hours turning the bones over and over, either with his hands or in his mind's eye, as the press stood watch daily outside the M.E.'s office. The case also brought to light some of Oklahoma's more unsavory characters. "I swore I'd never work on a case like that one again," investigator Forney remembers. "We had one hundred and thirteen calls the first day of the investigation. They all said that their brother or their uncle had molested them or their sister at one time or another. I didn't know there were so many child molesters out there until this thing happened."[6] And there also were two families hanging on every new piece of information.

From a strictly forensic point of view, the case had one thing in its favor — it was "closed." That is, there was a suspected victim against whom the bones could be compared. In open cases, with no putative victim, there are no dental records, photographs, or descriptions to use as yardsticks.

Little literature on estimating the height of children from bones existed; measurements of cadavers had been performed on what was available in morgues, but these were most often adults. However, studies of prehistoric populations and some European research provided enough data to suggest strongly that the bones were Brenda's, who was 51 inches and 6.7 years of age when she disappeared. Anna, short for her age, stood only 42 inches at 5.8 years of age.

But one thing about this case made Snow hesitate. Two girls had

37

disappeared, perhaps kidnapped and disposed of by the same person. What if both girls had been killed and buried together? Was there any way to tell?

Snow tried a bit of mathematical sleuthing. He reckoned that there are only about forty-six bones from a six-year-old that are sufficiently large and rugged enough to be recovered in these circumstances and assigned correctly to their position in a skeleton. He had before him twenty-two of these bones, and no two were the same. Adding the four vertebrae found by the search parties to the equation, he had over half the number of bones that could have been found. What were the odds, he asked himself, that these bones actually came from two girls if he had over half the "findable" bones in a child's skeleton without a single duplication? By Snow's calculation, the chances were one hundred to one — good enough to posit that these were almost surely the remains of only one child.

One more question remained. Brenda could have been dead only a maximum of four and a half months. How could everything but hair and bone have disappeared so quickly? Snow knew from a pair of previous local cases involving two sets of skeletonized remains that flesh decomposes quickly in the heat of Oklahoma's summer. In fact, he had calculated that one of these two bodies had been stripped of tissue at a rate of 2.9 pounds per day, the other, exposed during the more forgiving coolness of spring, at a rate of 0.9 pounds per day. The forty- to fifty-pound body of a child would be skeletonized within six weeks at that rate, certainly fast enough so that these could be Brenda's bones.

Brenda had disappeared the previous summer; her skeleton would not have spent a winter in the open. Nor had the bones on Snow's examining table. They showed none of the lacework of cracks that freezing temperatures etch on the surface of bone. Moreover, there were no signs of the delicate gnaw marks of rodents. While they occasionally feed on carrion, rodents generally ignore bones until they are at least a year old. And those cobwebs and dessicated insects that Snow had seen when he first looked inside the skull now had new meaning. The skull would have to have been skeletonized early enough in the year so that spiders and insects could have moved in, ruling out death in autumn.

Three weeks after he saw the first bone, Snow handed in his report to the M.E.'s office. Although it was the M.E.'s job to declare the results, Snow was confident that the hunters had in fact found Brenda's remains. It was the most exhaustive forensic investigation he had ever undertaken. Two other findings resolved the question of identity. The hair they recovered from the grave was long, except for a small portion that measured only about three inches in length. Brenda's mother recalled that a few months before she disappeared, Brenda had fallen off her bicycle and cut her head. The wound required stitches, and the doctor had shaved the hair over the cut. Furthermore, a photograph of the girl, smiling, showed a set of front teeth that matched the teeth in the skull.

As is often the case in forensic science, the satisfaction of sealing a case with calipers and calculator was no occasion for joy. No suspect had been apprehended, nor was any sign ever found of Anna. Whatever value could be wrung from the episode was the affirmation that science, when all else fails, could serve as ombudsman of death. Being of poetic mind, Snow later would draw not on scientific metrics to remember the Oklahoma child disappearances, but the meter of poetry, by quoting from "Time in the Rock" by Conrad Aiken:

> . . . what can we learn from you
> pathetic ones, poor victims of the will,
> wingless angels who beat with violent arms . . . ?
> O patience, let us be patient and discern
> in this lost leaf, all that can be discerned;
> and let us learn, from this sad violence learn,
> all that in midst of violence can be learned.

By the end of the 1960s Snow had married and divorced three times, fathering four daughters. As he sometimes says of himself, "I remain loyal to the end, but I reserve the right to change my mind at the last minute." In 1968 he was languishing in one of his unmarried periods, spending a good deal of time at the university. One February day, sitting and smoking in the student union in his blue workshirt, faded denim jacket, and khaki pants, he was discovered by the woman who would be the fourth (and present) Mrs. Snow. He could have passed for a student as he hunched over a book, *Field Guide to the*

Birds of Texas. A mutual friend, who had met Snow when she found the wallet he had recently lost, introduced the two. What he saw was a vivacious, dark-eyed graduate student engulfed in waist-length brown hair, fur-trimmed jacket, boots, and several pounds of Indian jewelry around her neck and arms. She called herself Jerry, and was one quarter Native American, from the Sac and Fox nation.

Jerry misunderstood the introduction, and thought this burly fellow with the lashless, hooded eyes and long sideburns was with the "FFA" — the Future Farmers of America — instead of the FAA. He looked a bit old to be starting a career in farming, she thought. They smoked and talked, and it became clear to Jerry that he was no farmer. On the other hand, he didn't say just exactly what he did. Nor did she tell him much about herself, not even her last name. After about an hour of sizing up one another, Snow offered to drive her to wherever she happened to be going. She accepted and he drove her home, but when he asked for her last name and phone number, she replied breezily, "It's in the phone book."

Snow tracked her down of course — he liked nothing better than a mystery to solve, especially when the mystery was a woman. She accepted when he asked her out. Driving on their first date, he stopped the car suddenly and jumped out to race after a snake. He caught it and brought it back to the car as if to test her mettle, only to find that this woman wasn't much frightened by snakes, which further raised her in his estimation. They dated several times, including one date for which Snow turned up three days late, before Jerry Whistler discovered that this man was a professor at the university. She admired and shared his passion for local history, and took him to Indian powwows, where Snow was often pulled aside and warned that Sac and Fox women possessed strong powers for both healing and hexing. It didn't put him off any. He was charming, she thought, even if he forgot to cut his hair for months at a time and constantly brought lost animals back to his house.

Clyde and Jerry were married in 1970. Snow forgot to buy a ring, so Jerry suggested before the ceremony that he might go down to the local jewelry store and pick one up. He returned with a gold ring that wouldn't have stayed on her thumb. After the wedding she went back to the store and traded it in for one that fit.

The Snows moved into a house in the country that had been built as an experiment by architecture students at the university. It wasn't too expensive and placed them in splendid isolation on the prairie. Animals turned up at the doorstep regularly, often with Snow's assistance, as if the place were some kind of Ellis Island for the wayward. They named the dogs after towns in Texas, such as Burkeburnett and Paducah. Cats got the names of movie stars; their first was Vincent Price. Snow would sit at the dinner table and pick the white meat off his chicken and feed it to the assembled throng. At various times there was an opossum that had been hit by a car, assorted snakes, and turtles. He once adopted a tarantula that he named Coalgate, after a town from which the police had brought him a skeleton. Snow had removed a boot from the skeletonized foot but before reaching into it to retrieve some loose bones he decided to upend it. Out fell Coalgate.

2

CORPUS DELICTI

Blunt trauma.
Shotgun wounds.
Hypothermia.
Electrocution.
Hanging and strangulation.
Autoerotic sadomasochistic sex hangings.
Incisions, chop, stab, or laceration.
Drug overdoses.
Poisoning by ingestion or inhalation.

SO many ways to die. Many of us do so under suspicious circumstances; the list above names only a few. And just because death follows life as surely as ashes a fire, we nonetheless demand an explanation whenever there is some doubt as to the cause and manner of its coming.

Forensic scientists have become our archivists of death. They record how many of us spend our final minutes on Earth. The popular conception of the forensic pathologist mirrors Yeats's advice, inscribed on his tomb: to cast a cold eye on life and death and "pass by." Because the circumstances of death can imbue even the drabbest lives with at least a few moments of high drama, however, the forensic scientist sometimes plays the liveliest role, sweeping in at the moment of greatest confusion to help solve the mystery. In theatrical terms, he or she might be the "fifth business," a sort of human catalyst who ties together the loose ends of an unraveled plot.

Perhaps the earliest forensic scientist can be found in one of the many apocryphal tales of the Roman empire. In A.D. 66, Nero's mistress demanded that the head of the emperor's wife be brought to her on a silver platter to prove that she was indeed dead. When the head appeared, an adviser to Nero's court convinced the doubting mistress by pointing out the discolored tooth that was the empress's salient facial characteristic. Centuries later, at the dawn of another empire, the American hero Paul Revere similarly identified the body of General Joseph Warren. Besides being a horseman in the right place at the right time, Revere practiced dentistry. He confirmed the identity of the corpse through a silver and gold bridge he had fashioned for the general two years earlier.

Until the latter part of this century anyone who applied the principles of science to the law could claim the title of forensic scientist. Since no formal body existed under Anglo-Saxon laws to certify forensic specialists, almost anyone from the ambitious amateur to the outright charlatan could label himself an expert. The only formal title available to the death investigator was coroner (from the French *corounne*, for crown). As supervisor of the Crown's pleas, the coroner represented the king in legal matters. Among the coroner's duties was assessing and collecting taxes, including a death tax; even leaving the world had a price, at least for the deceased's relatives. Coroners were among the first to arrive on the scene when someone died, and took charge of investigating circumstances surrounding suspicious deaths.

Medical expertise was not required of the coroner, who was elected and usually a friend of someone in power. Thus coroners usually got their information from questioning witnesses rather than examining corpses. The system was haphazard and sometimes corrupt. Jürgen Thornwald, one of the most accomplished historians of forensic science, describes one such "hopelessly defective" system in the United States:

> Among the coroners elected in New York between 1898 and 1915 were eight undertakers, seven professional politicians, six real-estate agents, two barbers, one butcher, one milkman, two saloon proprietors, and so on. The undertakers were presum-

ably the most knowledgeable of the lot, but they were notoriously unwilling to spoil the bodies consigned to them by performing autopsies. After all, they liked to show the family a good-looking corpse. The occasional doctors among this motley crew were heavy drinkers or failures at their profession. Some Brooklyn coroners were reputed to make it worth someone's while to push the drowned bodies that drifted almost daily in Newton Creek between Brooklyn and Queens over to the Brooklyn side. For every inquest was worth between twelve and fifty dollars to the coroner.[1]

Boston was one of the first large jurisdictions to abandon the coroner system for a more scientific approach. New York City followed in 1918 with its Medical Examiner Bill. Medical examiners, many of them trained in Europe in both forensic science and pathology, managed to hold off the backlash from outraged coroners and established basic rules for on-the-scene investigation and autopsies in suspicious or violent deaths.

States and cities outside of the East were slow to follow Boston and New York out of the antiquated coroner system. To their credit, however, many coroners, especially in large cities, hired experts in pathology, toxicology, ballistics, and other specialties to assist them. Indeed, forensic subdisciplines proliferated like spring mushrooms. Meanwhile, courts and police departments were discovering that good science could aid them in winning convictions, and they helped build bridges between the forensic sciences, criminology, and jurisprudence. By the middle of the twentieth century, scientists became a common sight in the precinct house and the courtroom.

Most investigations involving a body begin with an attempt to determine the cause and manner of death. The distinction between the two terms is important. An autopsy may reveal that the cause of death of a man fished from a river is asphyxiation due to his lungs' filling with enough water to halt breathing. If, however, the cause also is found to have involved an obvious blow to the head with a crowbar, after which the unconscious victim was fitted with concrete shoes and stuffed into a burlap bag, the investigation takes on an added air of urgency. It also helps investigators determine the manner of death. There are five possibilities: homicide, suicide, accident, natural, or undetermined.

As with most scientific disciplines, no single incident marks the beginning of forensic anthropology. But as astronomy credits Galileo's demonstration that the sun does not revolve around the Earth or biology Darwin's and Wallace's theory of natural selection, forensic anthropology likewise records a handful of events in the nineteenth century that paved the way for modern practitioners. Unlike Galileo's calculations or Darwin's globe-trotting treasure hunt of species, however, it was murder and mayhem, beginning with the case of George Parkman, that sparked the advance of this science.

The week before Thanksgiving, 1849, in Boston, Massachusetts, Dr. George Parkman, M.D., a Harvard man and a distinguished graduate of the University of Aberdeen, Scotland, paid a fateful visit to a colleague at the Harvard Medical College. The tall, spare figure of Parkman, adorned in a stovepipe hat and a long coat whose tails fluttered behind his angular frame, was a familiar sight at the university, to which he was a benefactor. His reputation arose not from his medical practice, which was minimal, nor his writings, which had focused on lunacy and the humane care of lunatics, but from his real estate holdings. He spent much of his time collecting rents and lending money at interest. However, he had donated land to the university in 1846 on which a building for the new medical school was erected. He was brusque and officious, yet said to be generous with his considerable inheritance, not only to Harvard but to the poor. At the time, Boston was blooming with a rapidly multiplying population of immigrants, most of them Irish fleeing their country's potato famine, to whom Parkman dispensed medical care as well as money. Whether considered ruthless or philanthropic, however, Dr. Parkman was most commonly known by his physiognomy. Students and faculty alike privately referred to him as "Chin," a nickname derived from his strongly protruding jaw.

Parkman had a special mission on Friday, November 23: to collect a debt. His efficiency and meticulousness in bird-dogging his debtors was legendary and had even earned him a reputation as "aberrant."[2] His appointment that day was with Dr. John White Webster, another well-known Bostonian of apparent breeding. Webster was a burly, gregarious man, possessed of a massive forehead, broad shoulders, and a large appetite for the good life. He held a professorship of chemistry and minerology, had a medical degree, served as editor of several medical publications, and was a member of various learned societies. His respectability, however, thinly veiled a profligacy that nurtured some of the university's juicier gossip. He spent well but not wisely and consequently fell frequently into debt, borrowing what he could not earn on a professor's salary to live in the style that so many of his peers considered the norm.

Webster owed quite a bit of money to Parkman, and the Chin was not one to confuse business debts with charity. By 1849, Webster's debt amounted to $2,432, more than his annual income of about $1,900 from his salary and fees from students. Parkman, owner of mansions and scion of a wealthy family of merchants, might simply have bided his time had he not recently heard that Webster had tried to sell a portion of his mineral collection, which he had already mortgaged to Parkman to cover his debts. Professor and M.D. he might be, but Webster was not especially clever: the man he had offered to sell to was Robert Gould Shaw, Parkman's brother-in-law, who promptly informed Parkman of Webster's desperate gambit. Infuriated, Parkman vowed he would lay down the law to this spendthrift.

Parkman spent Friday morning shopping. He bought a head of green lettuce, quite a luxury at the time, and proceeded to Paul Holland's grocery store in the West End, where he bought more groceries. He left all his purchases at the store, promising to retrieve them shortly. He never returned. Apparently, the last people to see Parkman were two schoolboys, who spotted him striding in the direction of the Medical College.

When Parkman failed to return home Friday evening, his wife contacted Shaw, who quickly advertised his brother-in-law's uncharacteristic disappearance in handbills and the city newspapers. In one notice Shaw suggested that "some sudden aberration of mind" must have diverted Parkman's steps to parts unknown. Word of the disappearance of such a prominent personality spread quickly, and on Sunday, after taking his family to church, Webster called on Parkman's brother, Rev. Dr. Francis Parkman, to report that he had met the doctor by appointment the preceding Friday at Webster's office at the medical college. "I paid him the debt I owed," Webster insisted, after which, he said, Parkman had hurriedly left his office.

Certainly a man in Parkman's business would have attracted a healthy share of resentment, which could only have been fanned by his acerbic manner. But no one had such a ready-made motive for getting rid of him as Webster. Discomfort over his debt would have been especially distressing in Brahmin society, which tolerated a man who owed millions but disdained a petty chiseler whose most valuable asset was a collection of rocks. Yet throughout the week Webster showed no sign of guilt, dining as usual with his family, making holiday visits, and playing cards with his neighbors. He even experienced a rare moment of generosity, giving his janitor at the medical school, Ephraim Littlefield, a Thanksgiving turkey, the first he had ever given the man in seven years of service. Littlefield would soon repay the gesture in a most unusual way.

Naturally, the police had searched the laboratories at Harvard Medical College, including Dr. Webster's, located next door to the dissecting room and close to the river, from which, presumably, fresher breezes would carry the odor of chemicals away from the campus. They found no clues. The day after Thanksgiving, however, Littlefield conducted his own clandestine search. His hunch, formed over the previous few days, led him to the stone vault beneath Webster's office, into which the professor's privy emptied. While his wife stood watch, Littlefield hacked through the vault's brick wall and peered into the gloom. Impaled on a dissecting hook hanging from the vault's roof was what looked like the better part of a human body.

Littlefield immediately summoned the police. This time they conducted a more thorough search of Webster's office. They discovered a human thorax — the sternum and ribs that comprise the upper torso — in a tea chest. And in the stove in which the professor heated his chemicals, they found what would prove to be one of the most damning pieces of evidence against the professor: a set of false teeth. They also retrieved bits of burned bone and a shirt button. That evening the police arrested Webster, charged him with murder, and locked him in jail.

The police called on a team of physicians and dentists from Harvard to sort out the remains. Never before had such a stellar corps of experts been brought together, at least in this country, to help solve a murder case. Among them was Oliver Wendell Holmes, renowned anatomist, dean of the Harvard Medical College, and father and namesake of the Oliver Wendell Holmes who would become a justice of the U.S. Supreme Court. Alongside Holmes worked Dr. Jeffries Wyman, another graduate of Harvard Medical College and a professor of anatomy at the university. A scholar of some fame, Wyman had published works primarily about animals other than Homo sapiens. These included such papers as "Remarks on the Anal Pouches of a Skunk," "Remarks on a Bat," and the not-to-be-missed "Remarks on the Jet from the Blowholes of Whales."[3] Nonetheless, he was deemed best for the job of reassembling the 150-odd bones (out of the 206 in the human skeleton) or pieces thereof from Webster's cache.

The investigators concluded that the remains were clearly human and belonged to one person of about the same age, height, and build as Parkman. They estimated the age of the victim to be fifty to sixty years and his height to be five feet ten inches; Parkman in life had been five feet eleven inches and sixty years old. Could the parts simply have been sliced from a cadaver by medical students and then tossed into Webster's privy as part of a ghoulish prank? Not so, the experts said. They found no trace of embalming chemicals in the remains. As for a dissection, the team could not agree on whether someone with knowledge of anatomy had done the deed. Webster's skills at dissection were shaky; twenty-five years before, as a medical student, he had once dissected a body, but his trade was chemistry. The team did agree, however, that the state of decomposition of the unburned body parts found in the privy vault was consistent with the amount of time Parkman had been missing. Thus the inquest suggested that Parkman had died violently by Webster's hand, though the means was not clear.

The investigation and accompanying press coverage had whipped Boston into a frenzy. The trial opened to a packed house on March 19, 1850, in the city court house. Crowds squeezed into the courtroom for the biggest show in town. Every ten minutes, the presiding judge, Lemuel Shaw, the son of a minister and another Harvard graduate, instructed police guards to roust one set of viewers from the gallery and usher in another. At the trial's end, police estimated that at least fifty-five thousand had watched some part of the proceedings.

Webster told the court that he had paid Parkman some of his debt, then watched him stride back out into the streets of Boston. Witnesses called to Webster's defense said that they had seen Parkman in town the afternoon of the disappearance. The forensic witnesses did not address the veracity of these eyewitnesses, however. Rather, the anatomist Wyman focused the jury's attention on the more "terrifying material being," or what little had been scraped together. He awed the jury with his meticulous testimony, later described as his "catalogue of bones." Wyman had carefully classified each tiny fragment of bone found in Webster's stove. He concluded that they came from the head, face, neck, and feet of one person. The parts from the skull, he said, looked as if they had been fractured by "mechanical violence" before being burned. He also testified that the fleshy part of the thorax that they had found was the hairiest that he had ever seen on a human. And Parkman, the jury was duly informed, had been a particularly hairy man.

Oliver Wendell Holmes then took the stand to add the weight of his reputation to the prosecution's case. Eloquent and dignified, Holmes opined that the hands that had dismembered the body of the deceased knew where to place the saw, and that their owner certainly had had training in human anatomy. Nothing he observed in the remains, he told the jury, was dissimilar from the Parkman he knew.

The testimony of a dentist, Dr. Nathan Keep, solidified the scientific findings. Keep remembered his patients well. Four years earlier, Parkman came to him for dentures. He had insisted that he have them as soon as possible, in time for the upcoming dedication of the new medical school in 1846. Parkman said he didn't want to clatter when he spoke. (The historical record shows that either Keep did a bad job or Parkman changed his mind; when the former governor of Massachusetts, Edward Everett, called on Parkman at the dedication, the doctor simply stood, bowed, and sat back down.) Parkman — the Chin — had a strange lower jaw, so out of kilter that Keep had to construct a most unusual block, or cast, for dentures. When Parkman tried the dentures on for size he complained that he had no room for his tongue. So Keep filed the block down. On the witness stand, he held up the dentures to the jury and demonstrated that they not only bore these file marks, but they fit his molds exactly. The teeth probably were still in the head when it went into the oven,

49

Keep said; otherwise they would have exploded from the fierce heat.

Keep's testimony moved his audience. Being a close friend of both victim and accused, he wept almost continuously through his long ordeal on the stand. He recounted to the jury what he had said to his medical colleagues when examining the teeth from the oven: "After examination, I said, 'Dr. Parkman is gone. We shall see him no more.'" He then burst into tears, along with most of the audience in the courtroom. At this point, the proceedings took a tragicomic turn: the prosecutor called for a recess because his office was on fire and he wished to save some important papers.

Despite its persuasiveness, Keep's testimony did not go unchallenged. The nay-sayer was Dr. William T. G. Morton, another dentist. Morton was no ordinary puller of teeth. Less than three years before he had discovered ether, described as the greatest single breakthrough in the history of medicine, at least by patients who had lived through surgery without anesthesia. On the witness stand Morton turned the dentures over in his hands and explained to the jury that they were too badly fused to be distinguished from any other set. When given the mold Keep had used to make the false teeth, Morton reached into his pocket and produced another set of teeth, which he proceeded to fit neatly into the mold, just as Keep had done with some of the teeth from the oven. Holding the mold aloft to fix the eyes of the jury, Morton pointed to the teeth from Webster's oven and scoffed: "I could take this mold and find teeth which would better fit the mold than these."

Webster, against the advice of his attorney, finally took the stand in his own behalf. For fifteen minutes, he wooed the jury with a cogent, well-reasoned argument for a verdict of not guilty. He warned them not to misread his calm during the trial as a sign of frosty superiority, but rather evidence of his faith in God.

Better in God than with Justice Shaw, who set a major precedent in his charge to the jury. Traditionally, the prosecution had to establish that the corpus delicti — literally, the "body of the offense" and in this case the murder of George Parkman — had actually taken place. Although the scientific evidence had been laid before the jury by an intimidatingly professional squad of experts, it sizzled without completely satisfying. But Shaw told the jury that the crime itself and the guilt of the accused need only be proven "beyond a reasonable doubt." Furthermore, he stated that circumstantial evidence alone could establish the corpus delicti.

On the eleventh day of the trial the jury's foreman returned to the courtroom after deliberating only three hours. The foreman delivered the verdict with a single word — guilty. Webster's wall of calm crumbled. He closed his eyes, gripped the rail in front of him, and tearfully collapsed into his chair. The following day Shaw sentenced Webster to hang, which, despite tenure, he did on August 30, 1850, becoming Harvard's first professor so dispatched. Before he died, however, he reaffirmed his faith in God by confessing his crime to a Rev. Dr. George Putnam, whom he had come to know during the trial. The reverend reported Webster's tale thus: a wrathful Parkman had indeed upbraided Webster in the latter's room at the medical college, and in a crescendo of fury, Webster retaliated. He grabbed a thick stalk of dried grapevine and with a single blow knocked Parkman to the floor, killing him instantly. Remorseful yet fearing discovery, Webster dissected the body and disposed of it just as the experts had surmised.

Legal scholars have argued ever since that the forensic testimony didn't really live up to its historical billing. None of the experts could determine any more than that the bones and parts belonged to an older, tallish male who had not been markedly "dissimilar" to Parkman. The rest of the evidence was circumstantial: Webster's motivation, Parkman's visit to Webster's office, and the fact that body parts had turned up in an odd place.

True, Webster's counsel may have let the prosecution and the press get away with their own form of murder; to this day, jurists cite the Webster case as an example of unfair pretrial publicity, improper admission of evidence by the prosecution, and incompetent defense counsel. In fact, Webster's lawyer, in closing arguments, advised the jury that his client probably was guilty but should be convicted of manslaughter instead of murder.

Nevertheless, the case laid the planks for a methodology that forensic scientists still follow. First, a team of experts shared the job of identifying the remains, each contributing from his or her own specialty to the panel's conclusion. Although Oliver Wendell Holmes, the sometime poet, would have blanched at the word, modern forensic scientists have come to call this the "multidisciplinary" approach.[4] Second, then as now, the team reached out to engage whatever other experts might be needed, as in the recruitment of the dentist Keep.

Now a local medical examiner, usually a pathologist, leads such a team, as he or she has legal authority for determining cause and manner of death as well as the victim's identification for all unexplained or violent deaths in a local jurisdiction. Wyman apparently played this role in the Webster case.

The Harvard team also appears to have followed a now commonplace basic protocol in investigating the crime and presenting the evidence. Outlined as a series of questions, the protocol asks:

1. Are the remains human?
2. Do they represent a single individual or the commingled remains of several?
3. When did the death occur?
4. How old was the decedent?
5. What was the decedent's sex?
6. What was the decedent's race?
7. What was the decedent's stature? Body weight? Physique?
8. Did the skeleton or body exhibit any significant anatomical anomalies, signs of old disease and injuries, or other characteristics that, singly or in combination, are sufficiently out of the ordinary to provide positive identification?
9. What was the cause of death? (for example, blunt force trauma, gunshot wound, cancer, unknown, etc.)
10. What was the manner of death? (natural, accidental, homicide, suicide, or unknown)[5]

Webster may have paid dearly for hiring poor counsel, but his ultimate confession laid to rest any question of his guilt. For his part, Parkman helped put American forensic anthropology and odontology on the map with his undershot jaw and unforgettable dentures. And Wyman, who earned the most credit for piecing together the corporeal evidence, assumed the place of honor as the father of forensic anthropology, at least in the opinion of today's leading practitioners. However, Wyman did not take to the forensic side of anthropology. Like most of the pioneers in the field, he regarded himself as one of the anointed priests of scholasticism, not a traveler in the alleyways of crime. He could hardly have turned down the Parkman case, however, as it involved both a colleague and a patron. But there is no record of his having worked on another criminal case. Instead, he went on to become the first curator of the Peabody Museum of American Archaeology and Ethnology in 1866. Wyman is credited with giving physical anthropologists their first precise knowledge of the skeletal system of the gorilla and the incidence of platycephaly (having a wide, flat tibia) in Native Americans.

If murder galvanized the first team of forensic scientists in the United States and laid the foundation for forensic anthropology (even if then under the name of forensic medicine or anatomy), it was simple curiosity that motivated the second important contributor to the field. Thomas Dwight, born in 1843, followed in Wyman's footsteps, obtaining a medical degree from Harvard and in 1883 becoming a professor of anatomy. Although Dwight did participate in some medicolegal investigations, none was spectacular. Rather, it was Dwight's notion that human skeletons exhibited variability reflected in the physical traits of their owners — sex, age, race — that edged the new science away from anatomy and toward anthropology, that is, toward the study of groups of humans and what physically distinguishes them from each other. In 1878 he published a paper, "The Identification of the Human Skeleton: A Medicolegal Study," which won him an award and a good measure of respect from his older colleagues. With the passion of a young man possessed by a new idea, he spent the next few years laboring over Harvard's dissecting tables and collecting skeletons from the steady flow of cadavers that passed through on their way to oblivion.

Dwight produced a stream of papers that for the first time sought systematically to show that an expert could measure a single bone or a set of osteological features and reliably conclude from them certain facts about their owner in life. For example, Dwight believed that the sternum, commonly known as the breastbone, varied according to sex, age, and height. In 1894 he wrote that the length of a skeleton's vertebral column could reveal the living person's height. Later, he would show that one could divine a person's sex from the articular surfaces, or ends, of the long bones of the arms and legs. Dwight worked almost exclusively within the polite society of the academic laboratory. With his soft twinkling eyes, luxurious mustache, and old-fashioned whiskers that splayed out from his chin like a white cow-catcher on a steam engine, Dwight fit the image of senior professor like a weathered glove. Perhaps because historians of forensic anthropology prefer to cast the "purer" scientists in leading roles, Dwight often shares credit for paternity of forensic anthropology with Wyman.

Many anatomists and pretenders to the craft during the late nineteenth century came to revere the skull as some sort of Rosetta stone, whose various eminences, fissures, processes, symphyseal arches, tubercles, trabeculae, and tuberosities could be read like glyphs. For many, the temptation to inscribe their social biases into their interpretations of the body's bas-relief overcame their supposed objectivity. Harvard geologist and historian of science Stephen Jay Gould has noted in several of his books that human biology in the nineteenth century tended to be exploited for the defense of some of the period's flimsiest social theories. While Dwight, for example, carefully limited his observations on the skull's sutures — lines where the bones of the cranium have fused — others saw racial destiny bred in the bone. Said one French scientist, Gratiolet, in 1865:

> Has the long persistence of patent [open] sutures in the White race any relation to the almost indefinable perfection of their intelligence? Does not this continuance of an infantile condition seem to indicate that the brain may, in those perfect men, remain capable of slow growth? Perhaps it is this which makes the perpetual youthfulness of spirit in the greatest thinkers seem able to defy old age and death. But in idiots and in Brutish races the cranium closes itself on the brain like a prison. It is no longer a temple . . . but a sort of helmet capable of resisting heavy blows.[6]

This sort of induction in reverse reached its apotheosis in scientific racism embraced by Nazi visionaries such as Heinrich Himmler, who likened the extermination of Jews to the culling of unwanted plants by a plant-breeder in the process of creating a better strain.[7] Like visitors to the mythical castle of Procrustes, who were stretched or cut down to size in order to fit the host's bed, Jews and other undesirables were attributed with whatever characteristics were necessary to reinforce the pseudoscientific conclusion that the "survival of the fittest" demanded their elimination. Besides scientists of almost every stripe who volunteered or were drafted into practicing this form of scientific racism, doctors occupied the front lines. And none did so more effectively or with greater enthusiasm than Josef Mengele, the doctor at Auschwitz in whom science and death made their most unholy pact.

As for Gratiolet's sutures, anthropology has since shown that no reliable, significant difference exists among races or between genders in regard to when the various sutures close. Moreover, the rate at which sutures close varies so much from person to person that today's experts don't estimate age from sutures alone any more exactly than within ten years except to corroborate other readings.[8]

By the 1890s anthropologists in Europe had begun a serious application of physical anthropology to solving crimes. After all, it had been European scientists who had built a systematic study of fossils. From there it was only a half step on the osteological scale to the study of human bones, whether dug from a paleolithic burial mound or recovered from underneath the floorboards of someone's house. The first man to gain fame as a forensic anthropologist was in fact a European. A flamboyant dreamer and orator, he ended up leading the science down a dead-end street.

Cesare Lombroso, an Italian physician, had by the 1890s begun to establish a reputation as a modern thinker. Lombroso had absorbed Darwinian theory and embroidered a few of its tenets with his own designs. Lombroso believed that *l'uomo delinquente*, the criminal man, inherited not only the "ferocious instincts of primitive humanity and the inferior animals,"[9] but also certain physical stigmata that Lombroso could categorize and use to identify the "born" criminal. Criminals were throwbacks in our midst and it showed, said Lombroso, as clearly as the noses on their faces.

Thus were explained anatomically the enormous jaws, high cheekbones, prominent superciliary arches [brow ridges], solitary lines in the palms, extreme size of the orbits [eye sockets], handle-shaped ears found in criminals, savages, and apes, insensibility to pain, extremely acute sight, tatooing, excessive idleness, love of orgies, and the irresponsible craving of evil for its own sake, the desire not only to extinguish life in the victim, but to mutilate the corpse, tear its flesh and drink its blood.[10]

Lombroso's flair for language far surpassed his skill as a scientist. As Gould observes, Lombroso viewed anatomy as destiny. He believed these stigmata of criminality to be something evolutionary, like bipedalism or a large brain. The line of argument glittered with modernism. It was a time when scholars were funneling Darwin's ideas, like some swollen river, into backwaters of their own making to irrigate their frequently self-serving notions. Those who diverted the theory of evolution of species through natural selection into justifications of the social status quo came to be known as the "social Darwinists."

In his major work, *L'uomo Delinquente*, published in 1876, Lombroso reached into the animal kingdom and invested it with all sorts of humanlike nastiness in order to then deduce that criminals are truly throwbacks to the animals from which we have evolved. Ants are driven by rage to kill aphids, he said, adulterous storks murder their mates, and apes copulate with orgiastic abandon. Indeed, Lombroso observed, how like the apes are the most "savage" of humans. The Dinka of the Sudan, he wrote, had trilobed noses, like monkeys. Moreover, they endured painful rites of puberty with seeming nonchalance and freely tattooed themselves. Having assembled his information from the a priori reasoning of a few European scientists, Lombroso could easily stitch together his theory of delinquency with a single thread: from ape to ignoble savage to modern criminal. Finally, he claimed to recognize the living primitive in modern children, further evidence, he believed, of the base criminality that lies germlike even among the enlightened Europeans.

Unfortunately, Lombroso's ideas worked their way into the criminal court system in Europe. Uncounted numbers of people over the latter part of the nineteenth century faced prosecutors who, either themselves or with the help of Lombroso and his disciples, saw guilt written all over their bodies. For example, simply being big could get you into trouble: Lombroso listed large jaws, long arms, large ears, and a relatively large face in comparison to the head as signs of lurking criminality. A thick skull with a low and narrow forehead was a bad sign, as were darker skin, hairiness, and premature wrinkles. There were elements of superhumanness that marked criminals as well, as if Nature had blessed criminals with talents suited for their trade, such as greater visual acuity and a high tolerance for pain. Lombroso even saw atavism — the appearance in an individual of some trait of ancient ancestors — in prostitutes. At the Fourth International Congress on Criminal Anthropology in 1896, when shown tracings of the outline of prostitutes' feet, he commented that they looked prehensile and even more abnormal than those of criminals.

What little scientific method Lombroso brought to forensic anthropology was in his measurements of criminals. The systematic measurement of bodies, known as anthropometry, was in vogue at the end of the century and would soon become science's foremost means of identifying criminals. Lombroso measured 383 crania from dead criminals and general proportions of 3,839 living noncriminals. Among other things, he was looking for signs that criminals have smaller brains — how could they not? — and like any scientist prospecting for data to fit his bias, Lombroso was rewarded. He consistently claimed that the smaller skulls predominantly belonged to criminals, while good citizens more frequently owned the larger ones (apparently having large body parts wasn't always bad). Actually, Lombroso's frequency distributions showed almost no significant differences between the two groups, as Gould has observed. Also, a few of the law-abiders had particularly large skulls, which was not surprising since, in the experiment studied by Gould, Lombroso examined 328 of the righteous and only 121 criminals. A larger sample size almost guarantees a larger range of variation — the bigger the sample, the higher the chance of finding extremes. Thus the average figure for the law-abiders was higher.

Some scientists ridiculed Lombroso's brand of criminal anthropology and its numerous followers. Nonetheless, Lombrosians testified at criminal trials as expert witnesses. In one account, Lombroso recalls his reasons for believing that a man accused of murder named Fazio, who eventually was acquitted, had really done the deed:

> Upon examination I found that this man had outstanding ears, great maxillaries [jawbones] and cheekbones . . . division

of the frontal bone, premature wrinkles, sinister look, nose twisted to the right — in short, a physiognomy approaching the criminal type. . . . In every way, then, biology furnished in this case indications which, joined with the other evidence, would have been enough to convict him in a country less tender toward criminals. Notwithstanding this he was acquitted.[11]

Lombrosia, as this frothy pseudoscience might be described, even insinuated itself into debates about how severely to sentence criminals (Lombroso preferred isolating "born" criminals in penal colonies to killing them). But the turn of the century brought new ideas about the social conditions that contributed to criminal behavior. One didn't need calipers or statistics to discern that crushing poverty or discrimination or jealous rage might drive a perfectly decent person to commit a crime. Besides, lawyers and judges were, and often still are, loathe to turn over their courtrooms and their jurisprudential domain to white-jacketed experts spouting scientific jargon. Criminal anthropology, at least this version, faded away. Vestiges still exist, however, and modern biology's recent focus on genetics may give birth to new variations on the desire to justify prejudice, which, like some persistent and hardy mold, will settle and grow on most any idea.

While Lombroso searched for signs of savagery in criminals, an extraordinary experiment was under way in Paris. A lowly clerk in the police department had hit upon the idea that a more complete understanding of the variety of human shape could serve in the fight against crime. Lacking the lofty pretensions of the Lombrosian school, this seed of an idea grew slowly in the shadows. No one in a position of authority would take it seriously. Yet it eventually revolutionized police departments in Europe, bringing scientific method to bear on the vexing problem of keeping track of hard-core lawbreakers.

The lowly clerk, creator of the anthropometric "print," was a caustic, ill-tempered, and obsessive Frenchman, Alphonse Bertillon. While he won few friends in the course of his career, Bertillon claimed one of scholarship's greatest rewards — a scientific technique, Bertillonage, was named after him, and during his own lifetime, no less. For over twenty years, Bertillon enjoyed the respect if not the affection of

European scientists as well as their sincerest form of flattery, imitation. Had the English not upset his applecart by discovering fingerprints, Bertillon's system of body measurements might still remain in the practice of criminology.

Alphonse Bertillon was born in 1853 into a family steeped in intellectualism. His grandfather had been a chemist of modest success and a dabbler in experimentation who invented a method of purifying sugar. Alphonse's father, Louis-Adolphe Bertillon, was a physician with a taste for engineering. The two passions drew him into the nascent field of anthropology, specifically the measurement of humans. The Bertillon household crackled with scientific debate, and its rooms became the regular meeting place for visiting scholars, especially those interested in the application of the newer disciplines, such as statistics, to social problems.

As Alphonse grew up, however, he failed to fit the Bertillon mold. A tall, pale teenager with mocking gray eyes, he fell frequently into black moods or was unaccountably irritable. He was expelled from the first school he attended, then drove a private tutor out of the house. His father sent him to boarding schools, but he argued with his masters and worked only on those subjects, such as natural history and mathematics, that interested him and ignored everything else. He specialized in getting thrown out of schools and because of his obnoxiousness earned the nickname "Barbarian."

Bertillon's final expulsion, from the Imperial Lycée of Versailles, was a fiery one. He had created a miniature kitchen inside his desk, a large item of furniture that, in nineteenth-century French schools, could practically have concealed a bathtub. A spirit lamp provided heat, while a dozen carefully sectioned eggshells served as saucepans. While his classics teacher droned on about Thucydides, Bertillon prepared hot chocolate and distributed it to his classmates. One day his pocket kitchen ignited and Bertillon's quietly frantic attempts to put out the fire failed. As black smoke and the unmistakable odor of burning chocolate seeped out from under the desk's lid, the master angrily marched up to Bertillon. He tried to open the desk, but the boy clamped it down. Suddenly, the desperate Bertillon rose, grabbed a weighty Greek dictionary, and smacked his enemy over the head with it.

So ended the boy's formal education. With tutoring from his maternal grandfather, however, he earned a baccalaureat. He professed no interest in a career, however, and as was the custom in France when saddled with a foolish and useless offspring, the family sent Alphonse to England, where at least he might learn the language. Two years later military service called him back to France, where he was a reluctant and exasperated conscript. But he began reading anatomy, a decision made out of boredom but one that eventually changed not only his life but the future of forensic science.

At age twenty-six, Bertillon secured a clerk's job with the Paris Prefecture of Police. He started low — his duty was to copy out forms. The tedious task kept his hands busy but left his mind idle. Around him he saw a police system without the slightest hint of scientific thoroughness. To keep track of professional criminals, the French police relied on informers and *agents provocateurs*. The latter were detectives who masqueraded as criminals, sometimes pretending to serve time in prison to keep abreast of their quarry. A brilliant criminal turned policeman, known simply as Vidocq, had created this fifth column in large part by recruiting other criminals to join the force. To identify recidivists, Vidocq encouraged his colleagues to do as he did — commit their physiognomy to memory. It was a haphazard process at best, prone to error and corruption.

Bertillon scorned the idea of memorizing human features. He decided that he could do better, and as he dutifully copied his police reports, he devised his methods. Photography had by then been introduced to the police system, and Bertillon spent hours cutting photos of felons into pieces, pasting noses on one piece of cardboard, ears on another, mouths on yet another. He measured each and reduced the measurements to formulas that could be systematically applied to every person who walked into police headquarters. While principles of physiology based on photographs rather than flesh and blood didn't qualify as ironclad, it didn't take long for Bertillon to realize that every human thus measured was unique. This method, he was sure, would transform police identifications into a scientific technique.

But when Bertillon, a mere junior clerk with only eight months on the job, presented his proposal to the prefect of police, Louis Andrieux, he got a dressing down. "Monsieur Bertillon," Andrieux said to the awkward fellow standing before him, "you are a young man in a junior position in this department, and with no experience of it.

You have no scientific qualifications, and you produce an incomprehensible report which you cannot explain. I warn you that if I am troubled again I shall take a serious view of it."[12]

A distraught Bertillon turned to his father, who by then was president of the Society of Anthropology and well connected in Parisian society and government. An angry letter from the prefect of police arrived at the doctor's house before Alphonse, however. Dr. Bertillon was not amused by his son's stab at assertiveness and showed him the letter, which suggested that Alphonse should have "his mind looked into." Inarticulate as usual, Alphonse could do nothing but dig in his pocket and proffer his notes on his new method.

To the eye of a trained anthropologist, the calculations and drawings showed an understanding of the principles of statistics and the human form. Perhaps this was not simply another of Alphonse's spasms of rebelliousness after all. What began as a reprimand turned into a panegyric. "Of course, I knew you were interested in anthropology and statistics," the doctor told his son, "but I never dreamt that you were going practically to apply what you have learnt from us in a new field." He went on enthusiastically: "You are going to identify lawbreakers with your measurements. Good! But we are also going to be able to prove that every man and woman born into this world is a unique specimen."

Had enthusiasm been enough to put Alphonse's hypothesis into action, criminal science would have been re-created that winter of 1879 in Paris. But Dr. Bertillon's entreaties on behalf of his son failed to move Andrieux. The only thing he could do, the doctor told Alphonse, was to bide his time until, eventually, the bureaucracy would thresh Andrieux from the system and plant a replacement.

So the young Bertillon returned to his desk to continue the farcical filling out of forms, with their amateurish and subjective descriptions of criminals' faces, bodies, gaits, and dress. His peevishness acidified into bitterness and the never-popular clerk, considered by his co-workers as too ambitious for his station, found himself shunned. No matter, he thought. He would continue his own work in spite of the ignorance around him. His superiors relented only enough to give Bertillon a somewhat longer leash to make a few experiments, perhaps thinking that he would entangle himself in his own dithering calculations and eventually stumble off somewhere out of sight.

Now that he knew what to measure, Bertillon set out to measure it. He bought some calipers and pincer gauges and experimented on whomever would submit. Eleven measurements were all that would be necessary, he concluded. These included the length and breadth of the head and of the right ear, the length from the elbow to the end of the middle finger, the lengths of the middle and ring fingers, the length of the left foot, the full body height, the length of the trunk, and the length of the outstretched arms. He added to this anthropometric map a written description that focused on a list of physical traits, plus an instruction to note anything peculiar or unique. He called this subjective description a *portrait parle*, or "spoken portrait," which he eventually augmented with photographs in full face and profile for every accused man, woman, and child brought in for questioning.

The anthropometric analysis did not impress Andrieux. Bertillon, who had done his statistical homework, argued that the odds that two people possessed exactly the same eleven measurements were only one in several million. But he couldn't get the idea across to Andrieux, who, like most policemen of the time, was suspicious of scientific double-talk in the prefecture. Moreover, Andrieux had staked his prestige on discounting Bertillon's claims. To reverse himself would cause loss of face. But Bertillon's break came in 1882. Andrieux resigned and was replaced by another political appointee, Jean Camecasse, who proved to be more receptive to if no more enlightened by Bertillon's system.

"From next week on we shall introduce your method of identification on an experimental basis," Camecasse told the querulous clerk after their first meeting on the subject.[13] "Two assistant clerks will be assigned to you. I give you three months' time. If during this period your method fishes up a single recidivist criminal . . ." Camecasse left Bertillon to guess at what that success might bring.

Three months! The task of making a positive identification within that time seemed impossible. Each measurement had to be exact, something a trained technician might accomplish consistently if done with care and enthusiasm. To Bertillon, his assistants were clods, stupid at best and even obstructive if given the chance.

Bertillon compensated by throwing himself completely into the task. At night he took his measurements home to his small apartment, which he shared with a nearsighted, shy young Austrian woman, Amelie Notar. She transcribed Bertillon's notes onto file cards, each containing the vital statistics on a single suspect or criminal. Each day Bertillon and his assistants would descend, calipers, tape measures, and a great box of a camera in hand, on another group of con artists, drunks, prostitutes, thieves, murderers, kidnappers, and other flotsam from the Parisian underworld. His subjects were incredulous of the sharp-faced doctor, with his stiff white collar, deep-set eyes, and bizarre demands. The man looked them over as if he were a butcher making ready to cut up a side of beef. Bertillon's assistants often had to pinion the hapless suspects while this "paleface of the prefecture," as he was sometimes called, measured various parts of their bodies. All he needed was one match from the hundreds of previously detained subjects recorded in his card files. Each night he returned home to Amelie, his disappointment and anxiety erupting in violent attacks of migraine headaches, to brood over his vanishing chances for scientific immortality.

With only two weeks remaining in which to prove to Camecasse that the technique could work, Bertillon's mood was as gloomy as the dank streets through which he made his way to work. The work on February 20 passed like most others, one face and body after another, until his assistants brought in a man named DuPont. The name meant nothing; it was a particularly popular alias at the time, as common among criminals as straight razors. However, Bertillon thought he recognized this one. Then again, how many times had he told himself that he had a match and rushed back to his files only to come up empty-handed? He finished his measurements and maneuvered through the cluttered desks of the documents department to his cases full of cards.

Had Bertillon never satisfied Camecasse's demand, he probably would have at least given forensic anthropology its first efficient system of categorization. By February 1883 he had about one thousand eight hundred file cards, each describing a different individual. To locate those likely to match a person in custody, Bertillon had divided and subdivided the cards according to a hierarchy of measurements. He would begin with a range of head sizes that was divided into large, medium, and small. M. DuPont — the sixth DuPont he had measured that day — was in the middle group. That eliminated about two thirds of his files. The breadth of DuPont's head further narrowed the search and the length of the little finger again reduced the number of candidates to the contents of three files. Within minutes Bertillon held before him a single card. Every one of the eleven measurements matched DuPont's. Only the name on the card was not DuPont, but Martin. He had been arrested on December 15, 1882, for stealing empty bottles.

Bertillon rushed back to the measuring room and confronted the prisoner. "I've seen you once before," he told him confidently. DuPont denied it. But his resolve crumbled when Bertillon calmly explained that the police had brought him in two months before for stealing bottles. "At the time you called yourself Martin," he smugly told the prisoner, who confessed his true identity on the spot.

Bertillon had finally vindicated himself. Paris's newspapers carried the story of the identification and the scientific process behind it. The young scientist won grudging praise from Camecasse and his colleagues, and a guarantee that he could continue his work with a larger staff and more money. One successful identification followed another as the pace of measuring quickened. During 1884 Bertillon identified three hundred suspects who had been convicted previously on other charges. He refined his technique, adding new descriptions based on carefully posed photographs of ears, the irises of eyes, deviated bridges of the nose, the size and shape of nostrils, and dozens of other spectra of the human form. He never found two people with exactly the same set of measurements. The French police and the prison system embraced this revolutionary discovery of their now favorite son of France.

Over the next decade, Bertillon won himself the title of Director of the Police Identification Service. In 1892 he solved his biggest case and became a household word by identifying Ravachol, an anarchist suspected of murdering several people and bombing restaurants and the home of a judge. Police in other European cities adopted Bertillonage, and the great man's office in Paris drew a long list of visiting dignitaries who came to pay their respects and learn from the man now labeled as the "genius" of nineteenth-century French forensic science.

Bertillon's triumph, like his desk at the lycée, burned but briefly. Even as his system was revolutionizing prison systems and police departments in Berlin, Moscow, Vienna, and Rome, a new idea that would replace it was germinating in London. Dactylography, otherwise known as fingerprinting, had caught the attention of Britain's Home Office. William Herschel, a British administrative official in Hooghly, capital of the district of that name in India, had discovered that the pads of fingers, if sufficiently grimy, left unique prints on glass or paper. These appeared to vary from person to person. Other investigators, in their characteristically cautious British way, spent over a decade toying with the idea.

But it was in Argentina that the beginning of the end of Bertillonage took place. By 1891 a copy of a scientific paper discussing fingerprints reached an unusally inquisitive and ambitious young Argentine. Juan Vucetich, thirty-three years old and a member of the provincial police in Buenos Aires, had already heard a great deal about Bertillonage and how it had made over the practice of criminal investigation in Europe. Like many Argentines, he was a recent immigrant, having been born in the Croatian village of Lesina, in what is now Yugoslavia. He wanted to set up a system of Bertillonage in Buenos Aires. But he also started taking fingerprints, as described by the Englishman Francis Galton, who was popularizing this new technique. He spent long hours in the morgues of Buenos Aires fingerprinting corpses, and even got prints from mummies in the museum of natural history at La Plata. Much as Bertillon suffered the scorn of uncomprehending skeptics, Vucetich got little but suspicion and wisecracks from his colleagues. But also like the Frenchman whom he revered, and whom he would help ruin, Vucetich's chance eventually came in the form of a protesting criminal.

On June 19, 1892, on the outskirts of a town of huts called Necochea near La Plata on the Atlantic coast, two children were found murdered. Their frantic mother, an unmarried woman named Francisca Rojas, had run screaming through the village, accusing a man named Velasquez of the deed. She claimed that Velasquez was angry because she had spurned his amorous attentions and so he bashed in her childrens' heads in revenge.

Velasquez had an alibi. The police from La Plata suspected that the mother had really committed the infanticide because her lover complained that the children were an annoyance and made marriage impossible. But proof was lacking, and Rojas stood by her story.

Several weeks after the crime a police inspector who had worked with Vucetich on his fingerprinting system visited the scene of the crime. He found a bloody thumbprint on the half-open door of the bedroom. The inspector lifted the print. Inexpert as he was, the print he took clearly and indisputably matched a print taken from Rojas's thumb. Confronted with this seemingly magical evidence that the police seemed to have spirited right off the wooden door, Rojas confessed.

A debate ensued in Argentina over which method to adopt, Bertillonage or fingerprinting. Perhaps encouraged by the fact that an Argentine had chosen the latter technique to solve a crime, the provincial police chose fingerprinting. Argentina became the first country officially to adopt the method. Ironically, the Argentine fascination with the technique would lead to widespread fingerprinting of the population and, eighty-four years later, would help the country's military pursue, imprison, and kill thousands of innocent citizens who challenged its dictatorship.

Dactylography created Vucetich; it destroyed Bertillon. The Frenchman had experimented with fingerprints, even including photographs of them in his records of criminals and using them in a few criminal investigations. But he was suspicious of them, and belittled their veracity and supposed infallibility. Years later when fingerprinting was replacing Bertillonage through most parts of Europe, France, true to form, clung longest to its hero's invention. Vucetich, meanwhile, was lionized in Argentina and enjoyed the privileges of travel that came with his notoriety. He even made a pilgrimage to Bertillon's office at the prefecture. According to an account by Bertillon's niece,[14] Vucetich arrived one morning in 1913 and was admitted to Bertillon's waiting room. After a lengthy period, the door of the great man's office swung open. Bertillon emerged, stood on the threshold, and pinned the visitor with a glare.

"Sir," he finally said, "you have tried to do me a great deal of harm." He then turned back into his office, slamming the door behind him. Vucetich never saw him again.

A year later, blind and incapacitated by pernicious anemia, Bertillon died. He was buried with national honors before a huge crowd of admirers. In addition to a scientific method, a short street in Paris's fifteenth arrondissement bears Bertillon's name.

A more gracious man might have accepted the inevitable replacement of Bertillonage by fingerprinting. After all, Bertillon had also helped to create scientific criminology, perfected criminal photography, and built the first criminological laboratory. But he fought the introduction of fingerprinting to the end. When he died, he died as Bertillonage's last adherant, and the technique died with him.

A final note on Bertillon: his place in history might have been loftier had he not curiously forgotten his hard-nosed objectivity and leapt across the boundaries of his science in the celebrated Dreyfus case.

In 1894 Captain Alfred Dreyfus, a French military officer, was arrested and accused of passing military secrets to German enemies. The strongest piece of evidence against Dreyfus was a treasonous document purportedly in his handwriting, called a *bordereau*, a thin sheet of paper favored by correspondents because of its light weight. Bertillon, who had written scholarly articles on handwriting analysis, but who had little faith in the graphologists of the day, was asked to compare the writing on the bordereau with that of Dreyfus. After a typically meticulous examination of the document, in which Bertillon measured spacings as well as the letters themselves, he concluded that the differences between the bordereau and Dreyfus's script were simply the captain's attempt to cover himself. Dreyfus, Bertillon testified, had attempted an "auto-forgery" but could not completely hide the intrinsic uniqueness of his handwriting. Dreyfus was convicted and sentenced to life imprisonment.

Dreyfus was a Frenchman, bad enough when the charge is treason. But he was also a Jew. The Dreyfus affair became a rallying point against the injustice wrought by anti-Semitism. His conviction inflamed the camps of Dreyfusards who continued to defend his innocence. Four years after the captain's conviction, he was vindicated: the real author of the bordereau confessed. Suddenly Bertillon plummeted from his perch among the eagles and landed in a heap with charlatans and quacks, at least in the opinion of the Dreyfusards. Even the legal establishment, which had no reason to doubt Bertillonage because of a single blunder, nonetheless viewed the great man now as something less than monumental.

Bertillon's clumsy performance in court may have caused his speculations to be misinterpreted as fact. Or perhaps the strength of French anti-Semitism would have overpowered any attempt at objectivity. Whatever the case, Bertillon, like others who would follow in forensic science, wandered or was enticed beyond his ken. Mastery of the arcane is hard, tedious work, often attained without much reward. If the public suddenly wants an expert, the temptation to satisfy them can be irresistible — in Delphi everyone's favorite sound was his own voice. Forensic science in the latter half of this century has academies and credentialing to weed out the haruspices and flim-flammers, but there always remains the urge, sometimes stoked by the attorney, the victim's grieving family, or that irrepressible hunch, to venture a little beyond what one knows. Forensic scientists watch for it like a sailboat's skipper checking a shoreline for submerged rocks.

3

DEAD RECKONING

IF Thomas Dwight cast the first light on forensic anthropology, Chicagoan George Dorsey generated the most heat. Like Dwight and most of the redoubtable crew that helped solve the Parkman mystery, Dorsey was trained at Harvard — but as an anthropologist. No course in the subject had even been given before 1890; Dorsey earned his Ph.D. four years later.

Dorsey apparently contributed little to the scientific literature. He gained his reputation instead from a sensational murder case. Although he performed like a trouper on the witness stand, the experience apparently rattled him, for he never again worked on a major criminal case. However, his participation as an anthropologist in the investigation and trial paved the way for others to follow — and illuminated some of the pitfalls awaiting them as well.[1]

If Boston had thrilled to the day-to-day unraveling of the Parkman-Webster drama, Chicago practically gagged over the case of Adolphe Louis Luetgert. Luetgert's grisly crime fit Chicago, "hog-butcher for the world" as Carl Sandburg described the city, as neatly as a feud between two dons from American aristocracy fit Boston. Luetgert, a native of Germany, was a stout, oily man who, at fifty-two, had made his life's work the processing of meat. At various times a tanner and a butcher, with a short digression into saloon-keeping, Luetgert had by May of 1897 elevated himself to proprietor of a sausage factory. Despite Luetgert's reputation as a wealthy man, his business had been struggling. The factory, a stained carcass of a building marred by peeling paint and broken brick, stood bleakly in a rundown neighborhood. Luetgert had abandoned his sausage-making operations, and only a small retail operation on the premises kept the debt collectors from closing the place down.

Adolphe, his diminutive wife, Louisa, and their two small children, Louis and Elmer, lived in a house adjoining the factory. The Luetgerts didn't get along very well. In fact, Adolphe slept in a room in the factory, kept company by his dogs. So it was somewhat out of the ordinary when, on the evening of Saturday, May 1, he invited Louisa out for a walk by lantern light. That was the last anyone saw of her, at least in recognizable form.

Three days later, Louisa's brother came to the Luetgert house. Asked about Louisa's whereabouts, Adolphe replied, "I don't know. Ain't she at your place?" When told that she was not, Adolphe nonchalantly suggested that she had run away. Several days later, the police were called in. They searched the sewers, dragged the river, and interrogated relatives and friends. Eventually, on Saturday, May 15, they got around to the sausage factory. A watchman there suggested that they investigate a large steam vat, one of three commonly used for dipping sausages, located in the cellar. According to a contemporary account of the investigation, this is what they discovered:

> This vat they found about half full of a reddish-brown liquid, emitting a sickening odor. A plug on the outside, near the bottom, was withdrawn by one of the police, and some gunnysacks (found near at hand) were spread on the floor at the bunghole. As the liquid passed out, a slimy sediment and a number of small pieces of bone were deposited on the sacks. The vat was then further searched, and at the bottom, besides other bone fragments, there were found two plain gold rings, stuck together (one inside the other) and covered with a slimy, reddish-gray substance; the smaller was a guard-ring, the larger a wedding-ring, and on the inner surface of the latter was engraved in script "L.L." and "18 karat."[2]

Near the vat the police found more suspicious material: a twelve-inch strand of hair, a piece of leather, a piece of cloth, some pieces of string, a hairpin, and the apparent half of an upper false tooth. In the street outside the factory, where, it was later found, Luetgert had ordered workers to dump ashes from the smokehouse, the police found fragments of burned human bones as well as some pieces of burned corset steel. The Monday after they inspected the factory (apparently they preferred not to disrupt the Sabbath), the police paid Luetgert a visit at home and hauled him, protesting all the way, off to jail.

Luetgert's trial in Cook County Criminal Court opened on August 30, 1897, before Judge Richard S. Tuthill. The charge — that Adolphe had killed Louisa and boiled her away in the sausage vat — assured a feverish level of public interest, even for a public somewhat hardened by the rough-and-tumble life in the Midway City. Newspaper reporters came from a thousand miles away, competing for ever more sensational accounts. The trial consumed almost two months and seethed with lurid accounts of Luetgert's cruel treatment of his wife. In jail Luetgert further scandalized the citizenry by writing love letters to a Christina Feldt, a rich widow with whom he had had financial dealings. And a certain queasiness suddenly overcame many Chicagoans at the mention of sausage, practically a staple in a town full of Poles and Germans.

It fell to George Dorsey to perform the expert examination of what were reputed to be Louisa's remains. His testimony probably influenced the course of forensic science and expert testimony in criminal trials more than it actually furthered the prosecution's case. The circumstantial evidence against Luetgert brimmed over, but at the same time, Dorsey's analysis of the bones found in and near the vat strained credibility.

First, Dorsey and colleagues from the Field Museum, where he was employed, examined the bones and bone fragments that the police had gathered from the scene of the alleged crime. They identified part of a femur, or thigh bone; a rib; a sesamoid, an extra bone that sometimes forms over tendons, especially near the joints in fingers and toes; a phalanx, or toe bone; a fragment from the temporal bone of the skull; a metacarpal, or finger bone; and part of a humerus, the bone of the upper arm. Other specialists determined that the reddish-brown liquid that oozed from the vat contained traces of hematin, a decomposition product of hemoglobin normally found in blood.

Before Dorsey took the stand a parade of witnesses served up a bruising history of marital discord in the Luetgert household. Several

71

female friends of Louisa's recalled that Adolphe often bullied his wife and occasionally beat her for good measure. He reportedly was sleeping with the maid as well and made no effort to hide it from Louisa.

Then came the story of how Luetgert had ultimately diminished his wife. According to smokehouse helper Frank Odorowsky, Luetgert had on March 11 bought and received at the factory 378 pounds of crude potash. On April 24, Luetgert ordered Odorowsky and "Ham" Levandowsky, another of his employees, to empty the potash into barrels alongside the vat. The potash, Odorowsky recalled, "burned like fire" when it touched his skin, and even though he put rags on his hands and face he still was scarred. Later that day, Luetgert and the factory's watchman poured the potash into the vat and filled it with water, where it simmered for a week. On Saturday, May 1, the day of Louisa's disappearance, Luetgert turned on a steam line that led into the vat to get the mixture to boil. He then sent the watchman on two errands that took him out of the factory, leaving the place empty most of the day and that night — except for Luetgert, who kept the vat boiling vigorously until about three o'clock in the morning, napping now and then in a chair in his office.

Sunday afternoon and into Monday morning, the vat bubbled away. Various workers helped Luetgert clean up some of the slimy residue that boiled over the top of the vat. Luetgert himself scraped up the solid material from the drains and the overflow and buried some of it, burned more of it in the smokehouse, and dumped yet more next to a nearby railroad track.

Luetgert was as sloppy a murderer as he was a businessman. He involved so many people in the goings-on in the vat room — he claimed he was making soap to clean the factory in preparation for selling it — and warned them so often to keep quiet about it, that suspicion clung to him like a sweaty shirt.

The prosecution also employed a bizarre but graphic demonstration to support its case. The authorities insisted on testing whether the hot potash solution that Luetgert had cooked up could actually reduce a body to the lumpy residue found in and around the sausage-dipping vat. They acquired a human cadaver and followed Luetgert's alleged recipe to the letter. They got much the same results.

Suppose Luetgert had been making soap? the jury was asked. What about the bones, then? Were they, as he insisted, merely animal

72

bones, as innocent in a sausage-making operation as pine shavings in a woodshop? The prosecution called George Dorsey.

Dorsey was an adventurer as well as an academic. He had spent several of the previous few years on the west coast of South America, excavating burial grounds at Ancón, Peru, and in Alaska, where he studied Native American cultures and physiology. He had hauled back a large collection of mummies from Peru and arranged to have them displayed in the museum for the four hundredth anniversary of the discovery of America by Europeans. Yet for a man more accustomed to digging waist-deep in muddy graveyards, Dorsey charmed the courtroom audience, according to accounts of the trial.[3] With the ruddy complexion of an outdoorsman, a compact physique and square jaw, Dorsey exuded quiet confidence. He could have been the model for Indiana Jones.

Dorsey carefully guided the jury through a series of comparisons between the handful of burned, bony remains to boxes full of specimens from the museum. He assured the court that the bone fragments, which together could fit onto a quarter, belonged to a human female. One observer, columnist Julian Hawthorne, wrote of Dorsey's testimony in the September 17, 1897, issue of the *Chicago Tribune*:

> Professor Dorsey was generally admitted to have made the strongest showing of any of the many strong witnesses of the State. He was as fresh when the day was over as when it began, and perhaps even more alert and poignant. Every statement he made helped the case against the prisoner, and yet it was abundantly evident that his sole concern was to present the exact truth as he knew it, exaggerating naught, and setting down naught in malice. His voice was distinct and his exposition so clear that even the technical character of many of [his statements] did not prevent them from being understood by the jury. His knowledge was so well systematized, so well in hand, so sound, precise and broad, that it was a pleasure to listen to him; it is not often one comes in contact with a brain of so fine a fiber, so vigorous, and so sane.

Had the adulatory Hawthorne been in charge, the trial might have been over in a matter of hours. The defense, however, called their own expert, W. H. Allport of the Northwestern University Medical

School. Unlike Dorsey, Allport was strictly a medical man and did not command a vast knowledge of bones. He simply argued that his general understanding of them was sufficient to say with confidence that Dorsey's identification of these pebble-sized pieces as Louisa was ridiculous. Allport didn't hold up as well as Dorsey under cross-examination, however. Again, through Hawthorne's eyes:

> It began very quietly yesterday morning. . . . But it gave us time to prepare our minds for what we knew must be coming. Dr. Allport was to be offered up as a sacrifice; his time was ripe. He sat in the chair looking resolute but somewhat pensive; McEwen [the prosecutor] and Professor Dorsey sat side by side with bones all about them. Dr. Allport had been at the trigger end of a cross-examination on sesamoids a couple of weeks ago; now he was to take his turn in front of the muzzle. . . .
>
> He was presented by his agreeable interlocutor with a bone of some animal's leg, which he immediately identified as that of a monkey. He explained to the jury, in an interesting discourse, its various characteristic points, when Mr. McEwen gently said, "I am informed by Professor Dorsey that that is the leg of a dog."
>
> The jury looked embarrassed, and a passing shade of despair crossed the doctor's features. At last he said:
>
> "There is a class of dog monkeys."

Looking back on the evidence, anthropologists doubted that Dorsey really could have made a determination of humanness, let alone sex, from the corpus delicti. Nonetheless, Dorsey won the confidence of the jury. The wedding rings found in the vat probably clinched the prosecution's case. Luetgert's account, in contrast, was laughable, if anyone at that point was able to laugh. Making two thousand pounds of soap, enough to scrub down the factory several times over at a cost far greater than if he had simply bought soap off the shelf, and then boiling it up in the middle of the night while he watched over it like a fretful chef, made a singularly unconvincing story. Luetgert admittedly hated his wife and didn't even try to find her after she allegedly ran off. The image of the cellar, the vats, the steaming potash, the slimy floor, and Luetgert, the husband, stirring the cauldron at midnight while his wife slowly seethed to jelly, no doubt had as visceral an impact on the jury as it did on the public who read the daily newspaper accounts. When the prosecutor finally proposed to the jury that Luetgert had spirited Louisa to the cellar, struck her down, and dumped her (mercifully dead, one would hope) into the vat, the jury believed him.

Luetgert got life in prison. His place in criminal history has been neatly summed up by Clyde Snow: "Unable to dissolve his marriage, he decided to dissolve his wife."[4]

The Luetgert case illustrates two problems that may explain the reluctance of some scientists to volunteer for legal duty. First, the Anglo-Saxon judicial system customarily recruits scientists for court-room appearances much the way the police shop for attack dogs — they look for signs of good breeding coupled with a willingness to take a bite out of an adversary. Most scientists, physical anthropologists included, believe that scientific data should lead to only one objective conclusion. But a courtroom battle between equally qualified pit bulls with Ph.D.s can leave the jury wondering whether science is settled on anything.

Indeed, Dorsey shrank from the practice of appearing in court. The Luetgert case was his first and last forensic investigation. He was later stung as well by criticism from his colleagues, including the embittered Allport, who had dared to dabble extemporaneously in anthropology in that Chicago courtroom. At a meeting of the Chicago Medico-Legal Society on December 3, 1898, where Dorsey discussed the treatment of the human skeleton in forensics, Allport struck back with a vitriolic petulance. Referring to the Parkman case, which involved Harvard, Dorsey's alma mater, Allport said to the assembled society:

It is to be noted that the papers of the day congratulated the Harvard faculty on their skill in identifying, placing and restoring Dr. Parkman's skeleton, some 156 bones being present. The advance made in teaching at this institution is remarkable, for a recent graduate of the same school [Dorsey] now identifies a woman from four fragments of bone the size of peas.[5]

The European system of jurisprudence shuns the shoot-out approach to expert testimony. The judge appoints an expert whose scientific report provides the grist for subsequent legal interpretation in a case. While this might make complicated subjects easier to fathom for the judge and jury, it ignores the fact that the practice of science is as porous as a sponge. While it does the job asked of it — for example, inferring from fossilized bones a theory of how humans evolved, or classifying humans according to bone structure — it is honeycombed with dispute. Over time even the surest of theories is replaced. The Anglo-Saxon approach at least ensures that both sides get a hearing, fair or otherwise. Furthermore, opposing experts often confer before the case comes to trial and frequently agree on the nature of the evidence. At such times the evidence in question may simply be dismissed or introduced without contest.

The second problem highlighted by the Luetgert trial still persists, and probably always will. Scientists don't view the world in black and white. Instead, they measure truth in gradations of probability. The probable, as Aristotle observed, is what usually happens. But scientists need a way to show that in numbers. Specifically, they need to illustrate the probability that the results they get might be an artifact of chance — an accident. In scientific papers authors carefully acknowledge this by appending in seemingly modest parentheses "($p <$ .05)," which is the P value. A P value of less than .05 means that the probability that the phenomenon the scientist observed really occurred by chance, and was not due to whatever hypothesis the scientist is proposing, is less than 5 percent. Or, in other words, the chances are less than five in one hundred that the phenomenon is simply random variation.[6]

Lawyers, judges, and juries, however, don't deal in statistical confidence, but in preponderance of evidence or reasonable doubt. Proof in civil cases need only satisfy the standard of preponderance of evidence in favor of one argument or another. The highest standard, applied to evidence in criminal cases, is similarly difficult to quantify: a jury may convict when guilt is clear beyond a reasonable doubt. These standards fall short of what scientists accept for judging their data. Yet once on the stand, as Dorsey discovered, the scientist must mix together all the shades of gray on his palette and bring forth an opinion. Were these "pea-sized" bone fragments those of a woman or a man, yes or no? There was no collegial panel of graybeards to review Dorsey's findings, as there would have been had he been

publishing in a journal instead of testifying in a murder trial. With
opposing experts and attorneys poised to pounce on the least slip, the
expert witness finds himself in the same pickle as Paris when he had
to choose which of three goddesses — Athena, Aphrodite, or Hera —
was the most beautiful: damned no matter which way he votes. (Paris,
at least, ended up with the beautiful mortal, Helen, in exchange for
giving Aphrodite first prize, rather a better deal than an expert witness's fee.)

The Parkman and Luetgert cases were extraordinary in that physical
anthropologists in America rarely ventured into court; the practice of
studying skeletons remained almost strictly within the walls of aca-
deme. In France, however, Bertillon had lent forensic anthropology
some legitimacy, and lawyers on the Continent frequently sought out
experts in the field. Consequently, scientists there turned their attentions more often to how the skeleton might be used to help solve
crimes, rather than simply as an object required for the study of
anatomy and physiology.

In 1888 Frenchman Etienne Rollet measured the long bones of one
hundred cadavers, seeking a way to deduce a person's stature from
the lengths of the long bones — the humerus, radius, and ulna of the
arm and the femur, tibia, and fibula of the leg. In 1892 countryman
Leonce Manouvrier, followed in 1899 by a German, Karl Pearson,
reworked Rollet's measurements and came up with additional formulas for determining stature.

All were pioneers in applying regression analysis to forensic anthropology. This now-common mathematical technique allows one to determine a value, such as a person's height, from several related values.
For example, if police find a femur from a human skeleton, a forensic
anthropologist would first measure its length on an osteometric board,
a simple device on which a long bone is laid flat between two boards,
like bookends, and its length read from a calibrated straightedge. The
femur's length in centimeters becomes the independent variable in an
equation involving multiplication and addition with standard values.
The product, plus or minus about three centimeters, is the height of
the person who once walked with that femur — the dependent variable. The heart of the technique lies in the standard values (they vary

slightly among some racial groups), which have been deduced over the years from countless measurements of bones from people of known height.

Rollet, Manouvrier, and Pearson began this process of deduction. They believed that some bones had to bear a consistent relation to a person's overall height. They proved which bones were best for this task and calculated the standard values, or coefficients. The process is similar to calculating the amount of paint needed to do a whole house based on the amount used to cover one wall. The three Europeans each published tables listing the bone or bones to be measured, the coefficients, and the corresponding statures. If one has more than one bone to work from, all the better, as the regression analysis then becomes "multiple" and thus usually more accurate.[7]

Margin of error, it turns out, varies according to which bones are available. Calculating stature from arm bones, for example, gives a stature that is slightly less reliable than leg bones. Furthermore, Rollet's one hundred cadavers numbered too few to take a good statistical bite out of the apple. And as modern anthropologists have discovered, skeletons now aren't what they used to be, even after less than one hundred years. The general level of nutrition and the prevalence of certain diseases can alter skeletal averages for populations. Racial mixing has also blurred distinctions that might have been clear-cut in the nineteenth century. Rollet's bodies might not even have been typical of the average Parisian of the time. They were available for his laboratory because they were drifters, criminals, or derelicts who had languished in the morgue unclaimed.

After the turn of the century physical anthropologists seem to have given the cold shoulder to forensics, although some of the leading scholars of the time, such as T. Wingate Todd at Case Western Reserve Medical School in Cleveland, occasionally assisted criminal investigators with an unidentified skeleton on their hands.

Todd drew up tables for roughly estimating age from the degree to which cranial sutures had closed. Eventually, he found a better measure for determining age at death. The right and left hipbones, also known as the innominate or pubic bones, meet to form the pelvis. Actually, the pubic bones never touch, but are separated by a small piece of cartilage.[8] The surface, or face, of each pelvic bone where it meets the cartilage is euphonically known as the pubic symphysis.

Todd noticed that the texture and shape of these symphyses change over a person's lifetime in a regular, predictable way. He carefully mapped the symphysis and divided it into five domains: a surface, outer and inner borders or ramparts, and upper and lower extremities. He also included certain subsidiary, topographical features, such as ridging and billowing, that changed as a person grew older. Todd then divided the human symphyseal record into ten epochs, starting with age eighteen to nineteen and ending with age fifty and above. Each epoch was associated with unique markings on the symphyses that could be read by anthropologists the way strata in exposed rock are read by geologists. At eighteen years its surface shows a mountainous landscape, traversed by horizontal ridges separated by well-marked grooves. Over the next four decades of growth the symphysis undergoes a variety of changes, developing plateaus, nodules, beveled edges, furrows, and rims, then losing much of its topography at later ages. Todd's technique, with refinements added more or less continuously, became the mainstay for aging a skeleton, and is still used even though microscopic analysis of the bone's cortex has eclipsed it in accuracy.

Anthropologists also tried to perfect the sexing of skeletons, that is, distinguishing male from female. One might think the differences are obvious: women are generally smaller, their bones lighter, their pelvic openings wider to accommodate the passage of children into the world. Sex differences can be seen even in the shape of the cranium and the facial bones, such as the brow ridge, which is usually more prominent in males.[9] But what about a woman who grows unusually large, such that her measurements cross over into the range of the smallest males? Such cases are not all that unusual. If an anthropologist wants to determine the sexual mix in an excavated paleolithic campsite, mistaking a woman for a man might constitute only a minor statistical oversight. But if the star of a women's Roller Derby team has been missing for a year and police find a skeleton and dismiss it as that of a smallish man, a solvable case might slip from justice's grasp.

Male and female skeletons actually differ surprisingly little to the untrained eye; one modern leader in the discipline, Wilton M. Krogman, who was to revive forensic anthropology in 1939 through his association with the Federal Bureau of Investigation, estimated that the difference amounts only to about 8 percent.[10] If they have only skulls to work with, for example, experts misidentify sex about 10 percent of the time.[11]

While imperfect, at least for legal applications, sexing skeletons has been less controversial than determining their race. The stereotypical notions about other races that nineteenth-century European and American anthropologists carried with them into the laboratory ensured that skeletons of whites would be made to fit into whatever mold was most flattering. Thus the distinguished scientist and physician Samuel George Morton, a patrician Philadelphian who began measuring cranial capacities of various races in the mid-nineteenth century, fiddled his data to guarantee that whites came out on top.[12] He made sure that subgroups of Native Americans who generally had the smallest crania, such as the Peruvian Incas, were overrepresented in his samples of American Indians. When measuring Caucasians, however, Morton conveniently excluded all but three Asian Indians in his collection of skulls, as their generally smaller crania would have brought the average size down.

Morton's experiments followed the conventional social wisdom of the time as closely as a train follows its tracks. As notions of racial character evolved to what we believe to be a more enlightened view, so has the position of physical anthropology. While certain structures in the skeleton vary regularly among races, they apparently bear no relationship to intelligence or character. For forensic anthropologists these differences are simply road maps that point them in the right direction. For example, about 80 percent of Native Americans have spade-shaped incisors. And most people of African descent have a wider nasal opening than Caucasians.

In 1930 Todd took a long look at 398 skulls of black American adults, 64 white Anglo-Saxon skulls, and 277 skulls of black Africans. He noted some typical differences between blacks and whites that still are helpful in identifying skulls. He found that skulls of blacks showed undulating rather than mesalike brow ridges; sharper margins at the top of the eye sockets, or orbits; a more rounded glabella, the most forward projecting midline part of the frontal bone; a slight difference in smoothness of the fronto-nasal junction, where the nasal bone that forms the bridge of the nose meets the frontal bone or forehead; and a wider gap between the eyes, called the inter-orbital distance. Other slight differences in shape can be seen from the lateral view, as well as in the overall shape of the head.

With the advent of more sophisticated discriminant-function analysis, in which different measurements are weighted in their ability to discriminate among skeletal features for race or sex, the accuracy of racial identification has improved. Anthropologists since the 1960s have been able to fix the race of an unidentified skull 90 percent of the time.[13] But the admixture of races in the United States has guaranteed enough blending to keep physical anthropologists busy remeasuring and recalculating, looking for better suites of measurements that will save them the headaches of dealing only with skulls.

From the turn of the century until 1939, physical anthropologists fought to establish themselves as something other than anatomists or bone collectors who enjoyed an occasional trek in the bush. One such fighter was a masterful if somewhat fractious Czech named Aleš Hrdlička. Hrdlička, a serious academic, put the stamp of respectability on the discipline in 1918 by launching the field's first journal, the *American Journal of Physical Anthropology*. Ten years later Hrdlička founded the American Association of Physical Anthropologists (in the culture of science an association proclaims a discipline's coming of age).

Forensic pursuits did not figure in the pages of the journal nor in the interests of the association, however. Hrdlička was trained as a doctor as well as an anthropologist, but he cared more for organizing his peers and directing scientific politics from the helm of the Smithsonian Institution's Museum of Natural History than for directing their abilities to more practical pursuits (although he was ahead of his time in trying to interest anthropologists in the physical and cultural anthropology of black Americans). Few anthropologists at the time, in fact, volunteered their services to the police, nor did the authorities often seek help from professors locked away in their laboratories.

Wilton Marion Krogman was an exception. An anatomist and physical anthropologist, Krogman spent a year with T. Wingate Todd at Case Western Reserve Medical School in Cleveland in 1928. Still of a mind to classify, Todd had begun collecting an unprecedented store of skeletons from known individuals, each of which was meticulously measured and duly recorded. Seeing that no one else in the country knew or cared as much as Todd about mapping the skeletal characteristics of populations, Krogman returned to Case after his first year there and stayed on at the medical school for ten more, in the process earning an associate professorship. During that time Krogman and Todd collaborated on a handful of forensic cases and found the work interesting enough to codify. The product, *A Guide to the Identification of Human Skeletal Material*, was one of those quiet contributions to human knowledge that the public never sees but the contents of which, like law books or symphonic scores, reaches them secondhand through a corps of interpreters. In this case the interpreters were at the Federal Bureau of Investigation, which by the bloody days of gangsterism during the 1930s had begun to sit up and take notice of what physical anthropologists had to offer. Krogman gave them their first lesson by publishing the guide in the *FBI Law Enforcement Bulletin*, thus inaugurating a special relationship between anthropologists and the FBI that endures today.

At about the same time, the FBI discovered a whole nest of anthropologists in the red gothic towers of the Smithsonian Institution, located only a few blocks from J. Edgar Hoover's office in Washington. Streetwise FBI agents began making the short trip across the green pastures of the city's resplendent mall to the Smithsonian's laboratories, lugging body parts to present to the museum's tweedy scholars.

As the G-men dumped more criminal cases on their desks, anthropologists realized the need for a broader data base in which to prospect for repeating patterns in the skeleton. For example, were there sets of measurements that would back up their own subjective judgments of sex and race? The need was especially urgent because the courts, where an expert won only as much respect from a jury as the skills of cross-examining attorneys permitted, required something better than "In my considered opinion this is indeed the pelvis of a Caucasian female."

Scientific theory sets like a custard when enough raw data from observations have been accumulated and analyzed. Such data may take the form of boxes full of dessicated beetles' wings for the entomologist or the spiraling tracks left by smashed atoms for the particle physicist. For physical (and forensic) anthropologists, bodies equal data. But since bodies generally don't keep as well as beetles' wings, they settle for skeletons. And forensic scientists prefer fresher skeletons: the bones of a two thousand-year-old Egyptian mummy don't reflect the norm of twentieth-century Homo sapiens. Diet and modern medical treatment have changed our bones. Thus the Todd collection, as the thirty-three hundred skeletons at Case Western came to be known, became the main laboratory for those who, as Daniel Webster was once described, were possessed enough by death to see the skulls of their fellow men beneath their skin.[14]

The Todd collection and one other, the Terry collection (after anatomist Robert J. Terry) at Washington University in St. Louis, with 1,636 skeletons, served as lodestars for forensic anthropologists until the 1940s. An hour's worth of battle during World War II produced enough bodies to outnumber the Todd collection. It was from the war's victims that forensic anthropologists were finally able to advance their knowledge in one fell swoop. In 1946 the Army's Office of the Quartermaster General hired an anthropologist to help identify war dead. The Graves Registration Service also required anthropological skills in order to repatriate war dead in Europe and subsequently in the Pacific. One of these anthropologists, a woman from St. Louis, saw a chance to turn this tedious and depressing task into something that could help the living.

Mildred Trotter was teaching anatomy at Washington University's School of Medicine in St. Louis when, in 1948, the Graves Registration Service asked her to set up shop in Hawaii. Bodies from Guadalcanal, Iwo Jima, the Philippine jungles, and the other battlefields of the Pacific were still in need of identification. The toughest cases fell to her: bodies, most without a trace of tissue or even hair, had to be matched with old X rays, physical descriptions supplied by relatives, dental charts, or the measurements taken when soldiers were conscripted. At the time, anthropologists still relied on the regression equations derived from Rollet's one hundred French cadavers to determine stature.[15]

Trotter's charge from the Army was simply to make identifications. Her bosses at the morgue in Hawaii didn't think much of this headstrong woman's idea of measuring almost all the bones of the bodies they had already identified. Trotter convinced them otherwise, pointing out that the charts and tables that she had to rely on to estimate height from long bones of the arm or leg were not only fifty years out of date but were French as well. She got her way.

Thus began the most extensive assessment ever undertaken aimed at estimating height from bones. Trotter and her assistants spent months measuring femurs, tibias, fibulas, humeruses, radiuses, and ulnas on osteometric boards. If they had both of a pair of bones from the same body, they averaged their lengths to reduce the chances of random variation. Military records assured them at least of the height of the skeletons in life. In all, they measured 790 male skeletons, 710 of which were from whites and 80 of which were from blacks.[16]

Trotter knew that the European regression equations didn't apply well to Americans. She already had tested them on the bones of one hundred white American males of known height and found that they miscalculated stature by as much as 4.38 centimeters. It was simply a matter of trying different numbers in the equation until she got one that reliably predicted height. Along with the war dead, Trotter measured skeletons from the Todd and Terry collections. She got the best fit — in which the mean error in her predictions of height from the length of the femur was only 0.02 centimeters — by multiplying the femoral length by 2.38 and then adding 61.41 centimeters.[17]

Trotter's unglamorous work replaced the standard of over half a century and remains the method most often used despite efforts by scores of anthropologists to improve on it. Only her own revisions a decade later, based on Korean War dead, altered what she established in the morgue in Hawaii. Because the Korea victims represented a wider genetic mix, including Mexicans, Puerto Ricans, and Orientals, these later measurements were more comprehensive.[18] (They also were generally less predictive, as it turned out, probably because racial mixing tends to blur osteological distinctions.)

That American soldiers of the mid-twentieth century were built differently from Rollet's Frenchmen should not have come as a surprise. Race and family alone do not predict anatomy; diet, a function of wealth as well as culture, also affects the way any animal or population of animals grows. Trotter also dethroned the notion that men's bones stop growing after age eighteen. In her sample growth continued until the early twenties. And she found that the relationships between bone length, especially of the leg bones, and height differs enough among whites, blacks, and Mongoloids to require different regression equations for each. Furthermore, Trotter's studies in the 1950s showed that contemporary white males with a given set of bone lengths were actually taller than they would have been a few decades earlier.

The Korean War drew the most attention from modern forensic experts. Not only were the equations for estimation of height rewritten, but also the means for estimating age. Never before had anthropologists in the United States had a chance to examine the skeletons of such a large number of young adults of known age.

The man who carried out the first extensive Korean War study was T. Dale Stewart. Every forensic anthropologist knows Stewart's name. He was to the discipline what Cecil B. deMille was to moving pictures. Of the old school, having first acquired an M.D. before moving into anthropology, Stewart shares only with Krogman the leading role in placing forensics in the firmament of physical anthropology. It was Stewart who tutored the FBI while he oversaw the anthropology division at the Smithsonian. A man of wit and formidable experience, he not only forged many of the tools of the science but helped others advance within their own specialties.

In 1954 officials of the Graves Registration Service asked Stewart to help them identify the war dead from Korea. As he had advised Trotter to do years before, Stewart took advantage of having hundreds of skeletons at his disposal to test some hypotheses of his own. His goal was to pinpoint changes in the skeleton as a person ages. The better one knows how bones change with age, the sharper the snapshot of death presented by the skeleton.

Stewart spent four months in a grimy industrial town called Kokura on the island of Kyushu in Japan. The place was a Mecca for anthropologists; nowhere had they ever had so many skeletons from known Americans to study. They labored daily in a stark warehouse stacked high with boxes of bones shipped back from Korea. Stewart's team examined 450 of them, mostly young men. Every day, boxes were unpacked, bones laid out in anatomical order on workbenches, and each one described in relentless detail under the scrutiny of the eminent professor from the Smithsonian. Although good-natured and jocular, Stewart insisted on a rigorous attention to method and an almost messianic devotion to the science.

The work both fascinated and depressed the small group of anthropologists. On the one hand, they were privileged to have the chance to test their ideas. Was dry bone weight an indicator of a person's living weight? Did age show on a person's vertebrae? Was bone continuously remodeled during a person's lifetime in a way that could reflect age at death? On the other hand, these were not the bones of some Iroquoian hunters culled from a three-hundred-year-old ossuary. These had been American boys who grew up on baseball diamonds and joined the Boy Scouts and danced the jitterbug on Saturday nights in the same towns and cities the scientists called home. And there were so many. Each day another femur, another shattered rib, another broken breastbone. Four hundred and fifty, and they were to all the dead of the war no more than a few fallen leaves in a vast forest. The scientific papers that flowed from the months in Kokura faithfully correlated age with symphyseal pits, the unions of epiphyses to diaphyses, the odontoid and transverse processes of the vertebrae, the femoral trochanters, the saggital sutures, the iliac crests, the medial epicondyles, and on and on like some Latin ode to an ancient hero. They did not record the late-night reflections on the fragility of life that disquiet the mind of anyone, seasoned professional or neophyte, who has held another human's bones in his hands.

The Kokura exercise, part of what the military called its Operation Glory repatriation program, in which war dead were exchanged across the demilitarized zone, sharpened the tools that now were proliferating within forensic anthropology. Stewart and a colleague, Thomas McKern of the Army's Quartermaster Research and Engineering Center in Natick, Massachusetts, established a new method for estimating age at death. Working with casts, drawings, and measurements taken in Kokura, they worked out a numerical scoring system for determining age. The best predictor, they found, was the degree of union between the parts of nine bones.[19] Until about the age of eighteen, the shafts of long bones, the diaphyses, are separate from their bony caps, the epiphyses. Some other bones, such as the centra — the central body — of the vertebrae, the collarbone (clavicle), the shoulder blade (scapula), the sacrum at the base of the spine, and parts of the pelvic bones, also have epiphyses. When a person reaches his or her mid-teens, the epiphyses begin to join the diaphyses, eventually forming a seamless union.

Because different bones complete this process at different times in a person's lifetime, they offer additional reference points that anthropologists can use to establish age at death.[20] For example, the epiphyses at the distal end (furthest from the trunk) of the femur joins the diaphysis at between fourteen and nineteen years of age (although the process may be complete slightly earlier in girls). The earliest union in a skeleton occurs at a part of the head of the humerus called the greater tubercle (tubercle being the name for a small projection or mound on a bone), at between two and four years of age. The clavicle is among the last to unify, doing so at its medial end, where it meets the sternum, between the ages of twenty-three and twenty-five.

Stewart had also taken careful note of another part of the human skeleton that, thirty-seven years earlier, Todd had discovered to be astoundingly regular and predictable in its evolution through a person's lifetime — the pubic symphysis. Stewart and McKern argued that Todd had oversimplified the range of changes in the symphysis. Like climbers diagraming an assault on a mountain face, Stewart and McKern described its every feature. To a layman it looked like a pockmarked, bumpy piece of bone no more regular than a chip of volcanic rock. To Stewart it possessed a dorsal plateau, billowy and grooved like a down quilt; a ventral rampart, beveled and porous; and a symphyseal rim, which over time gradually circumscribes the symphyseal surface until, with age, it begins to crumble like a Roman wall. Each section, Stewart found, changes independently of the others and at different rates. He and McKern assigned each section a number between zero and five, according to how far along it had metamorphosed. The numerical totals were correlated with the age. A total score of four to five meant that the person died at age eighteen to twenty-three, for example. The highest possible score, fifteen, indicated an age at death of at least thirty-six.

The Stewart-McKern method, distilled in 1957, proved to be the most accurate means ever devised to estimate age at death. Plaster casts of symphyses were manufactured, eighteen of them showing the six stages for the three sections. Forensic anthropologists, looking like itinerant chess players in search of a match, still carry them in felt-lined wooden boxes into morgues across the country.

Still, the symphysis tells little about a skeleton over thirty-six years of age. Again it was Stewart who brought back from his experience in Japan a new idea for identifying older skeletons. Working with the Korea casts and observations from the Terry collection, he observed a regular buildup of bony growths, known as osteophytes, on the centra of vertebrae. These start to form as early as age twenty and grow larger over time due to the ossification of cartilage into bone. Many joints suffer from similar growths, especially the elbow and knee. These growths help confirm estimations of age. So also do the ends of the ribs where they meet the sternum. They are rounded and blunt in youth, but ossification of the cartilage gives them a rough and ragged appearance, like the end of a badly rusted pipe, by middle age. Bones also become thin with advanced age as the central medullary cavity, which holds the marrow inside the bone, expands at the expense of the cortex, the dense outer wall of the bone. The cranial vault grows thinner with very advanced age. Bones also become pitted over time. And years of friction at the articular surfaces of bones wears away cartilage and polishes, or eburnates, the bone, another sign that a person lived to an advanced age.

Although Krogman in 1962 finally presented the state of the art in the first definitive text, *The Human Skeleton in Forensic Medicine*, Stewart became the guardian of the science. During his sixty years at the Smithsonian — he continued as a consultant through his eighties — Stewart created a cadre of experts and a body of practice that gave the discipline respect. He tutored not only two generations of osteologists and physical anthropologists there, but the FBI as well. His watchword was skepticism, not only of what the evidence suggests on first impression, but of one's own motivations. He cites his own backsliding as a warning:

> To cite an actual case, one day Dr. Newman [Marshall T., of the Smithsonian's staff] and an FBI agent came into my room and said, "Here are some burned finger bones. We want to know whether you think they are human." I feel that it is not surprising, therefore, that I examined these bones as phalanges [finger bones], opined that they were not human, and suggested that they be taken to the director of mammals for specific identification. The mammologist somehow avoided or overcame the same fixation because the report came back that instead of being finger bones, they were tail bones of a horse.[21]

Stewart frequently lectured his colleagues on ways to apply their science to the crime lab. He suspected many of his colleagues of boasting when they claimed the ability, for example, to distinguish sex correctly nine times out of ten on the basis of two measurements of the pelvis or one measurement of the mandible. "I suspect that there is a general tendency to become overconfident" of sexing abilities, Stewart said. This was something more than a polite criticism considering that one of the scientists he referred to was Hrdlička, his predecessor at the Smithsonian and a demigod in American physical anthropology. He also chastised Krogman, heavyweight (figuratively and literally at well over six feet and two hundred pounds) of the bone scientists, for describing the study of the skeleton in his 1939 article in the FBI *Bulletin* as an "exact science" whose practitioners apply "precise methods." Warned Stewart, "I feel that these statements are a bit on the optimistic side and create the false impression that skeletal identification is largely mechanical." While his laboratory was regarded as the standard against which others were compared, Stewart noted that although pulp magazines lavished attention on him as the Sherlock Holmes of forensic osteology, only three cases he worked on ever got all the way to trial.

The progress of forensic anthropology after the Korean War accelerated for several reasons. Besides the access to larger numbers of skeletons that war provided, scientific methodology, especially microscopy, led to new techniques. As is often the case in science, new tools whose usefulness appears at first dubious usher in new theories, rather than vice versa. Video cameras that can superimpose a photograph of a suspected missing person over the image of a skull have made identifications that could never have been accomplished otherwise. More accurate measurements of the thickness of the facial skin have given medical sculptors the information that they needed to recreate lifelike busts of the living person from nothing more than an anonymous skull.

Anthropologists have also learned the latest nuances of statistical analysis. They can quantify in cold numbers the subtlest turn of the ankle, the daintiest curve of the cheekbone, or the most shadowy crescent of the orbit. They put them down in tables and charts, submit them to mathematical cross-examination, and test them against new skeletons to scrape away the vestiges of opinion and guesswork.

But forensic anthropology still requires some artistry along with empirical measurement. Measurement techniques can be learned from books and professors; artistry requires years of close association with the bones, which only a rare passion for the human form and its evolution can sustain. Forensic anthropology to the journeyman could be called navigating by the book. To the artist, it is dead reckoning.

4

THE SKY ABOVE

A man's house reveals a great deal about the way his mind is organized. Besides being an animal shelter, Clyde Snow's cluttered rambler on the Oklahoma prairie serves as part library and part museum. Tomahawks, antique chess sets, portraits of Sac and Fox warriors, sketches of apes and monkeys and skulls, Navajo rugs, and an occasional bleached bone fill any space that isn't already occupied by furniture, animals, or pet paraphernalia. Open books lie about, the way books do when consumed by the restless scholar who reads until satisfied then drops a book where he stands and picks up another. Hardbound histories predominate, of the American West especially, but also on the British in Egypt and the Russian Empire. Torsos and faces, stripped of skin to show the graceful undulations of muscle and sinew, stare up from the pages of anatomy texts. The complete works of Shakespeare lie alongside the poetry of John Donne and manuals on crime-scene investigations.

Order, at least the kind in which objects or ideas are neatly shelved like items in a supermarket, does not rank highly in Snow's universe. His wife, Jerry, indulges his eccentricities. Over the years, Snow's bosses at the Federal Aviation Administration and the Civil Aeromedical Institute (CAMI) did likewise, if for different reasons.

Snow's controversial report on survival in air crashes lived to be published in 1970, Hippocratic allusions included, but the episode left both sides wary of each other. Snow's skill at his job in the protection and survival branch of CAMI, in a discipline whose practitioners could be counted in the dozens, counterbalanced his prickliness. It allowed him also to consult for various police departments, an outlet from the tedium of government work. The role of expert-on-call appealed to him, and his growing renown also reflected well on CAMI, whose directors gave Snow time away from the office to work on criminal cases. What began as a pastime would eventually absorb all his attention, focus his talents, and one day help him solve some of the century's bloodiest crimes.

The pathologist who assists police departments to investigate crimes exemplifies the classical character of a forensic scientist: a medical man, somewhat slow and methodical but wise within his narrow field, and a trusty Watson for the erratic genius of Sherlock Holmes. Well before Snow's forensic apprenticeship, however, the science had begun to change. Pathologists began to share their morgues with a menagerie of specialists — geneticists, entomologists, and now, anthropologists.

After the Oklahoma child disappearances case in 1967, the local and state police and the medical examiner's office started to bring skulls or pieces of skeletons to Snow's lab at CAMI. He would turn the bones carefully in his big hands and suggest that the splay of the pelvic bones indicated a female skeleton, or that the shape of the condyle on this femur indicated that the sheriff had dragged in part of a cow. As the number of consultations grew, Snow found himself going back again and again to the few texts that described how to view the human skeleton through the magnifying glass of forensics. His copies of Wilton Krogman's *Human Skeleton in Forensic Science* grew dog-eared with use. The *American Journal of Forensic Science* carried a few papers now and then about bones, and a careful search of the anthropological journals sometimes yielded clues that might explain an errant bone found in an irrigation ditch or down a well. The practical and scientific literature amounted to little more than dribs and drabs, however. As in most arcane pursuits, true expertise came slowly, case by case.

One of Snow's confidants during those years was a young doctor who in 1972 arrived at the doorstep of the Oklahoma medical examiner's office fresh-faced and as green as the forests of his native Maine. Slightly built, well-read beyond his medical texts, and painfully sensitive, Fred Jordan stuck out in this rodeo town like a debutante on a dude ranch. He'd never even owned a pair of cowboy boots. As an assistant to the chief medical examiner, Jordan's introduction to crime was as abrupt and shocking as a dive into a freezing pond. In Snow he found a mentor.

"Snow was an independent operator of extremely high reputation," recalls Jordan. "He was totally intellectually scrupulous. He does the science in its most pure, sterile form. And then he turns it from a sterile sea into a flower of compassion and understanding to the people who are left with the suffering that generated the case in the first place."[1]

Jordan and Snow worked together on dozens of cases, most of them murder investigations. For Jordan, who eventually became chief medical examiner for Oklahoma, the experience has left indelible marks that sometimes show through a protective layer of black humor:

> You are killed by the people you work with, the people you sleep with, the people you know, your family. . . . Today, most of the cases are of drug deals that have gone bad, domestic problems, fights in bars where bodies are taken out and dumped in a ditch. . . . The type of work we were doing here, and this may be part of my discontent, is that you are documenting man's inhumanity to man. But you are also documenting cases about which you can take no corrective action. I don't think that to put somebody in jail is corrective action. Well, it is, but it's not going to do anything. . . .
>
> It is one of the frustrating things about day-to-day work in a forensic office like this. Satisfactions are not with homicides. They are, for example, dealing with the suicides, that is, helping the families determine whether a death was a suicide or murder. In a way, we helped diagnose an epidemic when teenage suicides were becoming so common. Or it's satisfaction in finding an unknown disease that is in a family that they didn't know about. But most of the murders are just killings, you know, they're bad people, they're bad actors who have got themselves in trouble. They've gone out drinking, violence has erupted. . . .

Snow usually uncovered something intriguing in these criminal cases, however, something that flipped on the switch of curiosity while blotting out some of the horror. "When he was on a roll, you had to keep him busy," Jordan recalls. "It was a very revealing experience. If you asked him if he was depressed, then he'd say 'Hell, no,' because he is a different kind of person that way. If I'm depressed I'll be happy to tell you because maybe you can help me. That is a very real phenomenon in people who deal in the kind of work he was doing."

Few events in Snow's career would test this emotional mettle like those that took place in 1979 in Chicago. It was a tumultuous year. Although deadly accidents and shocking murders had become almost commonplace, the last year of the 1970s in Chicago was unusually calamitous, as if humanity, like the reckless Greek Phaeton, whose daring ride in the chariot of the gods earned him a fatal thunderbolt from Jupiter, needed a reminder not to presume it had mastered nature or even its own basest instincts. For Snow, it was a turning point in his career.

On the cloudless, sunny afternoon of Friday, May 25, 1979, American Airlines 191 took off from runway 32R at Chicago's O'Hare International Airport. Heading for Los Angeles, the plane lifted off the runway smoothly, heading northwest out of the airport's busy traffic. The McDonnell-Douglas DC-10 reached an altitude of about two hundred feet when the left engine and pylon assembly and about three feet of the leading edge of the left wing suddenly broke off the aircraft and plunged to the runway.

An air-traffic controller in the tower saw the engine fall, hit the runway, and skid along like a hockey puck for several thousand feet. He immediately radioed the plane: "American one ninety-one, do you want to come back? If so, what runway do you want?"[2]

No reply came. Scores of onlookers watched, transfixed and disbelieving, as the plane continued to climb to three hundred and twenty-five feet before it slowly began to roll to the left until it was flying sideways, its wings perpendicular to the ground. Describing an arc, its nose pitched further and further groundward until its left wing rent the earth in an open field near the runway. Less than a second later, the rest of the plane hit, exploded in a mushroom of flame, and scattered in innumerable pieces across the field and into an adjacent trailer park.[3]

Brian Pekovic, eighteen years old and a resident of the trailer park, gave this account:

"It [the plane] was leaning over so I knew something was wrong. It was shaking . . . going up and down, up and down. Then its nose just went straight down. All the area was full of black smoke. And then the heat. It must have been over 100 degrees blowing across the trailer park."

Two hundred and fifty-eight passengers, thirteen crew members, and two people on the ground were killed instantly. Flight 191 entered the history books as the deadliest crash in American aviation.

Little could be done until the flames and heat had dissipated. That evening and into the next day, crews picked through the rubble looking for bodies. Bruce Arbeit, a fireman in Chicago's Norwood Park, described the scene to a reporter: "We didn't see one body intact. Just bits and pieces. We haven't been able to see a face or anything, just trunks, hands, arms, heads, and parts of legs. But we couldn't tell whether they were male or female, whether they were an adult or a child, because they were all charred." Sticks with numbers printed on them rose out of the ground like newly planted seedlings. Each represented a body or part of one. Lit up with floodlights and hastily fenced in to keep curiosity-seekers out, the field smoked like a corner of Hell.

The Cook County medical examiner's office set up a morgue at a huge American Airlines hangar. Nine-foot-long body bags were lined up on the floor until a refrigerated van arrived. The National Transportation Safety Board flew in a "go team," a group of crash experts from around the country who keep their suitcases packed in case they get a call, day or night, to fly to a crash scene. Engine specialists from General Electric Corporation arrived, as did representatives of the Allied Pilots Union and McDonnell-Douglas. Experts grouped themselves into committees: power plant, airframe, navigation, weather, human factors, and so on.

Identifying the dead was the domain of the human factors team. Cook County's chief medical examiner, Robert Stein, a dapper and well-traveled man trained in Europe, led the investigation. At least one hundred expert investigators set to work. Teams consisting of a pathologist, dentist, lab technician, medical investigator, and recorder concentrated on one set of remains at a time, laying them out on the dozen tables set up in a corner of the vast hangar. The FBI had sent experts to get palm prints and fingerprints, although it was doubtful that files would exist on many of the passengers and crew. On other tables, workers stacked personal effects collected from the wreckage and the field where it lay. Rings, bracelets, watches, cameras, wallets, and the like accumulated in small, forlorn mounds like forgotten belongings in a hotel's lost and found.

Stein insisted that everything possible, including autopsies, be done to identify biologically as many victims as possible. As crash investigators well knew, passengers sometimes aren't the same people listed on tickets and flight manifests. To settle an estate, the law requires a death certificate. And Stein, like most reputable medical examiners, didn't plan to write any without exhausting every effort to make a final identification.

The condition of many of the bodies was such that dentists were making more headway than anyone else in identifications. Among them was a loquacious odontologist from New York, Lowell Levine. Darkly bearded, intense, and outspoken, the forty-one-year-old Levine had made his forensic reputation as a consultant to the medical examiner's office in New York City and Long Island's Nassau County. He also advised American Airlines. As one of only 150 forensic odontologists in the country, Levine had his hands full. He had helped verify autopsy X rays taken of John Kennedy for the House Select Committee on Assassinations. He had identified Diana Oughton, twenty-eight, one of three members of the radical Weathermen group who were blown up in a Greenwich Village townhouse on March 17, 1970, presumably by their own bomb. His clues in that investigation consisted of a fragment of a jaw and three and a half teeth.

Levine had become a great promoter of odontology in forensic work and was quick to challenge pathologists and other old hands who regarded dentists as crime junkies looking for an outlet from the day-to-day boredom of staring into people's mouths. He had spent years trying to legitimize the craft, if that was the word for it, of bite-mark identification, that is, the matching of bite marks on bodies to the teeth of murder and rape suspects. In a paper he wrote on the subject, Levine reminded readers, "As long as there have been human beings, human teeth have been used as weapons. As weapons, they have a unique feature: the wounds left by teeth are specific to the person who inflicted them."[4] Levine's work paid off; in 1975 he helped convict a man who strangled a twenty-six-year-old woman in 1974 by matching bite marks he left on the victim's breast.

Edward Pavlik, a Chicago odontologist, took charge of the team of about twenty dentists working on the Flight 191 case. But the press found Levine a reliable source of information and good for a snappy quote or two. In the forensic community, as with most scientists, an unwritten rule says keep the press at arm's length. When a scientist discusses his or her work, understatement and restraint are the watchwords. But Levine didn't care much for this rule; he said what he thought.

Levine had been sitting at dinner with his family in a restaurant in Fort Lauderdale, Florida, the evening of May 25 when he overheard diners at the next table mention a horrible plane crash in Chicago. He skipped dessert and boarded a plane to Chicago. At O'Hare, he booked a room at the Hilton, then tracked down Stein at the American Airlines hangar. Within hours, he and others had assembled what he described as "probably the largest institute of forensic pathology in the world."[5] Besides eight "reefers," large refrigerated vans for the bodies, workers installed running water, lights, and telephones in the hangar. Safes were brought in as well. "In these types of accidents," Levine told the press, "there usually is cash, lots of valuables, and they often disappear right at the scene."

Stein put the medical types in a large room on the second floor of the hangar. Levine, ever dramatic, called it the "medical intelligence center."

We took everything off the walls and papered them with brown wrapping paper. We broke the space into three hundred large rectangles on one side and three hundred on the other. We weren't sure exactly how many were dead. As we gathered names, we'd put them up on one wall, then add to the corresponding wall, as pouch numbers [body bags] came in, records, reports, all evidence, personal effects, heights, weights, ages, clothing fragments.

The administrative setup involved thousands and thousands of little pieces of paper. Each scrap may become the single

97

thing that allows you to make an identification — fingerprints, medical records, and dental information.

Even a negative dental identification is useful. If you can't tell who it is, you can tell who it isn't. So the process of elimination helps. It's painstaking. You go through so many things one way, then reach an impasse. Then you start a whole different approach. . . .

Because of the fire, there were almost no clothing fragments. Those fragments that were found were covered with jet fuel and charred. They had to be hand-washed and air-dried so they wouldn't disintegrate from the heat. These provided a clue to labels and sizes.

Also, jewelry was hard to find. That, too, had to be cleaned. Even a quarter-inch fragment of gold chain might be distinctive enough to be helpful later on. Thousands of fragments of personal property were accessioned. If there are trousers on a torso, the wallet in the pocket becomes useful. If just a wallet is found, it is not really worth a lot.

Basically, all the people become detectives. One nurse found a ring with a faded inscription inside. There were two names and a wedding date. This provided good tentative identifications, which we confirmed with other physical findings.

Within a few days, the investigators had named the majority of the passengers and crew. But several dozen sets of remains eluded identification. At the medical command center, Levine took Stein aside and made a suggestion: call Clyde Snow.

Snow arrived at the O'Hare Hilton with a single duffel bag, a change of underwear, a set of calipers, and a wooden, green-felt-lined box containing casts of pubic symphyses. Levine had told him he'd probably only be needed for a few days. Snow would end up eating, drinking, and sleeping the DC-10 disaster for the next five weeks.

In the morgue at the hangar, fifty bodies or their parts remained to be identified. Presumably, among the scores of medical and dental X rays and personal descriptions of the passengers that filled the rows of gray filing cabinets along the hangar's walls, some clue to the contents of each of the remaining yellow body bags lay to be discovered. Matching records with bones would be a gargantuan job, Snow told the forensic teams, trying their skills and their patience. Strong coffee would become a drug, food an afterthought, and sleep their only respite.

They needed a good radiologist. Forensics had not attracted many to its ranks, even though some precedent for using radiographs to identify unknown bodies existed. The first such identification took place in 1927, when two radiologists, W. L. Culbert and F. M. Law, identified a body from radiographs of a skull's nasal sinuses and the shape of its mastoid processes, located just behind each ear. Culbert had operated on the man in question in happier times to cure his mastoiditis.[6] In 1925 his patient disappeared in India's Indus River. Two years later a skeleton matching his description was found in the river, and the two doctors made the positive ID from their radiographic records.

A more tragic event provided radiologists with their biggest breakthrough. On September 17, 1949, the steamship *Noronic* burned while tied to a pier in Toronto, Canada. The fire raged quickly and engulfed and killed 119 people, 107 of whom were burned beyond recognition. Radiographers tried an untested technique, focusing their efforts in several cases on a small bone called the sphenoid, shaped like a bat in flight, located at the front and base of the skull. The sphenoid contains a small depression, the sella turcica, which houses the pituitary body and is perforated with holes to allow vessels into the organ. More important, at least to forensic experts, the bone's shape varies from person to person, enough so that investigators were able to identify nineteen of the *Noronic*'s dead from radiographs of it.[7]

In Chicago, however, Stein's team had no formal list of radiologists from which to draw on short notice. Stein knew of one, however, right in the neighborhood: the sober redhead, John Fitzpatrick.

Stein called Fitzpatrick at his office at the Cook County Hospital, where he practiced. When his workday ended, Fitzpatrick loosened his tie, threw his jacket into the back of his green Mercury Montego, and drove out through the western suburbs, under the overpasses and around the concrete cloverleafs, past the warehouses and truck depots, and finally to the massive hangars ringing O'Hare. By early evening the first shift had finished its day and the second shift was drifting in through the pools of lamplight cast in the echoing depths of the American Airlines hangar.

"The first thing they had me do," Fitzpatrick remembers, "was to go through a list of passengers who had had gunshot wounds. I think there were ten people who supposedly had gunshot wounds." He scanned the antemortem X rays sent in by relatives and compared them with the ones taken of the still-unidentified bodies retrieved from the smoldering field. Snow had already weeded out the remains of pheasants, stray dogs, and other animals whose bones are often inadvertently mixed in with human remains in these types of field searches.

Fitzpatrick found a small piece of metal buried in one man's forearm, a couple of inches below the elbow. A few calls to families of as-yet-unidentified passengers led the team to the victim's brother. Yes, he recalled over the phone, his brother used to have people feel this bullet underneath the skin. He thought it had been a .22, the brother said over the phone. A youngster's voice cut in and said no, it was from an air rifle. "Where had the pellet lodged?" Fitzpatrick asked. Just below the elbow, the family agreed. Fitzpatrick had made another identification.[8]

It wasn't always so simple. Some families declined to cooperate. Many had been advised by their attorneys not to talk at all to anyone pending the outcome of lawsuits against the airline. Some were downright hostile. "And sometimes you ran into a ticklish situation," Fitzpatrick recalls. "I knew of one case where the investigators called someone's home about a woman. Let's call her Mrs. X. They thought Mrs. X was one of the bodies. Well, Mrs. X was alive. Her husband had been killed, and there were two tickets, for Mr. X and Mrs. X."

The team worked under the able guidance of Robert Kirschner, assistant medical examiner for Cook County. Five and a half feet of bustling energy, the moon-faced, wisecracking Kirschner wore his dark beard without benefit of mustache and tended to bounce on the balls of his feet when he talked. He treated the work at hand with the utmost respect, but away from the job he played *tummler* for the weary troops.

Kirschner had performed many autopsies. But the scope of this disaster taught him a few lessons, not as much about how people die as much as how they lived.

"There was the girl in the Liz Claiborne blouse," Kirschner recounts. She had a mouthful of gold. The team thought they knew who she was from the passenger list but they needed harder evidence. "It was very difficult to get records from her dentist in Rochester to confirm. This woman lived in a well-to-do suburb and had a lot of dental work done." When they finally got hold of the records, it was obvious why the dentist had been reluctant: the records showed far less work than what the team had found in the woman's teeth. "This was a characteristic of this air crash . . . he had obviously shown half of the dental work on his records so he could cut his income to the IRS. On the other hand, if you got a welfare dentist, you saw a person who actually has three fillings in their mouth, but the dental record would show ten. They were marking 'em down left and right so they could collect from Medicaid!"[9]

It fell to Kirschner to deal with an impossible demand from the U.S. Department of State. Apparently a family of Saudi Arabians of some importance had been aboard Flight 191, and the government wanted them identified first. And Kirschner took the call from the woman who insisted on coming to pick up her daughter's bones because she didn't want them to be buried next to any Jews.

Meanwhile, Fitzpatrick continued to search for radiographic matches. Many of the victims fit a single stereotype: the average businessman. They were white, forty to mid-fifties in age, about five feet ten inches tall, and rarely adorned with helpful hints such as tattoos (if the remains were not skeletonized) or wounds that would have marked their bones. The less variety, the harder the job.

Fitzpatrick struggled. He had seen death close at hand, first in autopsies in medical school, then in Vietnam, where he had first put his medical training to work. He had also performed a radiological analysis in a "Jane Doe" case in North Chicago. But he'd never been exposed to a mass disaster like this. Quiet, even reticent, he was slow to warm to the others. "I felt a little bit like an outsider with people who had been in these things for a long time," Fitzpatrick remembers. He found in Snow a laconic partner with an unhurried pace, quite the opposite of Levine.

"I had almost no experience. I was out of my field. It took a while for me to get courage to start asking these guys to go pull a body out again and, say, take out the spine. But when they started doing that and cleaning them up, it helped quite a bit."

The spines in many cases were twisted or bent out of line. They certainly were not in the same anatomical positions shown in the antemortem films, as they had been when the people had been X-rayed at hospitals or the doctor's office. The individual vertebrae held clues, however. Each had its own terrain. Pedicles, transverse processes, and spines set them apart from one another just as bluffs, escarpments, and ravines define a landscape.

Three young girls, all in their teens or late twenties, all unidentified, presented a particularly difficult task. Snow had established their sex and age. That was about all the team had to go on. Antemortem chest X rays didn't show the spines well enough to distinguish much. None of the girls had had an extra rib or an injury or anything else to distinguish them. But Fitzpatrick had the clavicles, or collarbones, of two of the girls.

Like a collector checking the authenticity of a masterwork, he compared the angles and shapes of each slender bone with the X rays. In the epiphysis of each he found enough that was unique to match them to an antemortem X ray, making a conclusive identification of two of the girls. The team consequently identified the third by exclusion.

Despite Fitzpatrick's successes, it quickly became apparent that the team needed a better system to keep track of antemortem and postmortem information. The investigators still had several dozen unidentified bodies, each one consisting of a different suite of bones. Some sets were almost whole; others amounted to only a few fragments. Against these, they had to match an array of antemortem clues, as concrete as hospital X rays or as ephemeral as recollections of family and friends.

Snow, who up until this point in the investigation had been preoccupied mostly with settling questions of sex, stature, race, and individuality, had tinkered with computers at the FAA. Perhaps the team could devise a program that would let microchips do the work, he suggested to the others.

No one had tried computerizing forensic data from a mass disaster to make identifications. When he thought about it, Snow realized that a computer suited their kind of problem. Like carpenters fitting together a dovetail joint, the team had to join one set of people, the "living" memories captured in X ray, photo, and description, with another set, the remains in the yellow body bags. In their mechanical relentlessness, computers could do that sort of matching faster and better than any human.

With the help of a programmer from American Airlines, Snow wrote a program on a computer set up at medical headquarters in the hangar. Into it went a complete list of the biographies collected from families of the passengers — injuries, appendectomies, illnesses, whether the men had been circumcised, even the kind of underwear they normally wore. Snow and his partner also entered an anthropological and dental portrait of each victim: sex, age, race, stature, fillings, and reconstructions in the teeth, and marks or peculiarities such as healed fractures, pierced ears, or left-handedness, that could distinguish one body from another.

The computer couldn't have arrived at a better time. The identifications had been coming more slowly, despite the team's eighteen-hour workdays, each spent hauling the grim substance of their work back and forth from the trailers as Kirschner arrived with new information on an unidentified passenger. Anything that could pick up what their bleary eyes might be missing was welcome.

Snow programmed the machine to bring up the description of one set of remains at a time. The program would then scan all the information on the unidentified passengers and print out the names of ten passengers whose descriptions most closely resembled the one set of remains. Fitzpatrick and Snow would then retrieve whatever antemortem X rays they had on the ten passengers, X-ray the remains in question, and set them up side by side for comparison. Sometimes they reversed the procedure, asking the computer to compare a single unidentified passenger's physical history with the whole data base on the remains and to print out the tag numbers of the ten sets of remains most like the missing passenger.

Snow worked during the day and into the early evening, while Fitzpatrick came in nights after putting in his eight hours at Cook County Hospital and on weekends. The two scientists spent what amounted to days sitting in front of the X-ray viewing screen, turning and adjusting films, tracing outlines of this bone and that, searching for the elusive signature of individuality that the computer told them must be there. Matches started to click into place. Within a few days, men and machine had made about a dozen identifications.

And that was all. As quickly as the rush of new identifications had begun, it ground to a halt. There just wasn't enough information to go further. What they had accomplished, however, surprised Kirschner and the old hands at the M.E.'s office. In five weeks, applying a combination of techniques as varied and imaginative as anything attempted before in a crash investigation, the team had identified twenty bodies out of almost fifty.

The scientific teams and work crews had dissolved by this time, their members back at their desks in their regular jobs. Flight 191 lay behind them. Snow and Fitzpatrick packed up their instruments and closed the door on the American Airlines hangar, having fought the rear guard in the campaign to make what restitution the living can for the dead. Twenty-nine bodies of the 273 killed remained unidentified, at least biologically. In the arcane history of mass disasters, Snow and Fitzpatrick had set a milestone of sorts, creating new methods with not-so-new technology to take their science a small step forward.

Snow remembers his five weeks in Chicago:

I'll tell you what, that was the most unpleasant experience in my life. Mass disasters are hard work and you don't really learn. I like to take a single skeleton so I can fiddle around with it a day or two or three days. I'm always running into something new, and you learn a little bit. With these things, you know, you don't learn. . . .

I was staying over at the O'Hare Inn, that was the headquarters. I would get up in the morning and get a cup of coffee, then to gate H1 and American Airlines would have a truck over there waiting for me. We would drive over to the big hangar. I tried to get there at eight o'clock. They would have the crew, with the pathologists, the dentists, the policemen, the medical investigators, the American [Airlines] people. Fitz would get there at about five in the evening. We worked essentially two shifts. . . . I don't think I have ever worked or put out more physical effort in my life. Not heavy work, but it was sustained, just grinding.

I'd get back to the hotel, go up to my room and order from room service, just before midnight, when service stopped. I had a standard thing. I'd have them bring a martini, a split bottle of wine, and a steak. Some dessert and coffee. I would eat and try to do this, that, and the other, but no TV. I'd go to sleep about two or three in the morning, then get up at seven o'clock and try to get out and catch the truck again. . . .

That went on essentially for five weeks. The last three or four days, I was so tired that — and this has never happened to me before or since — I started to drift sideways when I walked. It was some sort of loss of equilibrium.

Had the Flight 191 crash been the only job at hand, Snow might have easily shaken off the somberness and fatigue that dogged his summer of 1979. But he was doing double duty. Between trips to the hangar, he had been called in by frustrated investigators working on a bizarre murder case, one so gruesome as to make old sausage-maker Luetgert's dissolution of his wife seem a prank by comparison.

5

THE MUD BELOW

THE incident that first lifted the lid off the murders in Des Plaines, Illinois, involved fifteen-year-old Robert Piest. On December 11, 1978, Piest called his mother to fetch him from the drugstore where he worked. When she arrived, her son asked her to wait inside while he went out to talk to a contractor about a summer job that would pay more than the $2.85 an hour he was earning at the pharmacy. Mrs. Piest waited for several minutes, then checked outside. Robert had vanished. His mother would never see him again.

Mrs. Piest drove home and called the police. Over the next two days, their inquiries focused on the contractor, who had done some remodeling work at the pharmacy. On December 13, the police visited the man's home and found evidence that Piest had been there. They checked the man's background and learned that he had once served time in Iowa for sexually molesting a young boy. They kept the burly contractor under surveillance for a few days while they secured a search warrant. When they returned to the ranch house at 8213 West Summerdale Avenue, the man calmly admitted that he had killed Piest. In fact, said the contractor, he had killed many, many other boys, usually after having sex with them. If the police looked under his house, said John Wayne Gacy, they could see for themselves.

The next day investigators ripped up the floor of Gacy's house to reveal a muddy eighteen-inch-high crawl space. Under two feet of soil

106

and lime they found one decomposed body and parts of two others. Gacy took the police out to his garage, spray-painted a spot on the cement floor, and told them to dig. Underneath, they found another body. Gacy said they would find about sixteen bodies under his house, and another twenty or so elsewhere, including a lake and a river where he had dumped them.[1]

Gacy's astonished neighbors reported that the man had seemed to be an all-American straight arrow. Outgoing and friendly, he excelled as a salesman for his construction business and seemed to take great interest in his community. He even ploughed the snow from the sidewalks in the neighborhood without being asked. In Iowa he was remembered as an outstanding member of the Jaycees. In Des Plaines he spent much of his spare time entertaining children in a clown costume.

Investigators reported that the thirty-six-year-old Gacy used his clown act as a way to kill. He would say, "Let me show you this trick," such as how to get out of handcuffs. Once the cuffs were on his victim, he would say, "Now let me show you another trick," and get behind the boy. Using a rope or sometimes a board, he would strangle him.

Cook County Medical Examiner Robert Stein arrived at Gacy's house the morning after police discovered the first four bodies. Stein had seen many casualties of Chicago's mean streets. But nothing in the city's history, even the country's, if Gacy's claims proved true, equaled this. Grim-faced, Stein donned overalls, lowered himself through a trap door in a closet inside Gacy's house, and wriggled into the crawl space. The beam of his flashlight illuminated freshly dug earth, pools of stagnant water, and, protruding from the mud, two human arm bones.

Back outside, Stein told reporters that the crawl space would have to be excavated with the same care given to an archaeological dig. "We are going to have my anthropologist over to examine all the evidence that may come up. It's camel-hair brushwork for sure."

Charles Warren, an anthropologist at the University of Illinois' Chicago Circle campus, and forensic odontologist Edward J. Pavlik set up shop at the Cook County M.E.'s office. Over the next few days police brought body after body to the morgue. Gacy's accounts of sex and strangulations were proving chillingly true. Young men and boys who had known Gacy, including some who had had sex with him but escaped, filled the newspapers with stories of orgies and violence.

By December 29 authorities had found twenty-eight bodies, all more or less where Gacy said they would be. Gacy's toll surpassed that of any serial killer in American history. And it kept climbing.

Police found personal items belonging to two of the boys in Gacy's house. For the rest, no tangible clues to their identity existed. Many had presumably been drifters, runaways, the kind of kids who regularly disappear into the night and never return home. The forensic team faced a daunting task. Police called on families who had a missing child to send X rays and dental charts. But by December 30, fewer than a dozen families had contacted the M.E.'s office.[2] And although Gacy had led police to some of the bodies, he could not or would not name most of his victims.

By January 5, 1979, authorities had identified six youths from dental charts and X rays. By January 26, the forensic team had identified four more, two from fingerprints. But Stein was disappointed with the pace. Few dental charts or X rays of missing youths had come in; investigators said they thought families were reluctant to admit that their sons had run away and involved themselves with Gacy. As months dragged on with no further identifications, Stein decided to call in outside help.[3]

Clyde Snow arrived in Chicago several months after the discovery of the first bodies. He had consulted for Stein before and the M.E. knew he didn't have to spell out procedures for the professor from Oklahoma. Stein took Snow straight to the morgue, where fourteen of the thirty-three young men killed by Gacy lay in body bags still marked "unknown."

Snow took over from Warren and teamed up with the radiologist John Fitzpatrick. Fitzpatrick was green when it came to forensic cases. Stein tested him with some of the X rays they had taken of the victims, asking, for example, if this one had the marks of a healed skull fracture or that one a broken elbow. The radiologist soon won Stein's trust and got the job working with Snow.

The final identifications, of course, were the hardest; it was like picking up a crossword puzzle someone has abandoned and trying to fill in those last few spaces. Fitzpatrick first examined the X-ray films that families and police departments had sent in from around the country. He alerted Snow to anything on the films that might show up on the skeletons in the morgue. Meanwhile, Snow started a by-the-book inventory of everything on each skeleton that would paint a picture of its owner in life.

To determine the victims' ages, Snow noted the stages of closure in epiphyses and cranial sutures and whether molars had erupted. He confirmed that the skeletons were male from the relative narrowness of the sciatic notch, a small V-shaped indentation, about the width of a thumb, on the edge of each hip bone; the relative acuteness of a curve on another portion of the same bone, called the subpubic angle; and the overall narrowness of the pelvic opening. Large brow ridges and robust mastoid processes, the latter being the pyramid-shaped promontories of the skull that project down behind each ear, also helped to confirm maleness. Discriminant function analysis of the skulls, in which several measurements are multiplied by standard numbers and then summed, produced a score that indicated that the victims were white. Snow could see as much just by eyeballing them: the cranial vaults were relatively high and narrow, as were the proportions of the face; the nasal openings were narrow; and the alveolar arches (the roof of the mouth) were wide rather than horseshoe shaped.

The sameness of the victims — aged fourteen to the mid-twenties, male, white — made the job of identifying individuals that much more difficult. Gacy had buried some of his victims on top of one another, and it fell to Snow to make sure that bones from different bodies had not been mixed up by the excavation crew. He drew up charts listing thirty-five characteristics of the skull alone for each of the fourteen bodies. Like a ballistics expert looking for grooves on a bullet to trace the gun barrel from which it came, Snow compared every characteristic of each skeleton to the photographs, descriptions, and the few X rays of missing boys that had trickled in to Fitzpatrick. Whenever a promising clue turned up, Snow would climb aboard a plane in Oklahoma City and return to Chicago, to the windowless basement of the morgue on West Polk Street where he and Fitzpatrick would compare the new information to their sets of now all-too-familiar bones. Usually each examination amounted to an exercise in exclusion: something on the skeleton, perhaps a dental restoration, or its height or age, would eliminate it from a match with the new candidate.

In November 1979 the scientists got a break. Their list of missing youths included David Paul Talsma. Talsma had been reported missing from the Chicago area on December 9, 1977. At the time of his disappearance, Talsma would have been nineteen years of age. His family had described him as an ex-Marine, five feet eleven inches tall, with a narrow face.[4]

One further detail — the family's recollection that the boy had once broken the upper bone in his left arm several years before — led them to one of the Gacy skeletons. Snow clearly recognized the signs of such a fracture on the left humerus of skeleton number 1378, the seventeenth dug up at Gacy's house. The fracture was of the supracondyle, a ridge of bone to which muscles are attached at the bottom of the humerus near the elbow. Young children often fracture that part of the arm in a fall in which the elbows hit the ground first. The fracture appeared old and well-healed, and had formed a callus.

But the family also insisted that their son had once injured his head and that doctors had put a metal plate in his skull. The skeleton in Chicago bore no metal plate nor signs of one. So the forensic team had eliminated Talsma from their list.

"But Clyde looked at the skull again," Fitzpatrick recalls.[5] "He thought that the posterior lambdoid suture looked like it had closed earlier and was a little bit flatter, so maybe this guy *had* had a head injury." The suture begins behind each ear and arches across the back of the head. It separates the cranium's occipital bone, just above the top of the neck, from the two parietal bones (from the Latin word *paries* for wall) that form the sides and roof of the cranium.

Fitzpatrick had X rays of Talsma's chest and abdomen from the family, but nothing of the head. Snow leaned on Cook County investigators to find out whether Talsma might have been treated for a skull fracture sometime in his short life. The police tracked down X rays and medical records from a hospital in Kentucky. There was no sign of a metal plate; it had simply been a figment of the family's imagination.

"So then Clyde took the bones, put them in anatomical position, and we radiographed them," Fitzpatrick recalls. "Then I sat down and compared the films of the skeleton with those from the hospital. Everything matched."

The scientists found final proof in a ridge of bone on a part of the scapula, or shoulder blade, that surrounds the glenoid cavity, where the head of the upper arm bone fits. Like a ball and socket, the elegant arrangement of bones allows the arm to swivel. However, when a person extends an arm, the humerus's head comes into contact with the bone at the back margin of the cavity. Over time, the posterior margin takes on a more beveled appearance because of the greater use of the joint on the dominant side. Regularly extending the arm to throw a baseball, for example, would change the shape of the bone, and a lifelong preference of one arm over the other — handedness, in the anthropological vernacular — would be noticeable. In addition, using one arm more often causes the bones of that arm to grow longer, sometimes by several millimeters.[6]

The left scapula in Snow's laboratory in Chicago clearly showed more beveling. And the left arm bones measured several millimeters longer than the right. David Talsma, the family had reported, had been left-handed. Snow and Fitzpatrick had finally made a match — no cause for celebration under the circumstances, but a hard-won success.

At the end of 1979, the two scientists tallied five identifications, bringing the total of named victims to twenty-four. Nine bodies remained. By now the trickle of antemortem records from families had dried up. Gacy was in jail forever but remained silent on the names of any more of the boys he had killed. It looked as if the time had come to pack up the dossiers, photos, X-ray films, and calipers and head home. The remaining skeletons would simply have to be buried as John Does.

Snow, however, wanted to try one more thing.

Betty Pat Gatliff didn't look much like the other government workers who occupied the warren of offices in CAMI's sprawling headquarters near Oklahoma City. She wore her dark hair to her shoulders, sometimes tied into a loose ponytail with a silver clasp of Indian design. Born and bred in Oklahoma, her open, friendly features radiated frankness and simplicity. Like many natives of the Southwest, she regarded turquoise not just as decoration but also as an emblem of her corner of America, and the azure stone emblazoned the large belt buckles and bolo ties she wore like an Oklahoma coat of arms. Otherwise, she dressed plainly, without pretense, much as she lived. Although her knowledge of the human form and structure, and especially the skull, had few peers, she had no scientific degree. In her own way, Gatliff conjured the human form. She was a medical artist.

When Dr. Snow — she almost always called him Dr. Snow, even though she had known and worked with him now for almost two decades — sat down in her studio in the fall of 1979 to chat, she played along. She suspected he had a job for her; he had a way of sidling up to his real topic, especially when he had something he wanted done. Not that she minded working with him; she always learned something. But sometimes the experience could be frustrating. He set his own "time frame," as she diplomatically calls it. Sometimes he would wait until the last minute, then expect a drawing of a figure or a skeleton right away. But late or not, what he did he did well.

This time Gatliff did not have to wait. Within a few minutes, Snow got to his subject: John Wayne Gacy. Gatliff knew Snow had been commuting back and forth to the Cook County M.E.'s office for the past several months. Now he had brought a skull from one of the bodies found in Gacy's house back to Oklahoma City.

Could she sculpt a face onto the skull?

Snow had asked Gatliff that question many times before. In fact, the two of them, anthropologist and sculptress, had earned a reputation over the years as the perfecters of an unusual and fascinating craft, part science and part art, known as facial reconstruction.

The face is an unlikely piece of work. Wildly divergent curves, prominences, orbs, and bulges bunch together in an oval space that is too small, really, for all that detail. Examined dispassionately, it looks like a bowl of jumbled fruit. Each arrangement is unique, however, providing an infinite array of markers by which we can distinguish among ourselves. There is no mistaking W. C. Fields's face for that of Grace Kelly. But Fields won his laughs and Kelly her prince not so much because of their flesh but their bones. Beauty is *not* skin deep; it reaches down to — or up from — the skull.

A German anatomist, Wilhelm His, first tried to reconstruct the features of a face from nothing but a skull in 1895. He took measurements of the thickness of the facial muscle and skin from twenty-four male and four female cadavers by thrusting an oiled sewing needle through their skin. When the needle's point hit bone, a rubber disk on the needle's shaft marked the depth of the muscle and skin.[7] He discovered that the skin's thickness varies significantly from place to place on the face. But these thicknesses remain remarkably consistent from person to person. Much of what makes one face differ from another, then, is carved into the contours of the skull. The face may be read like an open book, as Shakespeare once wrote, but it fits the skull like a glove.

A sculptor promptly translated His's measurements into a face over a skull, making sure that the thickness of the clay used matched each skin measurement. The reconstruction might have gone unnoticed outside the small circle of German anatomists interested in such things had His not chosen a skull claimed to have been that of Johann Sebastian Bach. It was indeed Bach's, and the reconstruction made His and his method famous.

Since that time many anthropologists have undertaken their own measurements of cadavers to refine the tables of skin thicknesses from which reconstructionists work. For whites, the numbers have changed little, although some practitioners believe that the flesh of modern Caucasoid Americans has plumped up some due to a fattier diet.[8] The thickness of skin on the face ranges remarkably: on a white male the thickest spot, eleven and a half millimeters, lies at the middle of the philtrum, the bridge of flesh between the bottom of the nose and the upper lip. The thinnest measures a mere two millimeters, at the end of the nasal bone, about one-third of the way down the nose. The glabella, the point on the brow ridge just above the bridge of the nose, is also thin, just four-and-three-quarter millimeters in most white males. The gonion, the point on the jaw down from the earlobe where the mandible takes a sharp turn upward toward the cranium (and the part of the male's jaw that the designers of razors have yet to conquer), is especially fleshy, at ten and a half millimeters.

That women's faces generally are softer than men's hardly needs confirmation from needles stuck into cadavers. But exactly where they are softer greatly interests the facial reconstructionist. The flesh of a woman lies closer to the bone than that of a man's at mid-philtrum and at the bridge of the nose, for example. Beneath the chin, however, a woman's flesh is thicker than a man's, as it is at the midpoint of the suborbital — directly beneath each eye — and back along the cheekbones. Relatively recent research shows that the average thicknesses on the faces of blacks generally runs deeper than on whites but is thinner among Orientals.[9] In fact, in some spots, such as below the eyes and over the cheekbones, the skin of black males measures twice the thickness of European males. (Many of the measurements for the Europeans, however, were performed before the turn of the century and employed relatively unsophisticated techniques. Current scholars suspect that these measurements may underestimate modern skin thicknesses and give some reconstructions an inaccurately gaunt appearance.)

Wilton Krogman's book on forensic anthropology had helped to revive interest in facial reconstructions in forensic cases. Krogman himself had helped sculpt a face from the skull of a known black man in 1946, which he claimed was readily recognizable. The method failed to convince everyone, however. Dr. M. F. Ashley Montagu of Hahnemann Medical College in Philadelphia typified the response of many in a monograph with the patronizing title, "A Study of Man Embracing Error." Wrote Montagu: "From the skull it is quite impossible to reconstruct the character of the hair, eyes, nose, lips, ears, eyebrows, skin creases, fullness or expression. . . . It is highly desirable that [reconstructions] be dropped, for they do real harm."[10] Many other scientists regarded reconstruction as sort of a parlor trick, fine for re-creating scenes of paleolithic Indians squatting around a campfire in museum dioramas but not accurate enough for forensic investigations.

Certainly one's hair, eye color, eyebrows, ears, skin creases, and other facial ornamentation do not leave traces on the skull. But Montagu's criticism missed the point: could an anthropologically careful reconstruction of a completely unknown skeleton not render a likeness of the living person that was good *enough* to bring forth relatives or friends bearing better information from which to make an identification?

In 1948 Krogman found a case on which he could try a reconstruction. Late in August 1947, some men fishing on Salt Creek at the northern edge of Menard County, Illinois, found part of a skeletonized human body in the lower branches of a tree where floodwaters apparently had lodged them. The skull and several of the bones testified that the skeleton had belonged to a white male in his late teens who had stood about five feet five inches tall. Nothing more could be gleaned and no one came forward with knowledge of a missing person who fit these characteristics.

Artist Bartlett Frost and colleague John McGregor, both with the Illinois State Museum, teamed with Krogman to create the mystery man's face. They glued the mandible back into position and made a cast of the skull. At fifteen points on the cast, which now replaced the skull, they affixed small dabs of clay. The thickness of each dab corresponded exactly to the skin thicknesses for European males measured fifty years before by His and his German associates. Then, keeping in mind the location and size of muscles, the team filled in the intervening spaces with graduated strips of clay.

They tried also to add their own touches to the technique. For example, Krogman determined from living models that the apex of the eye's cornea, when viewed from directly in front, lies at the juncture of two imaginary lines: one drawn from the edge of the eye socket nearest the nose to the widest point on the socket's outer margin; and the other vertically bisecting the socket. Krogman also knew that eyeballs don't vary significantly in size, ranging between twenty-five and twenty-six millimeters in diameter from birth. Only the size of the sockets, or orbits, varies.

The human nose might be described as a tent stretched over those flexible plastic rods that have now replaced the wooden tent pole. Instead of nondegradable plastic, however, cartilage supports the nose. Cartilage decomposes quite quickly after death, leaving that gaping hole one associates with a human skull. To reconstruct the dead man's nose, Krogman relied on the skull's nasal spine and the width of the nasal opening. The spine is a sliver of bone shaped like a narrow arrowhead that juts out of the face from the bottom of the nasal opening. Like a horizontal girder, it forms the foundation of the nose and generally measures one third the length of the base of the nose. As for width, the nose on a white person measures from wing to wing about one third wider than the nasal opening.

Lips were unpredictable, Krogman knew, but mouths stretched about as wide as the distance between the pupils of the eyes. Nor could an ear be read from the bone, although its height from lobe to tip could be approximated as equal to the length of the nose from the nasion, the indentation at the bridge, to the tip.

A photograph of the finished sculpture depicted a fair-complexioned young man with a large, prominent chin, almost nonexistent brow ridges, and a slight bulge of the forehead just above the nose. The lips were pressed together and the left orbit sat slightly lower than the right.[11] By intention or perhaps due to some empathy with the subject's unfortunate fate, the team gave the face a serious expression.

It wasn't art. Art, as Aldous Huxley once observed, transports the mind away from reality, while this sculpture sought to re-create reality incarnate, or at least in clay. Nonetheless Krogman was impressed with his work and had a photo of the reconstruction printed in local newspapers, hoping that someone would recognize the face and come forward to identify it. Wire services picked up the story and gave the photo nationwide circulation. Krogman received reports of several missing men who looked similar, but none fit all the other characteristics of the skeleton. When Krogman published an account of his experiment in mid-1948, an identification still had not been made.

Over the next two decades various forensic experts tried facial reconstruction with mixed results. Some, working with artists, skipped the reconstruction altogether and simply tried to sketch what they believed the living face must have looked like from the features of the skull. No one ever attempted to verify the technique scientifically until 1970.

By that time, Snow had read all the accounts of reconstruction he could find. He decided to test the technique objectively. Snow had already introduced Gatliff to Krogman's literature, and she had tried her hand at a few reconstructions while at CAMI.

The test Snow planned would require the skulls of several known individuals for whom he had antemortem photographs. Gatliff would build faces onto the skulls according to the rules laid down by Krogman, without being allowed to see the photos of their living owners. Snow would then ask unknowing observers — staff at CAMI, many of whom, Snow felt, fit the "unknowing" category to a T — to see if they could match the reconstructed bust with the antemortem photo, which they would have to pick out from several photos of people of similar age, race, and physical makeup, as in a police lineup.

Getting the skulls was easy enough. Snow had access to four that might work. One had belonged to a full-blooded Cheyenne male, aged twenty-six, who had died of unknown causes, tumbled into a farm pond, and decomposed before his body was discovered. Another came from a fifty-six-year-old white female whose bones were found in a wooded area where she had been strangled. The third had belonged to an elderly woman, a retired college professor, who had donated her body to the University of Oklahoma Medical School. And the last was the skull of a thirty-six-year-old white male, an ex-convict, whose body had been found in a roadside ditch where it had been concealed by his murderers. Except for the retired professor, the bodies had been identified at the M.E.'s office, and Snow had found photographs taken of all four before their deaths.

Gatliff followed Krogman's reconstruction techniques for all four skulls. When she completed the first, the Cheyenne, Snow asked friends of the victim if they saw a reasonable likeness, which they all did. With the second reconstruction, the strangled woman, the only antemortem photo had been taken twenty-five years before the woman's death, and the resemblance did not impress. Acquaintances of the woman said Gatliff's reconstruction missed the mark.

The real test depended on sculptures three and four. Snow located the retired professor's university yearbook and extracted photos of six other women of about the same age. The photographs were arranged alongside each other, including the yearbook photo of the professor. Below these Snow attached a photo of Gatliff's reconstruction. He repeated the process with sculpture number four, the murdered ex-con, whose photo and the photos of six other white men of similar age he took from a police file. He tacked up the montages, along with instructions to choose the photo that best matched Gatliff's reconstruction, on bulletin boards at CAMI, other FAA offices, and three police stations.

Former students of the professor and police officers who had known the murder victim had already told Snow that Gatliff's reconstructions closely resembled their living subjects. Snow was startled, however, by the responses from strangers who viewed the montages. Only twenty-seven of the 104 people who viewed the professor's montage correctly matched her photo with the reconstruction. While that number exceeded chance, two of the wrong photos had been picked twenty-five times apiece, almost as frequently as the correct choice. Women and police officers scored somewhat better than civilian men.

Gatliff's reconstruction of the murdered criminal fared much better; 135 of the 200 who tried to match the photos picked the right one. The photos of two other men were chosen about half as often, a frequency one might expect simply by throwing darts at the photos while blindfolded. This time, policemen did far better than civilians, and civilian women slightly better than their male peers.

Snow and Gatliff learned several things from the experiment. First, in the case of the professor, the woman was sixty-seven years old when she died, but the photo from her yearbook had been taken when she was in her early forties. The bone of the skull remodels itself throughout life, and changes wrought during later years would have shown on the reconstruction but not on the photo. Second, the old photo was taken in a professional studio, where the ability to flatter photographically rewards the photographer with repeat business. Thus, what showed up on the print might have differed significantly from the real face. In contrast, the police photographer who took the picture of the criminal in case number four had neither interest nor need to flatter to keep his business flourishing. Finally, most of the skin-thickness measurements taken up until 1970 were of male cadavers; mean values for women were suspect.[12]

Snow concluded that a positive identification of a skeleton should not rest only on a facial reconstruction. It might be used to *exclude* a match, however, or be added to other skeletal signs to identify someone by weight of evidence. In any event, facial reconstruction most certainly was not just a parlor trick.

In fact, Gatliff was eventually to prove the value of the technique beyond the dreams of Krogman and even Snow with a reconstruction that amazed police in Oklahoma and shattered any doubt that a face is worth a thousand words.

It was six years after Gatliff's experiment with Snow when detectives called on the pair to help them solve a case that had mystified the police. In the early morning of June 13, 1976, two squirrel hunters stumbled across a human skull deep in the woods on the outskirts of Stillwater, Oklahoma. A search turned up most of the skeleton, which apparently had been dragged by scavengers from a shallow grave in a gully. Some human hair, a pair of panty hose, a cross-your-heart bra, and a dress, noticeably out of fashion, were also discovered. No jewelry or other belongings that might help identify the body could be found.

Snow was called onto the case. Clearly, he told the investigators, the rectangular shape of the pubic opening, its delicate structure, and its wide sciatic notch indicated a female. She had been between twenty-five and thirty-five years old at death and about five feet tall. The skull looked like that of a white, a finding supported by mathematical formulas applied to several skull measurements. She probably had been a rugged-looking woman, Snow suggested, with a broad face and prominent cheekbones.

There was something more, however, something unusual. Her lower jaw showed a massive fracture, healed well before her death, and several other poorly knit fractures of the lower face. And Snow found a healed compression fracture of the first lumbar vertebra.[13] "She apparently had been in some type of accident, probably an automobile accident," Snow told detectives. "Maybe that might jog someone's memory."[14]

It didn't, at least for the next two and a half months. With no leads to go on, the Payne County Sheriff's Department asked Gatliff for help.

Gatliff sculpted a face on the skull, adding a wig that matched the color of the hair found near the grave. As Snow had predicted, she was not a conventional beauty, with a jaw and cheeks slightly out of kilter, a robust brow ridge, a blunt nose, and a small mouth. A local paper ran a picture of the re-creation, and detectives crossed their fingers. They were soon rewarded; an informant called the police. He said he had seen her in the company of a local man at a bar in Stillwater back in April. Her name had been Jeanett and she had come from California. That was all he knew.

The man at the bar was Elmer Clayton Finin, an ex-con with relatives in the area. Finin had recently jumped bail on a weapons charge, but he had held a job near Stillwater for two days. There, he had listed his beneficiary on insurance forms as Jeanett Bodard. Officer Joe Staley did some legwork and discovered that Finin had recently been in prison in Chino, California. While imprisoned, he had received mail with a woman's name on the return address. Her name had been Jeanett María Bodard, from Crescent City, California.

In Crescent City, Sergeant Roy VanDerpool closed the circle. He found a friend of Bodard's who recalled that the woman had been seriously injured in an automobile accident when in California. "She was thrown into the dashboard and window and cut up pretty bad," VanDerpool reported. At the city hospital, he found her medical records, including the one piece of evidence that Snow needed to nail down the identification: X rays.

The match was almost perfect. Bodard was white, thirty-five years old, and four feet eleven inches tall. And, as Snow had predicted, she had borne children, something the anthropologist had inferred from marks on the skeleton's pelvis. Staley was astonished at what Snow had been able to deduce. "It's almost spooky when you compare Snow's description and the medical records," he said. As for Gatliff's reconstruction, Staley said simply, "Amazing."

Finin, Bodard's common-law husband, was tracked down in Arkansas. The slightly built, brown-haired thirty-three-year-old confessed to killing Jeanett, in anger, with a single blow to the throat and was sentenced to serve ten years to life for second-degree murder. He too had been impressed by Gatliff's work; when he first saw the re-creation printed in the newspaper, he skipped town.

So it was with a mixture of hope as well as healthy scientific skepticism that Snow asked Gatliff, three years after their success in Stillwater, if she would apply her skills to the boys in Chicago. A year had passed since the police had torn up the floorboards of Gacy's suburban rambler. Nine bodies found there remained to be named. The chance of scoring a match from a reconstruction was a long shot, he warned. The work might amount to nothing. Then again, as gruesome as the case had turned out to be, it presented a rare chance to test the technique outside the neat confines of the laboratory, where, Snow knew, the sound and fury of scientific promise often signified nothing of much use out on the streets. And then there were the boys. The anonymous make poor witnesses. Who else could could give them names? Snow felt that reconstructions, given Gatliff's track record, might identify at least two or three of them.

Gatliff said she would try it. Even one success would make the effort worthwhile.

Gatliff could count herself among the best facial reconstructionists in the country. After a twenty-year courtship with the skull, she had wed art and anthropology. What the skull only hinted at she could complete. She knew, for example, what happens when the skull grows a high nasal bridge, the top third of the nose, and a short nasal spine. The nose starts out from the bridge with high expectations but must somehow curve back to meet the short spine. The result is a hump. When the situation reverses the opposite obtains: a low-slung bridge and a long nasal spine — the unmistakable salutation of a Richard Nixon or a Bob Hope.

The technique seems quite matter-of-fact when Gatliff describes it. "Things tend to agree. If you've got a wide, flat bridge and a wide, maybe even divided nasal spine, it is going to support a bigger bulb on the nose than, probably, a very sharp one. . . . You're not going to have a wide, flat bridge and a pointy nose. They just don't go together."

Gatliff also tries to compensate for what she believes are comparatively better-nourished Americans than the cadavers whose skin thicknesses His measured in the 1890s. She also worries about the position of the bodies when they were measured. "If you hold your head to the side or are lying down, the soft tissue shifts. I think the measurements right around the jaws seem too thick. I think it's because when people die they don't die sitting up. They die lying down. I've mentioned this to [researchers] and they say they don't know how to get around that. We can't ask people to die sitting up!"

A clay re-creation of a human face requires more than just millimeter-by-millimeter precision. Gatliff usually gives her reconstructions a smile. It's not that the dead should be cheerful; the smile shows the teeth, whose shape or arrangement often are unique. And few things live as long in the memory as a loved one's smile.

"But you don't just smile with your mouth," Gatliff explains to the students in the reconstruction classes she teaches. "Your eyes smile too. Your cheek rises. Put your hand on your cheek. Smile. Does it rise? And little puffs come under your eyes. It softens the eye, and your eyes smile." Gatliff dutifully re-creates these little puffs under the eyes of her reconstructions, a grace note without which, even though it may not be noticed consciously, the face would ring false.

Shortly after Gatliff signed on to work the Gacy investigation,

Snow brought seven of the Chicago skulls to Oklahoma for her to reconstruct. The sculptress had by then added several refinements to Krogman's instructions. Instead of applying dabs of clay to the skull to establish skin thicknesses as Krogman did, she removed eraser heads from pencils, whittled them to the proper thicknesses, and glued them to the skulls. She had learned to calculate the fullness of the lips by measuring the distance from gum line to gum line, and she set the corners of the mouth at the juncture of the canine and the first premolar on each side. She acquired plastic prosthetic eyes from medical-supply companies. In the cases where hair had been found with the bodies, she added an appropriately colored wig.

When Gatliff had finished the seven faces, Snow photographed them and sent the prints to Chicago. He and Gatliff then flew there and Gatliff did two more reconstructions over eleven days. The final two were aimed especially at the press. Medical examiner Stein and his associates hoped that newspaper photos of the reconstructions would reach relatives or friends of the victims and give them some new leads.

Stein and Gatliff fared no better than Krogman had with his drowning victim. The response was dismal. "It was one of my most disappointing projects," Gatliff recalls.

> Not one was identified. Dr. Stein sort of put me at ease about it. He said, "Well Betty, don't worry about it. It is disappointing, but we've done everything we know how to do. And if the parents won't cooperate . . ."
>
> I know one day when I was up in Chicago, the first day that they took calls after the reconstruction, two girls from different suburbs gave the same boy's name and said he was their brother. But when it came time to list the parents, they said, "Oh no, I'm not going to tell you, because my mother just refuses to talk about this." Well, we asked, who was his dentist? They said, "We don't have any idea." We said, could you ask your mother? "Oh, no, she won't even talk about it." . . . And whether either one of the girls knew that the other one called or not, we never knew.[15]

By that time, Gatliff reckons, "the police knew who had killed them anyway and they had other cases that were more pressing than

tracing out leads with people who wouldn't cooperate with them. . . .
They had their man and that was their job."

For the five families whose sons Snow and Fitzpatrick had identified, a mystery had been solved, albeit with a sad ending. Gatliff's
efforts, as it turned out, would also pay off. Several years after the
Gacy investigation was closed, a local newspaper reporter tracked
down the identity of one of the nine young men whose faces Gatliff
had reconstructed. The rest were buried unidentified. Photos of Gatliff's casts remain the closest thing to a memorial they have.

At the end of 1979, Snow had a choice to make. The FAA asked
him if he wanted to take early retirement. The agency needed to cut
back on personnel to save money and was offering full benefits. Snow,
whose talents were coming into more demand all the time, considered
the offer for a couple of weeks. Several police departments and M.E.'s
offices around the country could provide enough freelance work to
keep him supplied with Camels, new books, and a steak now and
then, he thought. He flipped a coin. Heads he stays, tails he goes.
He had to flip it twice for it to come up the way he wanted. He left
the FAA at age fifty-two in 1980 and set out his shingle. The time
had come to have some fun, he told his wife. And maybe, he thought,
to chase bigger game.

6

—————

THE OUTLAW IN
ARSENIC

F ORENSIC work, at least as practiced by Snow, had its lighter
moments. Not every investigation followed a tragedy. Some
sought to uncover or re-create historical events that may have
been tragic when they took place but had been dimmed enough by
the years to arouse more curiosity than pathos.

Snow's youth engendered in him a lingering fascination with the
people who shaped the Southwest. Especially memorable were the
cowboys, Indians, and outlaws whose exploits were spun into an
American mythology not so different from those of Greece and Rome,
except that Western heroes rode into the same horizons and sunsets
that Snow knew as a child in Texas. The books piled in the back of
his father's Chevrolet during those long drives through the panhandle
had primed him on the tales of outlaws and Indian scouts. Snow's
dalliance with archaeology during his twenties also sharpened his pre-
occupation with this slice of history, so much so that sometimes, even
as an adult, it threatened to usurp his profession.

Snow's special skills with skeletons gave him the privilege to poke
his nose into all sorts of investigations. Granted, he wouldn't be seen
pursuing a case; ambulance chasing was the mark of an amateur. But
by 1977 his reputation was such that cases came to him, and he had
the luxury of signing on to one now and then for fun.

So it was with the case of Elmer McCurdy, the outlaw who wouldn't give up.[1]

On December 7, 1976, a television crew from Universal Studios was filming an episode of *The Six Million Dollar Man* at the Nu-Pike Amusement Park in Long Beach, California. As cameramen set up to film a scene in a darkened corner of the Laugh in the Dark Funhouse, they discovered a dummy hanging from a thick rope tied to a two-by-four in the ceiling. It was done up with red phosphorescent paint that glowed in the dark when a hidden ultraviolet light nearby was switched on.

The dummy didn't fit in with the scene to be filmed so a technician grabbed it by the arm to move it. The arm came off in his hands. Underneath, still attached to the dummy, was an arm bone.

The crew called the police and homicide detectives, who took the arm to the laboratory of Dr. Thomas T. Noguchi, the medical examiner for Los Angeles and famed "coroner to the stars." There Dr. Joseph H. Choi, deputy M.E., examined it and certified that it was indeed human. The dummy, it turned out, was a mummy.

The police went back to the funhouse, cut the dummy down, and took it to Choi for a full autopsy. Choi had never seen a body quite like this one. The abdominal and thoracic viscera and the brain were as hard as stone. A roughly Y-shaped incision marked the upper chest down to the abdomen. Choi also recognized two incisions on either side of the groin as the kind made when a body is embalmed.

As to the cause of death, the organs were too solidified to tell much at first. But a close examination of the upper chest suggested foul play. Choi found a gunshot wound about four inches to the right of the midline of the chest. He tracked the bullet's path downward and to the left, where it penetrated the right sixth rib, right lung, diaphragm, liver, and intestine. The bullet was nowhere to be found, but Choi dug out a copper bullet jacket, known as a gas check, from the pelvis. He sent it over to ballistics, who reported that the jacket belonged to a .32-caliber bullet of a type first manufactured during the 1830s but discontinued before World War I.[2]

The organs were extraordinarily well-preserved. Under a microscope, individual muscle fibers of the heart had retained visible nuclei and pigment. The coronary arteries were normal, and red and white cells could be easily recognized, as could neurons from the brain. The lungs, however, didn't look too healthy, suggesting that the man may have suffered from pneumonia at the time he was shot.

No one had any idea who the funhouse mummy could be. But Choi, ever thorough, kept after clues. When he pried open the mummy's mouth, he got not only a surprise but the first good leads on its identity. Inside was a 1924 penny and a ticket stub. On the stub was printed, "Louis Sonney's Museum of Crime, So. Main St., L.A."

The next day, December 10, after an account of the ghoulish discovery hit the newspapers, a man named Edward Liersch called the police. Liersch said that he had once leased part of the Nu-Pike Amusement Park and had owned a dummy that he got from the owner of the Hollywood Wax Museum, one Spoony Singh.[3] Meanwhile, a check of driver's licenses under the name of Louis Sonney turned up a Dan Louis Sonney of 906 South Stanley Avenue. Over the telephone, Dan Sonney said that his father, Louis, had acquired the mummy — Dan said he thought it had been a dummy — in the 1920s from an unknown source. The elder Sonney worked the sideshow business at circuses and amusement parks and charged the rubes twenty-five cents to see the "outlaw who would never be captured alive." When Sonney died in 1949, the assets of his company, Entertainment Ventures, went into storage until 1971, when lock, stock, and dummy were bought by Singh.

Singh had trouble turning a profit from his new acquisition. Thinking it was papier-mâché, he sent the dummy off to Mount Rushmore to grace a haunted house being built there as part of an amusement park. It was returned as "not being lifelike enough." Singh regarded it as "too gross to display" in his wax museum (although a security guard at the amusement park said he had seen it exhibited there in a casket) and gave it to a friend — a man named Liersch — to use in a museum Liersch had opened on Long Beach pier. This venture failed in 1972, and Liersch's landlords at Nu-Pike kept everything in lieu of back rent.

So the police, after several days' sleuthing, had traced the corpse back as far as the 1920s. Regardless of how old it actually was, however, homicide was homicide, and the trail had to be followed. Where, then, had Sonney got it?

Louis Sonney had once been a sheriff in Centralia, Washington.

126

In 1921 he captured a bank robber, and with the $5,000 in reward money he went into the road show business with an attraction he called "The March of Crime." According to one source, he pried the dummy away from a carnival worker who owed him $500.

The final piece of information that the police were able to add came from an old carny and former partner of Louis Sonney's, Dwayne Esper, then living in Arizona. At eighty-five, Esper had trouble recollecting all the details, but he was sure that he had bought the dummy for $1,000 from a retired coroner in Tulsa, Oklahoma. The story he had heard was that it was the dummy of a man who had robbed a bank or some such and that his name had been McCurde. He said that he and Sonney took the dummy on the road, explaining to curiosity seekers that McCurde had been a drug addict who had committed suicide in an open field while surrounded by a posse after he had robbed a drug store. Esper was shocked when he heard the thing had been real.

That was as far as the investigation got in Los Angeles. If Esper's story held any truth, Oklahoma might have been the place where this McCurdy's afterlife began. And in fact an historian from Oklahoma, Fred Olds, had called Noguchi after reading about the mysterious discovery in the newspaper to offer some help tracking down the mummy's identity. Curious to see where the thread would lead, Noguchi invited Olds out to take a look. Olds brought along an expert: Clyde Snow.

"At this point," Snow recalls, "a strong chain of evidence linked the dummy, or the mummy, to an Oklahoma outlaw. But there was no antemortem information, even a description, to go on to make a positive ID. Nor were there any next-of-kin. The mummy was faced with cremation under the name Doe, John, number 255, unless someone could identify the corpse.

"Now Oklahomans are rather a peculiar breed," Snow points out. "Traditionally, they have dealt rather harshly with local lawbreakers while they are still alive, but become uncommonly sentimental about them fifty years after they are dead."[4]

Olds and some fellow history buffs combed libraries and state records of convicted criminals. They turned up a suspect: Elmer McCurdy, alias Elmer McCuardy, Elmer McAudry, Frank Curtis, and Frank Davidson. Profession: outlaw. In the University of Oklahoma's

Western History Collection they discovered two postmortem photographs of McCurdy. They also located mug shots of McCurdy taken when he was jailed in the Oklahoma Territorial Prison. A physical description at the time put him at thirty-one years of age and five feet eight inches tall. The historians found no dental or medical records, but they dug up one gem: a note attached to the prison description said that McCurdy had a scar two inches long on the back of his right wrist.[5]

Snow flew back to Los Angeles at the request of the Oklahomans. With the help of Judy Suchey, a local forensic anthropologist, he spent two days examining the carnival corpse. They had no difficulty determining its sex, and it clearly was Caucasoid. Fixing its age at death, however, posed a problem: how to get at the telltale bones without literally taking the mummy apart.

Suchey, a petite and energetic strawberry blond, specialized in pubic symphyses and had compiled a vast collection, the world's largest, she said, which she kept in a wardrobe — the males in blue boxes, the females in pink.[6] She and Snow adroitly cut the two symphyseal faces from the mummy's pubic bones with a minimum of damage and conducted the classical McKern and Stewart analysis, fixing age by the physical stages of the symphyseal surfaces. Next, they devised a plan to get a look at some of the epiphyses, which would give further clues to age at death. By carefully making incisions in the skin over the collarbones at the medial ends, where they meet just below the neck, they found the epiphyses had fused, indicating an adult in his late twenties or older. Cutting through to the sacrum at the base of the spine, they also discovered that five segments of the sacrum had completely fused, reinforcing the age estimation from the collarbones. Also they could see that the vertebrae of the spine were clean, that is, there was no sign of the lipping and ridging that begin to show in a man by his mid-thirties.

So far, everything led to McCurdy. But when Snow and Suchey measured the mummy's height, the trail took a wrong turn. "When we laid the guy out and measured him he was only 160 centimeters," says Snow. That was about four or five inches shorter than McCurdy as described in the Oklahoma records. "But we reckoned that he'd shrunk some over the years. We couldn't remove the bones like we would in a normal autopsy because the skin was so damn hard. But we got a measurement, without having to do too much dissection, of the length of the femurs. The standard calculations, from Trotter and Gleser, gave us an overall height of 170.5 centimeters — five feet eight inches tall, give or take some. Bingo. It was a match."

Snow had mailed tissue from the mummy to a colleague in Detroit, Theodore A. Reyman, then chief of pathology at Mount Carmel Mercy Hospital. Reyman reported that the body was full of arsenic. Embalming with arsenic had disappeared in the United States around the turn of the century. In fact, most states had outlawed it by the 1920s.

The values for arsenic in the body were .270 milligrams per gram of tissue in the lung, .390 mg in the skin, .270 in the heart, and .659 in the bone. The brain was the most pickled: .700 mg per gram of gray matter. Whoever had done the job planned to keep the body around for a long time; it had several hundred times the amount of arsenic found in Egyptian mummies.

Then there was the scar that McCurdy reportedly sported on his right wrist. From shrinkage and weathering, the reddish skin had cracked like drought-dried clay, but Snow could make out the tracings of the scar, just as the prison records described.

One last test remained. Forensic scientists had long tried to compare skulls with photographs of alleged victims to make identifications. The method, first made famous in Britain in the case of Buck Ruxton, is notoriously subjective. When performed by a talented anthropologist with a good eye for detail, however, it has helped solve several criminal cases, as it did with Ruxton. But there was more to it than simply holding the skull up in one hand and a photograph in the other, like some latter-day Hamlet, and comparing the two.

How closely the mummy's face would match its image in life was unclear; time and the mummification process had given the skin and facial features a gaunt, pinched aspect, not to mention the festive coloration his owners had painted on. "All those years in show business — if indeed it was McCurdy, of course — would have taken their toll," Snow explains.

Snow had fiddled with photo comparison in his laboratory in Oklahoma and had added a little modern technology. He had tried mounting a skull in front of one video camera and a photograph of its living owner in front of another. He had eventually settled on a system using an electronic device known as a production switcher, or vision mixer. With it, Snow could take the images of the photograph and the skull and display them on a single video screen. From there, a technician can perform a variety of superimpositions of the two. First, one image is laid over the other, like a double exposure on the same piece of camera film. The technician then "dissolves" one image gradually while simultaneously enhancing the other. With the addition of a special-effects generator, the images can be "wiped" as well. For example, a wipe pattern blocks out a portion of one picture and replaces it with the corresponding part of the other. Or the technician can slowly wipe the overlaying photo from top to bottom or from one side to the other.[7] The technique creates a particularly eerie effect as the photograph of a living person is electronically peeled like tissue paper off the underlying image of the skull.

Snow had learned to compare landmarks on a skull, such as the location of the cheekbones or the nasal opening, to corresponding landmarks on the photo of the living person. In this case, he didn't have a skull but a mummified head. He worked with two photos instead of a skull and a photo. One photo was of the mummy in profile. As for the other, the cowboy historians in Oklahoma had the two photographs of McCurdy taken just after he had died, laid out in a black suit on a bier, also in profile view.

In Los Angeles, Snow and Suchey set up a video camera. The weeks of investigations, autopsies, and anthropological examinations all came down to this one "double exposure." When they superimposed the photographs, the answer was clear. Unless McCurdy had an identical twin, they had their man.

Meanwhile, the Oklahomans had put together a pretty good account of McCurdy's last days. "You could say that Elmer's career had two phases: antemortem and postmortem," says Snow, who knows the story as well as he came to know the man — inside out.

The antemortem story starts in the early 1900s in Oklahoma, where McCurdy worked variously as a miner and a plumber. He also served a term in the Oklahoma Territorial Prison. In the spring of 1911, he joined up with a gang that robbed a Missouri Pacific train near Coffeyville, Kansas. Later that year, he recruited two friends to rob a Missouri, Kansas, and Texas train, known then as the Katy train.

The intended target was a safe carrying several thousand dollars in payments to Indian tribes.

The gang struck on the night of October 6, stopping the train in an isolated stretch near Okesa, Oklahoma, and detaching the engine and baggage car from the passenger cars so they could collect the loot at leisure. It was then that their plans began to unravel.

The gang had nabbed the wrong train. The cash box yielded a paltry forty-six dollars. "Maybe, like many another traveler before and since, Elmer had difficulty reading railroad timetables," Snow speculates. The bandits' only consolation consisted of a shipment of liquor on board. As the disgruntled desperados made their getaway, Elmer grabbed two demijohns of whiskey.

The group split up. Within two days, however, when Elmer showed up at the Revard Ranch in the Osage Hills, he had a posse on his trail. The territory had a reputation as one of the wilder parts of the new state of Oklahoma despite the nearness of the oil belt, and there were few places available for a night's rest. So, according to an account in the Bartlesville *Daily Enterprise* of October 8, 1911, Elmer stopped at the ranch, drunk and tired. He gave his name as Frank Amos and said the whiskey had come off the train that had been held up near Okesa. He drank with the ranch hands for about an hour and asked for a place to sleep. He was led to the haymow. Shortly thereafter, at about two o'clock in the morning, three members of the posse rode up: Bob Fenton, his brother Stringer, and Dick Wallace. They'd been trailing Elmer all day. Informed of who was sleeping in the barn, they took up stations outside and waited for daybreak.

The versions of what happened the next morning differ somewhat in the details. An account attributed to "The 'Sage' of the Osage," Arthur H. Lamb, however, describes the ensuing battle with "Curtis" (one of McCurdy's aliases at the time) in the most detail:

> Curtis would not give up, he was drinking booze. When he was commanded to surrender, his reply was a rapid discharge of his six-gun, but thanks to the quality of the booze the express company had delivered on this Indian reservation, his aim was bad and the boys sought their rather inadequate breastworks in scattered stumps and trees. They returned the fire and the battle

raged for about an hour when the besiegers signalled G.H.Q. for a new supply of ammunition, declaring they would fight it out on the line if it took all summer, or words to that effect. They noticed that the besieged had also ceased firing but thought it unwise to charge across the open unless sure that his supply of ammunition had also been exhausted.[8]

A boy "volunteered" to approach the hay-shed fortress bearing a white flag and asked for Elmer's surrender. Elmer refused in no uncertain terms. The battle began anew, and during the next lull the boy was sent back in, only to be refused again. On the third trip, however, the boy's plea was met with silence. He climbed up into the loft and found McCurdy stretched out on a bed of hay, dead. A bullet had pierced his chest as he lay prone, firing at the posse through an opening in the loft. Three good-sized drinks remained in the jug, but McCurdy's six-gun was empty.

The body was taken to the Johnson Funeral Home in nearby Pawhuska. No next of kin were known; in fact, no one knew if McCurdy was his real name. All that was certain was that he meant business about fighting to the death. "He must have been a nervy fellow, and game too," Stringer Fenton told a reporter at the time. "[When] we sent the messenger to the barn with a request for the bandit to surrender, McCurdy sent back word that we could go to the Devil."[9]

Snow has his own opinion on the man's behavior. "It seems clear to me," he says, "that anyone who had spent a cold night in a hayloft after consuming the better part of two jugs of whiskey might be in an exceptionally quarrelsome mood if aroused at seven in the morning."

Since no one claimed McCurdy, Dr. Johnson, the undertaker, embalmed him with liberal helpings of arsenic. "Instead of burying him," Snow explains, "Johnson kept him in a back room of the funeral parlor for several years. For a nickel, local curiosity seekers were allowed to view Elmer, billed by now as the 'Bandit Who Wouldn't Give Up.'" Johnson, Snow says, was living proof that what H. L. Mencken said about the American public's intelligence applies equally well to its taste: no one ever lost money underestimating it. "But then our rural forefathers didn't have the advantage we have today," Snow adds forgivingly, "of being able to view violence and its aftermath in the comfort of their living rooms."

Thus was Elmer launched into his postmortem career in show business. Photographers even made postcards of him, some of which survive today, showing the now-wrinkled outlaw decked out in six-guns, dungarees, and cowboy hat, propped up in the corner of the funeral parlor and looking somewhat forlorn.

Historian Lamb's tales of the Osage describe the next development in McCurdy's career:

> His body stood in the corner of a small room in the Johnson undertaking establishment for a long time. Thousands viewed it but no one claimed it. Every showman or street carnival that came to town tried to buy it for show purposes but was advised it was not for sale, that it was being held in the hope that relatives would claim it. Letters of inquiry came from almost every state in the Union asking for descriptions and photographs without result.
>
> Finally, alleged relatives from California wired for details and shortly afterward two very nice-appearing men came to see him and one of them positively identified him as a long-lost brother whom he had not seen for several years. It was a pathetic story of a wayward son and broken-hearted parents, both of whom were sleeping in the Land of Golden Sunshine. The brother was anxious to obey the last request of his parents and take the body back to the old California home and deposit it in the family plot alongside the parents. Accordingly, it was shipped out on October 7th, [almost] five years after his tragic death.[10]

Months later, word drifted back to Pawhuska that the mummified body had become a showstopper in a street carnival show in western Texas. McCurdy's "brothers" had pulled the next best thing to cheating death — they cheated the undertaker. Various accounts over the next several years confirmed Elmer's performances across the West, including one from Bob Fenton, who claimed that showmen passing through Tulsa allowed him to view the outlaw and renew the acquaintance they had made seventeen years before at the Revard Ranch.

"So," Snow writes in his version of the saga, "like other contemporaries from Oklahoma — Will Rogers, Tom Mix, Gene Autry, Woody Guthrie — Elmer followed the sawdust trail to movieland, hanging around Hollywood for a few years before getting his big chance. Unlike them, however, when his moment finally came — a guest appearance in *The Six Million Dollar Man* — Elmer blew it and literally went to pieces on the set."

With the story cinched together by Snow and his fellow historians in Oklahoma, Noguchi was able to sign a California death certificate and clear the way for McCurdy's return to Oklahoma. The remains arrived by jet in Oklahoma City on April 14, 1977. A delegation from the Oklahoma State Medical Examiner's Office met the body and took it to the morgue to await burial. Funeral expenses were paid by the Indian Territorial Posse of Westerners, an organization of prominent Oklahomans interested in the state's history, and by the Oklahoma Historical Society.

The following week, on a rainy Friday morning, Elmer was carried to the Summit View cemetery in Guthrie by a glass-sided hearse drawn by two white horses. Two wagons and five men on horseback made up the funeral procession. Hundreds of spectators lined the way, snapping pictures as the last cowboy outlaw was taken to the raw, red grave in the Oklahoma soil. He was buried next to several other outlaws, pioneers, and politicians who had made names for themselves during Oklahoma's untamed days.[11] None, however, not even the politicians, had managed to prolong their notoriety quite as proficiently as McCurdy.

There was even an epitaph drawn up, though only privately. Snow wrote it and, of course, remembers it well:

> Rest in peace, dear Elmer,
> Beneath this Okie sky,
> Where many an outlaw slumbers
> And politicians lie.

At the insistence of the state medical examiner, two cubic yards of concrete were poured over the coffin before the grave was closed. "That was just to ensure," Snow explains, "that the restless Elmer would wander no more."

7

CUSTER'S LAST
STAND AND
FIRST RESURRECTION

IF "The Winning of the West" was America's longest running morality play, then several characters deserve at least equal billing to the train robber and desperado: the rancher, the Indian, the mountain man, the cowboy, and the lawman, for example. To an anthropologist with Snow's peculiar talents, each had something to say about the era.

In 1985, Snow got a chance to study the bones of some of the most legendary characters of Western history — the Indian-fighting cavalrymen.

Under the soil of the rolling plains of Montana, just west of South Dakota's Black Hills, are the remains of most of the 267 soldiers and civilians who fell with General George Armstrong Custer at the Battle of the Little Bighorn on June 25, 1876. Custer's Last Stand marked the greatest victory for the Sioux and Cheyenne in the war that the white man made against them in the 1870s. Its decisiveness also brought down the wrath of a nation and sealed the fate of the Plains Indian a few years later.

The battle has become legend, more so because none of Custer's troops lived to tell the tale, leaving historians to piece together the story from the memories of Indians and soldiers who were part of

Custer's larger regiment. Changing attitudes toward the conquest of the West now make Custer something less of a hero than an oppressor of Native Americans. At the time, however, he and his men acted heroically, which is the stuff of legend regardless of whether its characters served a cruel cause.

The course of the battle and its immediate aftermath have been debated from the day the bodies were found strewn across what now is Custer Hill. Each new piece of information stimulates a reassessment. The most recent development occurred in August 1983, when a range fire burned the prairie grass and sagebrush covering the battlefield. Archaeologists descended on the site and recovered a small store of artifacts from the bare earth, including the bones of some of the Seventh Cavalry's soldiers that had escaped discovery over the previous 107 years. Those bones have since led historians to new discoveries about the event.

Custer's Last Stand was the second of three major skirmishes with warriors from an encampment of some two thousand Sioux, Cheyenne, and Arapahoe on the south bank of the Little Bighorn River in what is now southern Montana.[1] Custer commanded a regiment of the Dakota Column, consisting of twelve companies of the Seventh Cavalry of the U.S. Army. His troops were part of a multipronged attack aimed at scattering and demoralizing bands of Indians who refused to gather on reservations to the east. Gold also played a part; prospectors had discovered ore in the Black Hills, which belonged to the Great Sioux Reservation in Dakota Territory, and pressure to wrest the lode-bearing land from the Indians had reached all the way to the White House and President Ulysses S. Grant.

The first battle was joined in mid-June by Brigadier General George Crook on the Rosebud Creek, a tributary of the Little Bighorn. Fighting with the help of Crow and Shoshoni Indians, Crook had expected an easy victory. That was one of the first of several errors of judgment the army was to make in its campaign. Instead of melting into the woods and wilderness, the Sioux and Cheyenne warriors spent almost a full day in battle and fought Crook's men to a standoff.

The army persisted. In the days following the first skirmish, several columns of soldiers closed in on what they believed to be the main body of Indians, perhaps eight hundred warriors, many under the leadership of Sitting Bull, somewhere along the Little Bighorn River. Despite the battle at Rosebud Creek, Crook didn't expect that the Indians, who never seemed able to ally themselves in large numbers for more than a few days, would pitch a serious resistance.

Custer, known for his zeal as well as his flowing blond hair and fringed buckskin jackets, was tapped as the one to close in first for the kill.

More skirmishes punctuated the pursuit up the Indians' trail along the Rosebud. Unbeknownst to the soldiers, however, Sitting Bull's eight hundred warriors had been joined by as many as a thousand new fighters from the Indian agencies. Several bands of Sioux, including Hunkpapas, Oglalas, Miniconjous, Yanktonnais and Santees, along with Sans Arcs, Blackfoot, Two Kettles, Brules, more Cheyenne, and a few Arapahoe, threw in their lot with Sitting Bull.

Counter to the army's assessment, the Indians were basking in the fullness of new resolve; nothing had so united them before as the white threat to their treasured Black Hills, full of game and fish and the bones of their ancestors. At a sun dance convened by the Sioux a few weeks before, Sitting Bull had described a visionary experience, prophesying that many white soldiers would fall that spring. As the sun rose over the Little Bighorn on June 25, a Monday, it shone on a vast encampment primed for war.

That day, from a hilltop several miles away, Custer spotted the Indians' village. He was unsure of how large it was, nor did he know the terrain and how to approach the camp. His orders were ambiguous; some say he was supposed to skirt the main force of Indians and seal off its route for escape until more troops arrived. Instead, he dispatched Major Marcus A. Reno to strike first, along the south bank. Reno's 140 horsemen were quickly repulsed, taking heavy casualties, and made a confused and desperate retreat through thick woods and across the river to the north bank of the Little Bighorn.

Meanwhile, Custer's own companies followed the ridge along the north bank. Unaware of Reno's rout, Custer sent two of his companies down a ravine to the riverbank. They were immediately set upon by Sioux and hastily rejoined Custer at Calhoun Hill. The Hunkpapa Sioux, led by the famous warrior Gall, now closed in on the soldiers from the south, while Crazy Horse of the Oglala attacked on the western and northern flank. They rarely chose to charge the soldiers.

Instead, they fired from behind sagebrush clumps, tall grass, and what little cover they could find in the wrinkles of the folded but treeless hills.

Custer and his last forty men drew themselves into a rough circle and shot their remaining horses to make breastworks of their corpses. Now vastly outnumbered and trapped, they fought to the last man.

Over the next two days, Reno and his remaining men and a third party of Custer's troops under the leadership of Captain Frederick Benteen, who had trailed a dozen miles behind Custer's battalion, held their ground in a saucer-shaped, earthen redoubt on what is now called Reno Hill. They had no idea what had become of Custer, though they hardly had time to ponder the general's fate. Dug in around their wounded, 350 of them endured withering fire from all sides, fearing that any moment a massed attack would overwhelm them. Surviving the first day with only eleven killed, they spent the night listening to the drums of the Indians' war dance in the valley below and watching the glow of their bonfires in the dark bowl of the night sky.

The next day saw more fighting. But late in the afternoon, mysteriously, the Indians broke off the engagement, rounded up their horses, rolled up the tepees in their valley emcampment, and scattered.

That night the troops buried their dead and, suspicious that the Indians would return, prepared for another day of battle. But the day dawned peacefully. And in the distance a thin blue line of soldiers could be seen snaking into the valley. It was the Second Cavalry, led by General Alfred H. Terry, Custer's commander. A forward patrol arrived shortly. Their first question: Where's Custer? No one knew.

Within hours, they discovered Custer Hill. Most of the dead had been scalped, dismembered, or mutilated. Custer's brother Tom had not only been scalped, but his head crushed and his body filled with arrows. The patrol buried the bodies as best they could and marked the shallow graves with crude wooden stakes. The soldiers identified those who could be recognized by writing the victims' names on slips of paper, which they inserted into empty cartridges and buried with the bodies.

The army and an infuriated public soon wreaked revenge on the Sioux and Cheyenne. The Indians never were able to re-create the solidarity that won them victory at the Little Bighorn. Over the next few months, they were divided and hounded into reservations. Late in 1876, they signed over the Black Hills to the U.S. government. Crazy Horse, Gall, and, finally, Sitting Bull, who had escaped to Canada but was barred by soldiers from hunting buffalo, turned themselves in.

During the years following the battle at the Little Bighorn, the army returned several times to the scene of its most notorious defeat. In 1877, a detachment of soldiers from the Seventh Cavalry went to recover the bones of Custer and his officers. Ten sets of bones, including those of Custer (who was eventually buried at West Point), were retrieved. Many of the others had been scattered by scavengers and the elements, as the original graves had been close to the surface. Over the next few years, visitors to the now-famous site reported further scattering of markers and exposure of the graves.

In 1881, the government dispatched another detachment of men to collect the exposed bones and inter them in a common grave at the top of Custer Hill. A granite marker now stands at the spot. All of the graves that could be located were exhumed and the bones added to the common grave, although numbered marble markers still stand in spots where the men were believed to have fallen. And the bones of the many horses that still littered the field were also gathered up and buried in another large grave near the remains of their former riders.

Over the next century, human bones occasionally surfaced on and near the battlefield. Those that weren't spirited away as souvenirs were stored in a museum at the battlefield, which is now a national monument. In 1958 archaeologists conducted excavations at the Reno-Benteen battlefield before a road was to be put through for tourists, and found the remains of three soldiers, whose bones were also placed in the museum.

After the range fire in 1983, an archaeologist found a human bone eroding from the ground near markers thirty-three and thirty-four along the Deep Ravine Trail. It was believed to have been the place where a troop of about twenty to thirty of Custer's men had been trapped and wiped out. Their bodies had reportedly been buried together where they lay. In 1984 detailed excavations began. A meager collection of artifacts turned up: a few river cobbles, a bullet, a lead shot, a rubber button, three trouser buttons, and a shank-type mother-of-pearl shirt button.

The anthropological fruits of the search were slightly more promising. Archaeologists Doug Scott and Melissa Connor of the National Park Service found three fragments of a cranium, a cervical vertebra, a vertebra from the coccyx (tailbone), a finger bone, a right greater multangular (wrist bone), and fourteen unidentifiable bone shards. The skull fragments included part of the maxilla, the bone just above the top row of teeth, and the left part of the cheek, known as the zygoma. Eight teeth remained as well.[2]

Scott and Connor wondered whether enough was left of the skeleton to identify its owner. They realized they needed an anthropologist, a forensic anthropologist, on the scene.[3]

Clyde Snow arrived at the battlefield in May 1985, enthusiastic for a new historical project. The sets of bones that the archaeologists had found were for the most part only small fractions of whole skeletons. But to Snow that just made the job more challenging. Moreover, the museum was full of bones from the battlefield. They provided a slice of anthropological history, a set of "osteobiographies," he told Scott. "Sometimes," Snow said, "these historical cases are a lot more interesting than modern murders. Besides, you don't have to testify in court, and you can speculate a little more."

Snow made several trips to the battlefield to examine bones that Scott and Connor and their little army of volunteers had uncovered. He called on radiologist John Fitzpatrick to X-ray most of the remains from the site. At the same time, Snow indulged his curiosity in the historical minutiae that had been collected on the men of the Seventh Cavalry, reading as many accounts of the battle as he could find.

Just over 40 percent of the men killed at the Little Bighorn were foreign born. The largest contingent from one country, twenty-eight, was Irish, followed by twenty-seven Germans and sixteen Britons. Three of the men were Crow Indian scouts: Bloody Knife, Bob-Tailed Bull, and Little Brave. The casualties also included a black man, Isaiah Dorman, an interpreter. Snow expected that a skull from any of these four men would show enough signs of its race to make a tentative identification. Another interpreter who died, Mitch Boyer, had had a French father and a Santee Sioux mother.

Median ages of the soldiers were somewhat higher than one might expect from the modern U.S. Army. For privates, it was about twenty-seven years; the thirteen officers ranged between twenty-two and thirty-six years of age. Average height, according to measurements made when the troopers enlisted, was five feet seven inches, almost two inches shorter than the average recruit in 1966. Snow noticed a gradient in stature and rank. Privates were slightly shorter than corporals, who in turn were shorter than sergeants by over an inch. Snow reckons that larger men had an advantage in promotion in an army in which sheer physical ability to impose one man's will on another was still an important factor in leadership.[4]

After eliminating some animal bones stored in the museum that had been misidentified as human, Snow put together twenty "assemblages," each representing a single skeleton, plus three collections of various bones taken from a wide area that may have come from as many as fourteen different people. Most parts of the body were represented, including vertebrae, ribs, the arm and leg bones, foot and hand bones, a few mandibles, and even a couple of tiny hyoid bones, found in the throat. Scott and Connor took the bones down to the M.E.'s office in Oklahoma City so that Snow could examine them in detail.

From the long bones Snow estimated the soldiers' heights. Vertebrae sometimes showed the lipping of osteophytosis, indicating an age above thirty. As might be expected, many of the bones showed signs of violence. Cut marks testified to the work of Indian axes and arrows, and some bones showed signs of bullet wounds. In some cases Snow could tell that the victors had dismembered parts of the bodies. A fragment from a cervical vertebra in one assemblage was clearly cut obliquely, in a single blow — a decapitation, Snow concluded. Many of the skulls, and sometimes other bones, were fractured and the rough edges and shapes of the fragments could only have been caused by what experts call "blunt-force trauma." When the fighting stopped, the Indians apparently moved in to dispatch those still alive with massive crushing blows to the head.

The most complete skeleton was found in 1985. Known as "Mike" to the archaeological team, the man had been about twenty-one when he died, with a strongly projecting chin and slightly bowed long bones, the latter indicative of a Caucasoid or perhaps a Mongoloid.

Some beveling of the glenoid in the right scapula suggested a right-hander, and pronounced muscle attachments on the long bones meant that he had been a strong fellow and probably stocky at five feet seven inches.

"Mike's" fifth lumbar vertebra added a little more information. It lacked a right lamina and inferior articular facet — a congenital deformity, Snow concluded, that may have caused some lower back pain, especially for someone who had to sit on a horse for long periods. The mandible had well-developed muscle attachments, suggesting a diet that required particularly heavy chewing.

Something of a horseman himself, Snow also looked for the telltale signs of a cavalryman. He found them: tubercles, or raised ridges of bone, on the femurs. These are the signposts left by a well-developed *adductor magnus* muscle, characteristic of riders.

From the condition of the mandible, which was broken in two places, it appeared that "Mike" had been hit with a hard object at or about the time of death. A cut mark on the left collarbone suggested that he had been wounded with a knife or a metal-tipped arrowhead. Several ribs were fractured in a manner characteristic of bullet wounds. It also looked as if the soldier had been shot at least twice in the chest and abdomen. The radius of the left arm showed a small fracture containing a piece of lead bullet, just above the wrist. Both thighbones exhibited chop marks that Snow recognized as coming from a moderately sharp instrument like a hatchet or ax. Apparently Mike had been dismembered.

Snow thought he could do more than sketch a picture of the typical cavalryman during the Indian wars and how he often met his end. Among the anonymous remains found at the site were a piece of skull, a part of an upper jaw with eight teeth, along with some vertebrae and a finger bone. They offered just enough unique features to tantalize. Perhaps he could actually identify one of the fallen.

What stood out about the skull fragment was the nasal opening. At twenty-five millimeters, it was rather wide for a Caucasoid. The nasal sill, the ridge of bone at the bottom of the nasal aperture, did not display the raised margins characteristic of Caucasoids either. The man may have been an Indian, or in technical terms, a Mongoloid type. Yet the incisors didn't show the shovel shape prevalent in Native Americans. Snow also had some vertebrae from the skeleton.

The lipping around the edges was advanced enough for the man to have reached at least thirty-five years of age before he died. And the mother-of-pearl button found with the remains suggested that the man had been a civilian, or at least dressed in civilian clothes.

Snow and the archaeologists checked the historical records of Custer's troops. Only one man fit the description: Mitch Boyer, the half-Indian interpreter and scout. He had been thirty-eight years old when he rode out with the Seventh, about the age indicated by the vertebral lipping.

Doug Scott gave Snow a photograph of Boyer from the archives at the museum. Boyer, a stolid-looking man with a firmly set jaw, downturned mouth, and headfeathers, stared out past the camera as if he were posing for a spot on Mount Rushmore. Now the photograph had become far more interesting than just another cameo from Snow's "longest running drama"; it presented a way to confirm that the bones excavated so carefully by Scott and Connor belonged to a half-Indian who fought for Custer.

After getting some instruction from Snow on how to do a skull-face superimposition, Scott took the skull fragment and the photograph to the studio of the Nebraska Educational Television Network, in Lincoln, where the archaeological team had its headquarters. Snow had practiced skull-face superimposition with several cases, but he wasn't sure that the piece of skull Scott had would be enough to make a comparison. It was only about four inches long and a couple of inches wide, comprising the maxilla into which the left-top row of teeth fit, the left side of the nasal opening and the bottom of the orbit of the left eye socket, and the left cheekbone. As abbreviated as it was, its shape was unique.

When Scott superimposed the image of the skull over the photograph, the match was as snug as a horse and saddle: the eye sat right in the orbit, the nose covered the nasal cavity the way it should, and the teeth fit exactly under Boyer's stiff upper lip.

Snow provided a final flourish to seal the identification. With the skull fragment back in hand, he perused the teeth under his hand lens. On the left incisor and canine, he found unusual arched wear marks. He'd seen that before; the marks were caused by a pipestem regularly clenched between the teeth. And Boyer had been an habitual pipe smoker.

Boyer's identification might not have held up in a court of law, but it served an historical purpose. Scott and Connor had found his bones at the crest of a small ridge of what was known as the South Skirmish Line. Indian participants in the battle, however, had told historians that they had seen Boyer's body in Deep Ravine. Others said they had seen him in the river, on the bank of the river, halfway between the Custer and the first of the Reno battlefields, and on a ridge. If the skull fragment indeed belonged to Mitch Boyer, said Scott and Connor, then several accounts on which the battle has been re-created in history texts had to be doubted.

Snow agreed. That was the sort of thing that digging up bones often accomplished — a revision of conventional wisdom. "Bones make good witnesses," Snow is wont to say. "Although they speak softly, they never lie and they never forget."

In the museum at the battlefield, Snow found something else that he believed could tell a story. It was a nearly complete skull. It had been there since 1958, when it was discovered by archaeologists at the site of the final Reno-Benteen battleground. The skull lacked the lower jaw, but it certainly was the most intact Snow had seen in the collection. A left arm, a rib, and two vertebrae found with it indicated that the soldier had stood about five feet eight inches tall, was of light to medium build, and probably was between twenty-five and twenty-seven years old when he was killed.

In 1986 the body, along with others found in 1958, was reburied. Before it was interred, however, casts were made of the skull. Snow asked if one could be sent to the facial reconstructionist Betty Pat Gatliff in Norman, Oklahoma.

Normally, Gatliff wouldn't do a reconstruction on a skull without a mandible. There were just too many variables in the chin that could grossly alter a person's looks. But she figured she could estimate the shape for a case such as this, where a criminal prosecution or a prison sentence for someone didn't hang in the balance, by using some calculations first suggested by Wilton Krogman.[5]

Scott sent Gatliff the cast, and she went to work at her office, the "SKULLpture lab" in Norman. She recreated a rather handsome young face with full, fleshy lips on a wide mouth, a strong jaw, eyes set slightly close together, and a broad nose. When Scott saw the reconstructed skull, the first he'd seen in person, he was astonished at the detail Gatliff had extracted from the contours of the skull. He compared photographs of some of the soldiers at the Little Bighorn that historians had collected over the years to the sculpture. He returned repeatedly to one picture. A rakish young soldier, his cavalry cap tilted casually to one side, his expression one of rough-and-ready enthusiasm, bore a strong resemblence to Gatliff's sculpture. The man in the photo was Sergeant Miles O'Hara. When Gatliff added a cap to her sculpture, partly to cover what she considered the rather crude head of hair she had made for it, the resemblance was uncanny.

Scott took the sculpture back to Lincoln and showed it to his colleagues. The records on O'Hara bolstered what their eyes told them. O'Hara had been five feet eight and one-quarter inches tall and twenty-five years and eight months old when he fought his last battle. Using the video superimposition technique again, they got an exact fit between the photograph and the skull. To test the technique's reliability, they superimposed photographs of three other soldiers killed near O'Hara. The skull clearly did not jibe with any of them. They had another match.

Again, the archaeologists found that the hard evidence before them contradicted historical accounts of the battle. O'Hara had fallen in the Valley fight. Yet his body, they now knew, was buried on Reno Hill. Snow suggests that he may have only been wounded and was evacuated to a field hospital.

In a waggish moment, Snow suggested that much bigger surprises might lie in wait among the bones of Little Bighorn. After doing some digging into records of Custer's burial at the battlefield and the subsequent exhumation of the body for removal to West Point, he wrote this account:

According to Sgt. John Ryan of M Company, who personally supervised Custer's interment, special care was given to his burial. In contrast to most of the other dead whose graves were barely deep enough to cover the body, the grave prepared for the General was dug to a depth of about eighteen inches. It was also made wide enough to hold the body of his brother Tom, and the two bodies were laid side by side. The general had been shot twice; one bullet had entered the left temple and the second struck him in the chest. There was also a wound in his right forearm which could have been due either to a third bullet or an exiting fragment of the bullet which had caused the chest wound. He had not been scalped or dismembered. . . .

Before the grave was closed with earth, the bodies were covered with blankets and some canvas tent sheets. Finally, an Indian *travois* [a stretcher pulled by a horse] found in the abandoned village was laid over the grave and weighted down with rocks. While far from Pharaonic, such an interment should have been sufficient to protect the bodies from the elements and animal scavengers which combined to expose the shallower graves of the lesser dead. One would expect, therefore, that the exhumation team would have found two complete sets of remains. . . .[6]

Instead, when the detachment returned in 1881 to retrieve the bones of the officers and some of the civilians, the grave they identified as Custer's contained only one body. After removing the remains from the earth, the diggers discovered that the rotting uniform blouse found with the bones bore the name of a corporal. So they tried another grave they thought might be Custer's. In it they found only one skull, several ribs, and a femur, apparently from one person. Despite doubts voiced by some at the exhumation, these bones were declared Custer's and sent off to West Point.

"It also seemed strange that they apparently found no remnants of the blankets and canvas sheets used to cover the bodies," Snow observed after studying the records. It just might be, he mused, that the man buried in General Custer's tomb is not George Armstrong Custer.

PART

II

8

THE FALLEN ANGEL
OF DEATH

ON the sixth of June, 1985, the Federal Police Chief of São Paulo, Brazil, stood at the edge of a hillside grave in a village cemetery where the people of Embú bury their dead. Arms folded across his chest, Romeu Tuma watched as three gravediggers hacked with picks and shovels at the weed-covered tomb. For nearly an hour the men had taken turns driving their spades into the hard ground and lifting large red chunks of earth from the widening trough.

One of the gravediggers' picks caught wood. Tuma leaned forward, motioning for another man to climb down into the hole. The men scraped clumps of dirt off the lid of a coffin and struggled to pry it open with a pick. It wouldn't budge. The latches, six years in the damp soil, had rusted shut.

Tuma ordered one of the gravediggers to smash the coffin open. His pick pierced the lid, scattering splinters against the sides of the hole. He struck it again and wrenched the lid free. Inside the coffin lay a jumble of musty bones poking through tattered clothing.

Tuma looked at the remains and then, out of the corner of his eye, at Lisolette Bossert, a tall, drawn woman with cropped gray hair and square shoulders, who stood by the grave with her husband, Wolfram. Her pale hand moved mechanically up to the corners of her eyes, and the tips of her fingers quickly brushed the tears away.

149

Two days before, Brazilian police, acting on a tip from West German investigators, had surprised the Bosserts at their home in Embú, twelve miles west of São Paulo. Wolfram spoke openly to the police at first, until Lisolette hushed him in sharp German tones. Eventually the police broke the couple's resolve and persuaded them to lead Tuma to the graveyard at Embú where, Lisolette confessed, she had arranged for a man to be buried in 1979 under the name of Wolfgang Gerhard, an Austrian expatriate and a friend of the Bosserts. Lisolette told the police that the man she had buried had died in a swimming accident. He had adopted Gerhard's name, but they had long known his true identity. It was Josef Mengele, the Angel of Death. He was the Nazi doctor who sent 400,000 people — many of whom he tortured — to their deaths at Auschwitz, and the world's most wanted murderer.

At the opened grave Dr. José Antonio de Mello, the assistant director of the police department's forensic laboratory, pushed his way through the crowd of journalists, photographers, and curious onlookers who pressed toward the tomb like filings drawn to a magnet. A rotund, bustling man, de Mello's shiny black shoes slipped in the dirt as he kneeled to reach into the coffin. He placed the bones in a long white plastic box, saving the broken skull, however, to hold up for the crowd to see. Within hours this image would flicker on television screens around the world.

Tuma stepped back from the grave and surveyed his audience. It was a fine moment for Brazil, for its police force, and for Romeu Tuma. He knew his next words would soon be cabled to newsrooms around the world. He spoke clearly and solemnly, a hint of a smile just visible under his bushy black mustache. "I can state categorically," he said, "that he is well and truly dead."[1]

Seven thousand miles away Ralph Blumenthal, a senior investigative journalist on the *New York Times*, tossed a slip of wire copy onto his desk. Looking up, he eyed the reporter who had just handed him the cable. "This is the most ridiculous thing I've ever heard," he said with a laugh. "It's so perfect. The guy's being looked for all over and they concoct these bones in Brazil. I mean, it's such an obvious ploy."[2]

Blumenthal had reason to be skeptical. Few journalists knew as much as he about the demimonde of Nazi war criminals. In the early

150

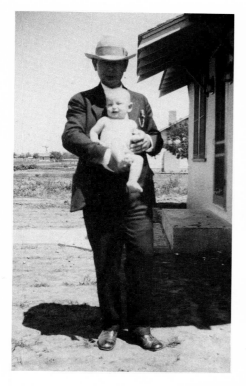

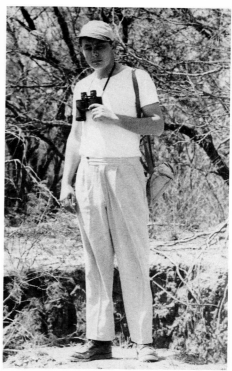

Photograph by Scott Rutherford/Black Star

Above left: "Sonny" Snow at age one with his father, Wister, in Ralls, Texas.

Above right: Clyde Snow bird-watching in New Mexico, 1952.

Right: Snow holding a piece of evidence, a mandible, from the anthropological collection at the Oklahoma City Medical Examiner's Office.

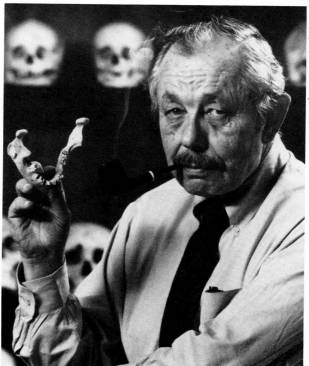

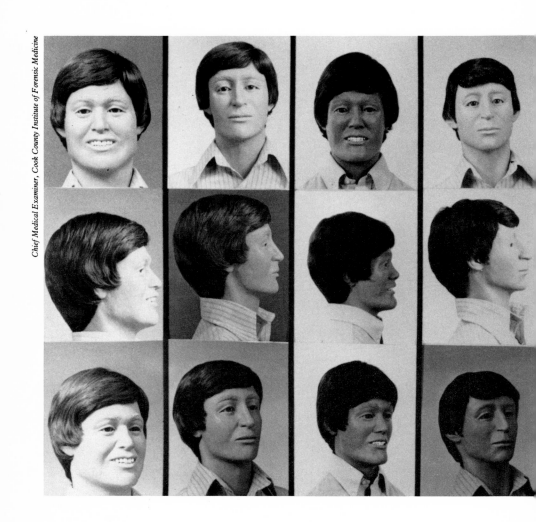

Oklahoma artist Betty Pat Gatliff's facial reconstructions from the skulls of eight of the anonymous victims of mass-murderer John Wayne Gacy, 1979.

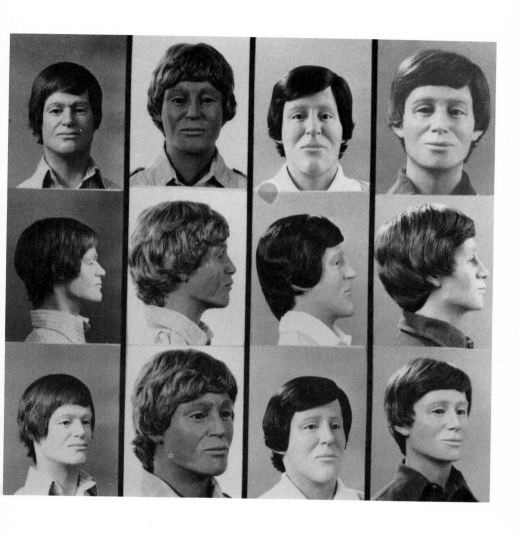

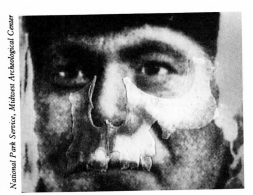

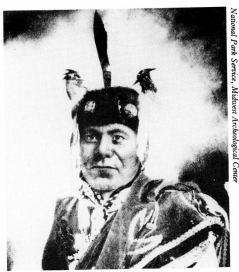

The photographic superimposition that gave a name — Mitch Boyer — to a skull found at the Custer battlefield.

Mitch Boyer, half-Indian, half-French scout for General George Custer, in traditional garb. The photograph served as a template for a superimposition using skull fragments found at the site of the Battle of the Little Bighorn.

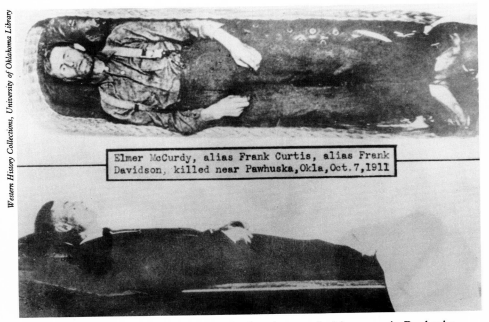

Elmer McCurdy, alias Frank Curtis, alias Frank Davidson, killed near Pawhuska, Okla, Oct. 7, 1911

Elmer McCurdy, the bandit who wouldn't die, photographed in repose in Pawhuska, Oklahoma, October 1911.

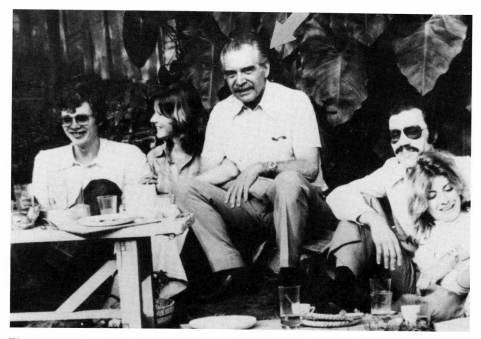

The arrow points to Auschwitz's "Angel of Death," Josef Mengele, at an outing with friends near São Paulo, Brazil.

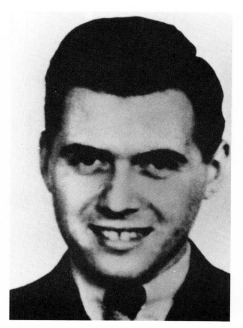

Mengele's 1938 SS photograph clearly shows the distinctive diastema between the two upper incisors that was also found in the skull from Embú, Brazil.

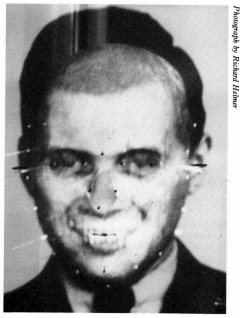

A full-face superimposition of the Embú skull with the 1938 SS photograph of Mengele. The dots on and around the face are markers on pins that guide the alignment between skull and fleshy outlines of the face.

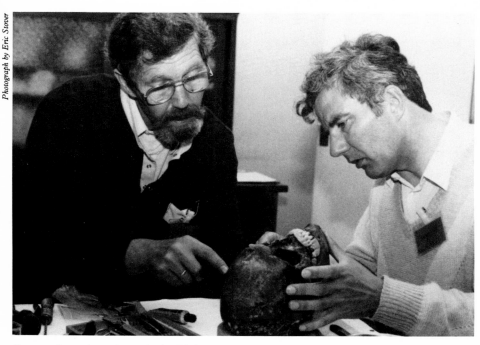

Snow (center), holding Josef Mengele's skull, with Brazilian anthropologist Daniel Muñoz (left) and a Brazilian colleague at the Medico-Legal Institute in São Paulo, Brazil.

German forensic anthropologist Richard Helmer (right) and an assistant apply the finishing touches to the reconstruction of Mengele's shattered skull.

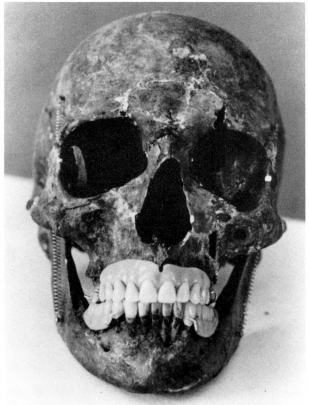

Mengele's skull, complete with reconstructed dental work, as assembled by Richard Helmer in Brazil during the summer of 1985.

Skull-face profiles from Richard Helmer's photo-montage of the living and dead Mengele.

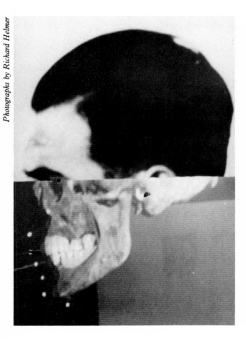

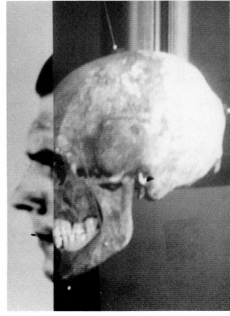

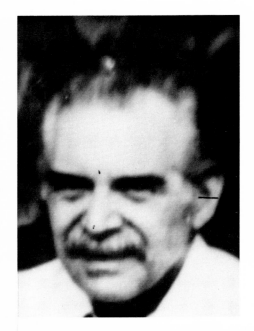

Photographs by Richard Helmer

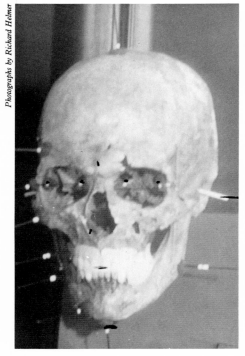

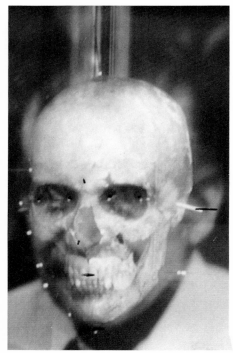

Richard Helmer's skull-face superimposition technique proved decisive in matching the Embú skull to photographs of Josef Mengele.

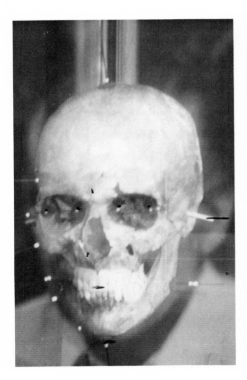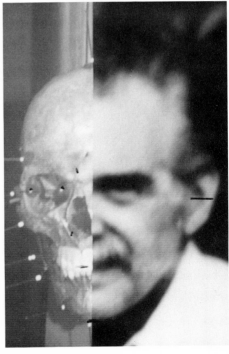

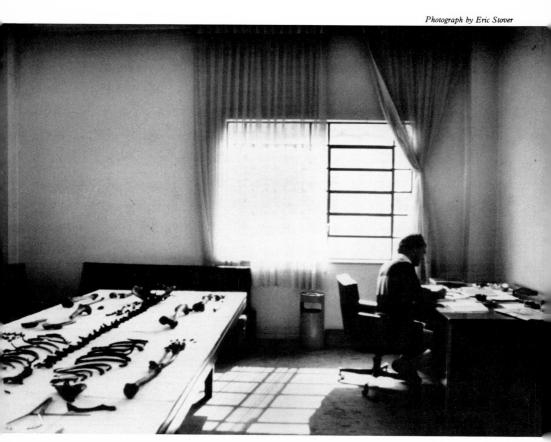

The Embú skeleton laid out in the examining room at the Medico-Legal Institute, São Paulo, Brazil, 1985.

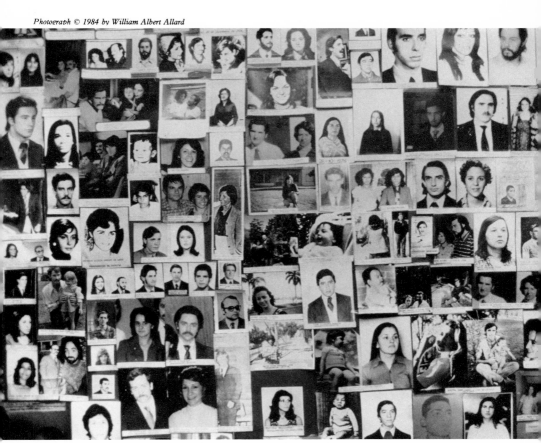

A montage of some of Argentina's disappeared displayed in the offices of the Mothers of the Plaza de Mayo in Buenos Aires.

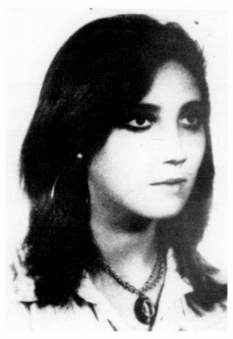

A photograph of *desaparecida* Liliana Pereyra, taken shortly before her disappearance in November 1977.

Dr. Laura Bonaparte, the mother of a disappeared woman, looks in vain for her daughter among remains removed from a mass grave by Argentine authorities in early 1984. A year later Clyde Snow began training Argentine medical and anthropology students in the proper techniques for exhuming and identifying skeletal remains.

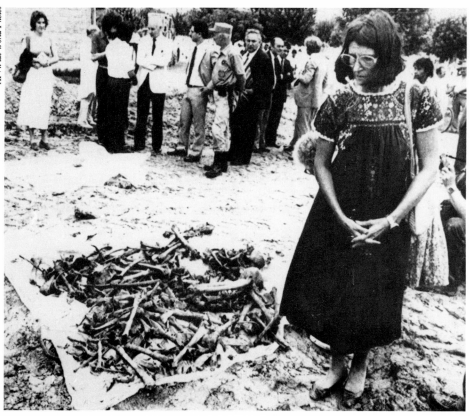

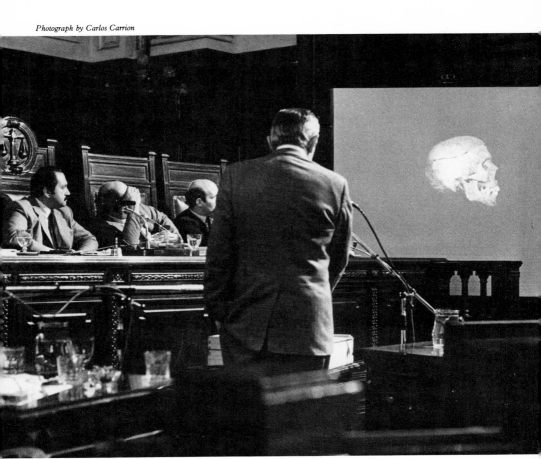

Snow offers scientific evidence on the identification of Liliana Pereyra at the 1985 trial of the junta members who ruled Argentina from 1976 to 1983.

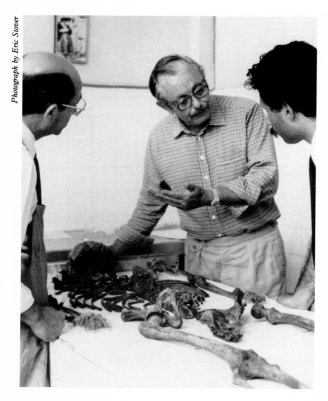

Snow examines the remains of one of the disappeared with the help of Argentine forensic specialists.

Argentine team members Luis Fondebrider and Patricia Bernardi working in a *cuadrícula* at the Avellaneda Cemetery, just outside of Buenos Aires.

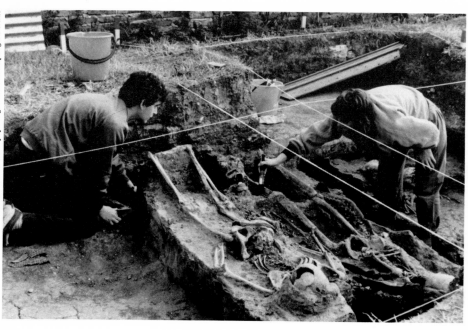

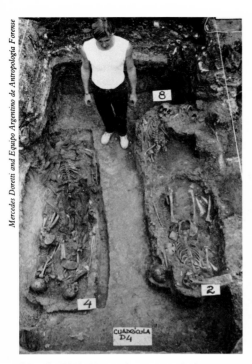

Morris Tidball stands next to skeletons uncovered after a year's work by the Argentine forensic team at Avellaneda, 1989.

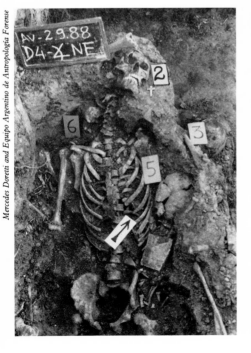

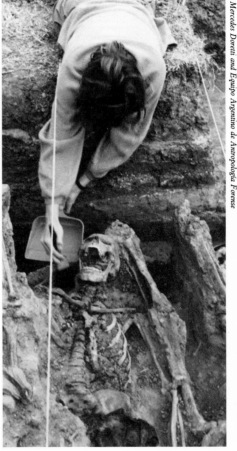

Mercedes Doretti of the Argentine Forensic Anthropology Team exhumes a skeleton from a mass grave at the Avellaneda Cemetery, 1989.

The carefully uncovered skeleton of one of the disappeared buried anonymously at the Avellaneda Cemetery.

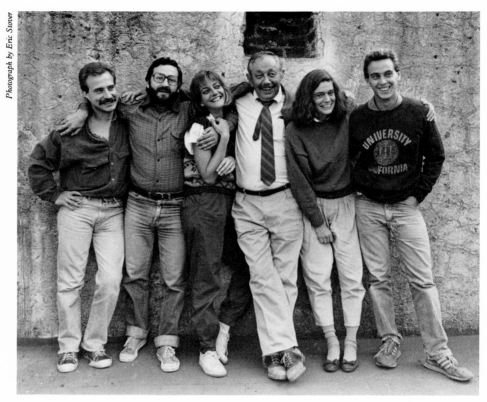

Clyde Snow with the Argentine forensic team outside their office in Buenos Aires, 1988. *From left,* Dario Olmo, Alejandro Inchaurregui, Patricia Bernardi, Snow, Mercedes Doretti, and Luis Fondebrider (Morris Tidball not shown).

1970s Blumenthal had written a series of articles about "Operation Paper Clip," the code name used by the U.S. Immigration and Naturalization Service when, shortly after the war, it allowed dozens of Nazi scientists to lie about their past and settle in the United States. Since then, he had made Nazi-hunting, and particularly the Mengele chase, his beat. The world's most wanted criminal couldn't be dead, he thought. His sources said Mengele was hiding in a German enclave in the jungles of South America.

Josef Mengele was one of the last surviving instruments of Hitler's *Endlösung*, or Final Solution, the plan to exterminate all the Jews in Europe. Born in 1911 to a prosperous Bavarian family, Mengele displayed a vaulting ambition. Someday, he once told a school friend, people would read his name in the encyclopedia. He developed a passion for classical music and art and fancied fast cars. But what excited him most was science.

Mengele left his family home in Günzburg in 1930 and enrolled as a student at the University of Munich, where he earned a degree in anthropology and later a medical degree. He joined Hitler's personal police and security squadron, the SS, or *Schutzstaffel*, in 1938 and later spent nine months in occupied Poland, attached to the Genealogical Section of the Race and Resettlement Office. Under direct orders from Heinrich Himmler, Mengele and other SS doctors were assigned to "cleanse the annexed territories of non-Germans" and to examine the racial suitability of those who would be settled there. In 1941 he joined the German troops in the Ukraine, where he was soon recognized as "a specially talented medical officer." By 1943 he had risen to the rank of captain and in May of that year was posted to Auschwitz, the largest extermination center in the Third Reich's genocide program.

Survivors of Auschwitz vividly recall the man who stood before them in the morning mist at the death-camp railhead. He was a handsome officer, upright in posture, well-groomed, with dark hair and a dark complexion. He always held his head erect, his SS cap raked to one side, a riding crop or silver-capped cane in his gloved hand. In summer he wore suspenders and a khaki shirt. In winter, even as icy winds and sleet swept through the camp, he always looked immaculate in his knee-length leather coat, his polished black boots glistening on the frozen mud. He rarely said a word. He just tipped his thumb. Death to one side, life to the other.

Mengele seldom changed his cool expression as he surveyed the new arrivals on the transport ramp. But occasionally, when his eyes fixed on a pair of twins, he would smile, revealing the distinctive gap between his two front teeth. "Zwillinge heraustreten! [Twins step forward!]," he would shout. Mark Berkowitz, who was twelve years old when he arrived at Auschwitz, recalls Mengele's fascination as he peered down at him and his twin sister. "He asked my mother one question: 'Your son is blond and your daughter is like a Gypsy; can you explain that?'"[3] For Mengele the anthropologist, these children were rare subjects for experiments that he believed would make his name in scientific history.

Mengele housed the twins in special barracks and gave them good food and comfortable beds. On some days he brought them chocolates. He took meticulous anatomical measurements of their heads, eyes, noses, ears, and limbs. As one twin survivor recalls: "He concentrated on one part of the body at one time . . . [one day] he measured our eyes for about two hours."[4]

Mengele's interest in human morphology dated to his university days. He had earned his Ph.D. with a thesis entitled "Racial Morphological Research on the Lower Jaw Section of Four Racial Groups." At Munich and later at the University of Frankfurt, he studied eugenics, a body of pseudobiological theory that regarded persons such as the feebleminded, the mentally diseased, and the deformed as inimical to the human race.

By the early 1930s eugenicists had sprouted like weeds on university campuses in much of the Western world. In the United States proponents of the theory had managed to convince legislatures in twenty-five states to enact laws providing for compulsory sterilization of the criminally insane and other people considered biologically inferior.[5] But it was the Nazi eugenicists who pushed the field to its most hideous extreme. They held that doctors should destroy "life devoid of value," so as to "purify" the Aryan race. This "life unworthy of life" theory led to Hitler's compulsory sterilization laws, enacted in July 1933, which empowered doctors to sterilize patients suffering from disorders such as schizophrenia, chorea minor, manic depression, and hereditary blindness. Beginning in 1934, hundreds of thousands of people were sterilized against their will or without their understanding. Hitler later used the theory to justify "mercy" killing for the supposedly incurably insane and for the mass extermination of Gypsies and Jews.

At Auschwitz, Mengele believed that his experiments on twins would prove his own theory that through appropriate selection and breeding, the quality of a race could be improved. He reasoned that those features that were identical between twins must be inherited and therefore could be genetically controlled.

Mengele received funding for his "research" at Auschwitz from the German Research Society and got encouragement from his mentor, Professor Otmar Freiherr von Verschuer, director of the Kaiser Wilhelm Institute for Anthropology, Human Heredity and Genetics, in Frankfurt. Mengele used the money to construct a special pathology laboratory in one of the crematoria. After completing his experiments on a pair of twins, he often had them killed and taken to the lab for dissection. He could then compare healthy and diseased organs to show the effects of heredity. These results, as well as others obtained during his twenty-one months at Auschwitz, were sent to the Frankfurt institute for further analysis.

Besides twins, Mengele selected other inmates to further his scientific ambitions. In the hospital blocks he weeded out the weakest patients and had them delivered to his laboratory. In his arrest warrants and indictments issued by the West Germans between 1959 and 1981, Mengele was charged with using electrical equipment on young women to test their endurance of pain.[6] He is also alleged to have subjected a group of Polish nuns to intense radiation from which they suffered severe burns. On other occasions he conducted bone-marrow transplants on healthy inmates for no other reason than to observe the results.

Immense red-brick chimneys greeted the first Russian soldiers who arrived at Auschwitz on the afternoon of January 27, 1945. As they passed through the camp gates, they could see fires smoldering in the furnaces. The Nazis had fled, leaving behind hundreds of corpses scattered about the camp.

On the night Mengele left Auschwitz, he paid a last visit to the camp anthropologist Martina Puzyna. "He came into my office without a word," she told writer John Ware in an interview years later.[7] "He took all my papers, put them into two boxes, and had them taken outside to a waiting car." From that night on, Mengele found anonymity in the growing exodus of German soldiers heading west. Although American troops captured Mengele in Bavaria in June 1945, they failed to identify him as an SS officer. Freed by the U.S. Army, he found shelter among Nazi sympathizers until he reached Munich. From there he traveled south to Rosenheim, near the Austrian border, where friends had arranged for him to work as a farm laborer. He stayed at the farm until August 1948 and then settled near his home-town of Günzburg. However, by spring of 1949 Mengele realized that the net cast by those who sought to avenge the Nazis' victims would eventually snare him. He fled across the Alps to Genoa, Italy, where he obtained an International Red Cross passport under the name of Helmut Gregor. Finally, in mid-July, clutching a small suitcase filled with notes from Auschwitz, *der Totenengel* (the Angel of Death) boarded the *North King*, a passenger ship bound for Argentina.

Thus began a thirty-year odyssey. During that time Mengele was posted as dead or alive in over ten countries. In 1968 a former Brazilian police agent said he had tracked Mengele to the Paraná River between Paraguay and Argentina and shot the Nazi doctor in the neck and chest in a gunfight. By 1979 Mengele sightings had even pushed UFOs off the front page of the *National Enquirer*. That year Nazi-hunter Simon Wiesenthal said that Mengele was living in a secret Nazi colony in the foothills of the Chilean Andes. Then it was Asunción, where he had taken up beekeeping and was frequently seen driving about town in a black sedan. In 1981 *Life* magazine published a sensational story claiming that the Nazi fugitive had moved into a private house in Bedford Hills, thirty miles north of New York City. Mengele's last "death" occurred in March 1985 when a man committed suicide in Lisbon and left a note saying, "I am Josef Mengele." The West German police examined the corpse and declared that he wasn't.

At the *New York Times*, Blumenthal had also been sucked into the slipstream of the Mengele chase, and at times it moved faster than the facts could follow. Early in 1985 Blumenthal picked up a lead that Mengele was flourishing in sybaritic splendor at a seaside villa in Uruguay. The *Times* sent Blumenthal to the Los Angeles–based Simon Wiesenthal Center, where he was shown photographs of Mengele lounging by a swimming pool. Blumenthal flew to Paris to share the information with Nazi-hunters Serge and Beate Klarsberg. Then he went to Frankfurt to question West German investigators.

The chase had begun in 1984 with a cloak-and-dagger tale recited by Herbert John, a West German journalist, and Saul Sztemberg, a retired Argentine policeman. They claimed to have been approached by an Uruguayan colonel who knew a prostitute who was Mengele's mistress. The prostitute had told the colonel that she visited the aging Nazi doctor, who went by the name of Walter Branaa, once a month at one of his several villas on Uruguay's Atlantic coast.

John and Sztemberg cut a deal with the colonel and then gave the information to the *New York Post*. In late 1984 the *Post* sent reporter Charles Lachman to Buenos Aires to talk to Sztemberg. When Lachman arrived at Sztemberg's house he found another writer, Richard White, already there. White was a reed-thin adventurer in his early forties who spoke fluent Spanish and had written two books on Latin America. He had plans to abduct Mengele, a.k.a. Branaa. After a long night of negotiations, Lachman finally persuaded White to take him along on a reconnaissance mission to photograph the playboy Mengele in his *palais de plaisir*. In return, White would be cut into the *Post* payroll.

Once in Uruguay, White and Lachman staked out one of Branaa's several estates. In some woods near the villa they jerry-built a duck blind and took turns watching. The waiting put them on edge, but they were reassured by their New York editor's promise that if they had trouble with the authorities he would have Senator d'Amato bail them out. They finally snapped four shots of Branaa while he was taking a stroll on his estate by the ocean. They rushed back to New York, had the pictures computer-enhanced, and, with great expectations, took them to the New York medical examiner's office. Their hopes fell when consulting anthropologist Peggy Caldwell said the pictures weren't clear enough to analyze.

Lachman and White returned to Uruguay, this time with *Post* photographer Dan Brinzac. They rented a van, fitted it with curtains, and hunkered down in a parking lot one hundred meters from the villa. Using a two thousand-millimeter lens, Brinzac snapped away as Branaa descended the veranda steps to his swimming pool. The photos show close-ups of Branaa, a gold chain dangling across his hirsute chest, staring in the direction of the camera. In another set of shots, he is sitting by a swimming pool, wearing a bathing suit and talking to a fleshy woman with short dark hair.

Convinced that they now had what they needed, the three operatives returned to New York. They made three sets of prints, leaving one set, along with a 1938 SS photograph of Mengele, with Caldwell; another with J. Lawrence Angel, the late distinguished physical anthropologist at the Smithsonian Institution in Washington; and a third with Ellis Kerley, a forensic anthropologist at the University of Maryland. So as not to prejudice his analysis, Angel told White, "I don't want you to tell me who this is."[8] According to White, he also didn't inform Caldwell or Kerley of the presumed identity of the man in both sets of photographs.

The three scientists conducted independent analyses on the 1938 and 1985 photographs. In her report Caldwell describes how she measured and evaluated characteristics such as "slope of the forehead," "adiposity of upper eyelid," and "mouth-nose 'worry' lines."[9] She found a diastema, or gap between the two upper front teeth, on the photograph of young Mengele but not on the later pictures. The discrepancy puzzled her, but she attributed it to "an age factor . . . due to mesial drift, which would have been considerable between 1937 and 1985!"

All three scientists reached similar conclusions. Both Kerley[10] and Angel[11] stated that there was a 95 percent probability that the SS and Uruguayan photos were of the same man. White recalled later that when he questioned Kerley's finding, the anthropologist told him, "Well, in a way I'm betting my professional life on this." Angel found the comparisons so striking that he told White he "would be willing to go to court if that is necessary." Asked to elaborate, Angel said, "It is pretty much like seeing an automobile coming down the street at about fifty feet away and saying, 'That is a Mercedes.' It is of that order. We ordinarily act on that kind of thing."

Caldwell concluded in her report "that there is at the very least a ninety percent probability that these photographs were taken of one and the same caucasian male individual at different times in his life."

White and Lachman rejoiced.

On February 4 White and Lachman flew to Israel, where they met with members of the Mossad, Israel's foreign intelligence–gathering service. According to White, the Israeli agents said that they agreed with the photographic evidence but said they would have to send their own people to Uruguay to check the story.

White and Lachman returned to New York. They spent weeks planning their next step — the kidnapping of Mengele. Meanwhile, however, Ralph Blumenthal had latched onto the story. So had NBC, which sent a film crew to Uruguay.

Then, like a sand castle in the rising tide, the story started to dissolve. The Israelis called Lachman. Walter Branaa, they insisted, was not the man the forensic experts said he was.

That might have ended the episode. But as White put it years later, "For the media, it was just too big a bet to lose." Maybe the Israelis were wrong. ABC's John Martin asked White what he knew, and White sold his information about Branaa to the network for $15,000. ABC confronted Branaa at his villa. Branaa was shocked. It was absolutely untrue, he said, producing his birth certificate and school records. He even spoke Uruguayan Spanish. His son was a local rock star. The networks were convinced. Once again, a Mengele myth had been created by Nazi hunters too eager for the kill to see the obvious.

Nazi-hunting was experiencing a revival in 1985. The year marked the fortieth anniversary of the liberation of Auschwitz, and camp survivors were pressuring officialdom to capture Mengele at any cost. The first surge came from the Simon Wiesenthal Center, which with great fanfare in December 1984 disclosed U.S. Army intelligence documents showing that American troops had had Mengele in their custody after the war but had let him go. The center followed its disclosure with an offer of one million dollars for information on the Nazi doctor's whereabouts. Other rewards soon followed, until the bounty on Mengele's head had reached a staggering $3,458,000.

On January 17, 1985, a group of camp survivors held a vigil at the gates of Auschwitz. As TV cameras whirred, the former inmates huddled against the cold and described Mengele's atrocities and their indignation that he was still free. A week later Simon Wiesenthal staged a mock trial of *der Totenengel* in Jerusalem. For four nights TV viewers around the world watched as dozens of survivors took the stand to describe Mengele's hideous experiments.

The politics of shame succeeded. Within days the American, Israeli, and German governments had announced that a new attempt would be made to find Josef Mengele. U.S. Attorney General William French Smith said that his government was concerned about the disclosure that Mengele may have been in U.S. custody after the war. He directed the Department of Justice's Office of Special Investigations (OSI) to spearhead the hunt in cooperation with the U.S. Marshal's Service. Established in 1979 by the Carter administration, the OSI was already tracking down and deporting Nazi fugitives who had lied about their crimes to gain entry into the United States at the end of the war. "Yes, I think we'll get him," OSI chief Neal Sher told the press after Smith's announcement. "I'm ninety-nine percent sure of that."[12]

Sher's West German and Israeli counterparts shared his optimism. "I'm sure he's alive and I'm confident he'll be caught," said Hans Klein, the prosecutor in charge of the West German investigation.[13] Sher and Klein, along with the head of the Nazi crimes section of the Israeli police, Menachem Russek, pledged to work together in the new push to find Mengele. What happened next, however, caught the American and Israeli investigators by surprise.

On May 31, 1985, without a word to the Americans or Israelis, the West German federal police, acting on a tip from a university professor, raided the house of Hans Sedlmeier in Günzburg. Sedlmeier was a childhood friend of Mengele's who later became the purchasing director for the Mengele family's farm machinery firm in Günzburg. The professor had told the police that he had dined with Sedlmeier and his wife, Renate, while on holiday in late autumn of 1984. Toward the end of the meal, the professor said, Sedlmeier boasted that he had funneled money to Mengele at his hideaways in South America.

At Sedlmeier's house police found an address book in code and photocopies of letters from Mengele that Renate had stashed under the floorboards. One of the letters was from Wolfram Bossert. It announced "with deep sorrow the death of our common friend."[14]

Six days after the Günzburg raid, in Washington, D.C., Morgan Hardiman strode into the office of Senator Alfonse d'Amato with an urgent message.[15] As a legislative aide to the senior senator from New York, Hardiman had spent the previous year investigating charges that Mengele had been in U.S. custody after the war and had been released in 1947 in exchange for intelligence information. Working hand in glove with the Simon Wiesenthal Center, Hardiman had uncovered previously classified documents that convinced a subcommittee of the Senate judiciary committee to hold hearings in February and March of 1985 on the role the U.S. Army may have played in allowing the Nazi doctor to escape.

The hearings failed to produce any conclusive evidence either to incriminate or absolve U.S. forces. Instead they devolved into a game of cat and mouse as tight-lipped Department of Justice and army intelligence investigators repeatedly dodged queries from the subcommittee. As one Justice Department offical told the senators, "This [investigation] remains a ticklish business, in the sense that we have a query in the field, and we would respectfully suggest and request permission from this committee that we not publicly go into any further details of the pending investigation, or its particular methodology."[16]

Now, three months later, Hardiman stood fuming in d'Amato's office. The Brazilian police, he said, had located Mengele's grave and were going to dig it up later in the day.

"Where's the Justice Department figure in this?" d'Amato asked.

"Well, I just now got off the phone with [OSI's] Sher. He called me from the airport where he's about to catch a plane to Brazil. He doesn't know any more than we do!"

"Get Leslie Lukash on the phone," d'Amato ordered.

Minutes later, Dr. Leslie Lukash, chief medical examiner for Nassau County, New York, took a call from Washington.[17] Lukash, a compact, soft-spoken man in his late sixties, was something of an institution in New York's medicolegal community, having practiced in and around the city for several decades. He had been a friend of d'Amato's since the 1960s and immediately recognized from the Senator's voice that something was amiss.

"Have you heard about the affair in Brazil?" d'Amato asked.

159

"No."

"Well, the Brazilian police claim they've found Josef Mengele's body."

Lukash cleared his throat nervously.

"Leslie, I know it sounds absurd, but it seems the Germans are taking it seriously. They've already sent down two investigators."

"What about the Americans and Israelis?" Lukash asked.

D'Amato said he didn't know all the details but it appeared as if the Justice Department hadn't even known what the Brazilians and Germans were up to until the day before. As for the Israelis, they were highly skeptical and worried that it might be a hoax. For his part, the senator said, he wanted the examination of the body to be handled properly. Lukash sensed what was coming next.

"Leslie, can you go down there?" d'Amato asked. "Just to keep an eye on things."

Yes, Lukash replied, he'd go down. But not alone. These were skeletal remains, he explained, and any scientific investigation worth a damn would require a team. He'd need an anthropologist, an odontologist, and a radiologist. Several names came to mind: Clyde Snow, for one. And Lowell Levine, the forensic odontologist. And a Chicago-based radiologist by the name of John Fitzpatrick. But pulling that sort of team together, Lukash said, would take some time. D'Amato understood; in the meantime, he'd work on getting clearances for the team through the Justice Department.

Lukash hung up the phone and leaned back in his chair. It sounded like a hoax to him. In his thirty-five years as a forensic pathologist, with a caseload of a thousand or more autopsies a year, he'd seen his share of false starts. Many of them led nowhere and eventually ended up in the "unresolved" file. Most of the successes, he knew, came about only because the best forensic scientists with the right combination of skills and experience had worked together. He reached for the phone and dialed Snow's number in Norman, Oklahoma.

"Why not?" Snow chuckled when he heard Lukash's proposition. "I haven't even unpacked my bags from a trip to Argentina, and Jerry says she'll be damned if she's gonna do it. . . . Yeah, it sounds good to me." Next, Lukash called Fitzpatrick, who was one of the finest forensic radiologists in the world. Fitzpatrick said he would have to check with his boss, but in principle he'd go. The rest of the afternoon, Lukash left a trail of telephone messages around the country for Lowell Levine, the dentist who had assisted the Nassau Medical Examiner's Office for the past fifteen years. Levine, as it turned out, was on active duty with the Naval Reserve in New Orleans. Several days would pass before he finally returned Lukash's call.

At six o'clock that night in Norman, Oklahoma, Snow turned on the evening news, slid into his leather armchair, and kicked off his boots. The lead story took the American viewer to the hillside cemetery in Brazil. The screen showed several policemen and onlookers milling about. A man, identified as a Brazilian scientist, stood next to a grave with something raised above his head. Snow leaned forward to get a better look. The screen flickered and a broken skull came into focus. "Christ," he muttered to himself, "they're making a goddamn carnival show out of this."

Lukash watched the same footage. He never forgot his first impression of the exhumation. "They exhumed that skeleton like a bunch of Keystone cops. The only thing they didn't do was serve drinks and hamburgers."

The following day, Snow drove to Oklahoma City and to the newsroom of KOCO, ABC television's affiliate station in Oklahoma City. A technician clipped a tiny microphone onto Snow's lapel and pointed to the monitor screen where in a few moments *Nightline* anchorman Charles Gibson would materialize to start the interview with the famous forensic anthropologist.

What worried Snow was the condition of the skeleton. Policemen, untrained in forensic techniques, had manhandled the bones. That kind of unprofessional hatchet job could ruin the investigation before it started. When Gibson began the interview, Snow, usually circumspect with the press, vented his feelings.

"Having a policeman dig up a skeleton is a little bit like having a chimpanzee do a heart transplant in this case," he told Gibson. "Skeletal remains are extremely fragile. As I indicated before, small items, such as teeth, bullets, other personal effects, which could be helpful in identification, do tend to get lost. And what you need to use is the same sort of painstaking, methodical technique that archaeologists have used for a hundred years in excavating prehistoric remains."[18]

Snow was right, of course. Only forensic scientists could determine if the Brazilian discovery was a hoax. And even they could be fooled, as the Uruguayan misadventure had shown just two months earlier. The Israelis were especially suspicious. When Israel's chief Nazi-hunter, Menachem Russek, heard of the Brazilian discovery he flatly dismissed it as another subterfuge carefully crafted by Mengele's family to divert the world's attention from his real hideaway in Paraguay. "He must be feeling himself cornered now," Russek commented. "He knows the American, German, and Israeli police are cooperating and the circle around him is closing."[19]

Back in Washington, officials at the Justice Department were dithering about whether or not to send a team of forensic scientists to examine the Embú skeleton. "Things just got a little mixed up," an OSI official said later. "Tensions between the OSI and the U.S. Marshals Service were high."[20] OSI wanted to lead the investigation, but the marshals flexed some muscle, claiming they owned the foreign rights in the Mengele chase. The marshals prevailed. "I don't know why," the OSI official said, "but the marshals ruled out Snow. Maybe what he said on *Nightline* had something to do with it, but I'm not sure." The marshals turned down Lukash and Fitzpatrick as well. Finally, on June 10, the Department of Justice asked Lowell Levine, an officer in the Naval Reserve, to represent the U.S. government in the case.

Although he had already been asked to join the group being assembled by Senator d'Amato's office, Levine decided to sign up with the Justice Department. "I had marching orders from the Attorney General," recalled Levine. "He wanted to know whether it was Mengele, or whether you couldn't tell one way or another, you know. That's all they cared about. . . . What went through my mind was, 'This has gotta be the biggest bunch of bullshit that ever existed. . . . [But] you know, I always wanted to go to Brazil.' "[21]

The Justice Department signed on two more scientists: Ellis Kerley, the forensic anthropologist who had misidentified White and Lachman's photos; and Ali Hameli, a forensic pathologist and chief medical examiner for the state of Delaware. The Department also retained three document examiners: David Crown, a retired CIA examiner of questioned documents; Antonio Cantu, a paper and ink specialist with the FBI; and Gideon Epstein, an examiner of questioned documents with the U.S. Immigration and Naturalization Service.

Senator d'Amato was dumbfounded when he learned that his list of scientists had been rejected. "Things were pretty hectic at our office," Hardiman recalls. "The senator works that way. He orders all his troops toward a goal. He wanted the best scientists, the very best team. Then he's snubbed. So we dug in our heels." Hardiman called Rabbi Marvin Hier, dean of the Simon Wiesenthal Center, and explained the situation. Hier agreed to send Snow, Lukash, and Fitzpatrick as a separate team representing the center.

The West Germans were also assembling a forensic team. Prosecutor Hans Klein arranged for two of his country's top forensic specialists to join the investigation. One was Rolf Endris, a forensic odontologist from Mainz. The other was Richard Helmer. A quiet, introspective forensic anthropologist from the University of Kiel, Helmer had a very special talent — he was the master of the video technique known as skull-face superimposition. At the time, no one could have predicted that this unassuming professor would hold the key to the world's most famous forensic investigation.

Ralph Blumenthal stood on a street corner in the heart of São Paulo, his eyes fixed on the backs of the two Americans crossing the street in front of him. Sweat streaked down his neck, largely due to his habit of wearing a tweed jacket and tie even in tropical Brazil. It was rush hour and cars and trucks sped past in a blur. A bus pulled up to the curb, momentarily blocking his view. When it finally moved, the reporter could see the two men had already made it to the steps of the headquarters of the federal police. Dashing across the street, he followed the men into the ash-gray building.

Blumenthal had finally succumbed to the lure of the story in Brazil and flown to São Paulo to cover it firsthand. Since his arrival the week before, he had spent most of his time roaming the hills around Embú. He had interviewed the Bosserts and many of Mengele's neighbors. He also learned that two American handwriting analysts, David Crown and Gideon Epstein, were in the city and working out of a room Tuma had set aside for them at the police station.

Blumenthal caught up with the two Americans just as they were entering their office. Crown and Epstein told the reporter that they were on assignment from the Justice Department to check handwriting samples, said by the Bosserts to be Mengele's, against documents the young Nazi doctor had written in Germany during World War II. Crown then took Blumenthal aside and said, "You know, we can't say anything yet, it's not official," he told the reporter, "but I think we've decided that it's authentic."[22]

The following day, June 14, the two Americans announced their findings at a press conference. Crown later wrote of the investigation:

> One subject overshadowing this case was the recent debacle of the forged Hitler Diaries. While the exact circumstances involved in that case are not specifically known, the outcome of the case was obviously a warning to all forensic scientists. It is easy to get involved in a case where allegedly misrepresentations regarding evidence are made and where there is pressure to reach a premature conclusion.[23]

Crown and Epstein told the press that they had independently examined fourteen documents discovered by the Brazilian police in several houses where the Bosserts said Mengele had lived for more than fifteen years. The documents ranged from several slips of paper to a set of thirteen pages of notes beginning with the date January 1, 1976. For comparison with the Brazilian documents, the scientists were given Mengele's original SS file, obtained from the Berlin Documentation Center, the central repository of Nazi war documents in West Germany. It contained biographical statements written by the Nazi doctor. At the time the German documents were written, Mengele was twenty-eight years old and, according to Crown, "had reached writing maturity." The scientists postulated that his handwriting would not have changed over the years "unless illness, drugs, or other such situations affected his writing."

The scientists determined that the fourteen Brazilian documents showed none of the classical signs of forgery such as hesitation marks, extra-movement impulses, or patch marks. As for the documents' contents, Crown said that they "seemed to be the personal musings of a ticket-of-leave man living on the fringes of society, scared that Israeli agents could show up at any time." One was a meandering and semiautobiographical essay called, in Latin, "Fait Lux," or "Let There Be Light." Another essay, also in Latin, "Verbum Compositum," or "Collected Word," was a somewhat featherbrained discourse on evolution.

More than twenty-five points of individuality matched in the Brazilian and German samples. The experts noted "agreements of individuality" such as "an extra dash near the top of the staff of the capital 'D,' the arcaded movement in the intermediate 'e' and 'o,' and the extra downward impulse in the eyelet of the initial 'e.' "[24] Twelve of the Brazilian documents, they said, had been written by the hand of Josef Mengele. "All we're saying," Epstein cautioned, "is that Mengele made the handwriting — what can be drawn from that as far as who the body is — that will have to be done by the pathologists and odontologists and other people who've arrived here. . . . "[25]

On June 14 a Delta airliner carrying Clyde Snow taxied away from a boarding ramp at the Oklahoma City International Airport. In a window seat in the smoking section, Snow slipped his pen from his shirt pocket and clipped it to the seat pouch in front of his knees. He had seen enough autopsy reports at the FAA to know that a sudden halt would catapult him into the seat in front of him and transform an innocuous ballpoint into an ice pick aimed at the heart. His forehead pressed against the window, Snow watched the last rays of sunlight slip behind the horizon. To the south, dark anvil clouds blotted out the sky.

Snow had recently heard about Kerley's blunder with the Uruguayan photographs. He respected Kerley, but his old friend should have known better. Although photo comparison had its merits, it was more of an art than an exact science. And now Kerley was in São Paulo. If the press made the connection, they could really go to town.

As soon as the No Smoking sign flicked off, Snow fished a Camel out of his jacket pocket. He shifted in his seat and looked down the aisle to the row where Lukash was sitting. Now, there's another problem, he thought. Earlier in the week Lukash had called Snow to complain about how Levine had betrayed him by switching to the Justice team at the last minute. Levine's move, at least in Lukash's eyes, was much more than just a professional snub. Snow knew that Lukash had nurtured Levine and regarded him as a protégé. He hoped the two of them would bury their hatchets. He wanted everybody together inside the tent pissing out, as the saying went, rather than having someone on the outside pissing in.

When Snow and his colleagues landed in Miami to change planes, a swarm of photographers and journalists intercepted them in the transit lounge. Hoax or not, the media was playing the Brazilian story like a bass drum. "How can we say what our thoughts are about the case when we haven't even seen the bones?" Snow shot back at one persistent reporter. Back in flight, the anthropologist couldn't sleep. Drinking shots of whiskey and smoking, he quelled his growing apprehension about the whole affair by sketching out a step-by-step plan for conducting the investigation based on the team approach he had learned to use in aircraft disasters. The diversion worked until the plane landed in São Paulo, where another mob of reporters swept after Snow and his teammates.

Police cleared a path through the thicket of microphones and shouting journalists and hurried Snow, Lukash, and Fitzpatrick into an old makeshift limousine. As they pulled away, Snow mopped his brow with a white handkerchief and looked around the car. It seemed oddly familiar. He tapped the driver on the shoulder and asked in broken Spanish, hoping it sounded enough like Portuguese to be understood, "So, amigo, digame, es una Chevy?"

"Why, yes, sir, it is," the man replied in perfect English. "It belonged to my father."

Snow smiled, remembering that his father bought only Chevys. Well, he thought, at least something down here was done right.

With over six million inhabitants, São Paulo is the most populous city in South America and the continent's leading industrial center. Until the 1880s, it was a sleepy, shabby little town of thirty thousand people. Now it is three times the size of Paris, sparkling with new skyscrapers and flowering parks and roaring with a febrile energy. Industrial districts spread and engulf villages and townships one after the other. From the port of Santos, forty kilometers to the south, cotton, sugar, fruit, machinery parts, and electrical supplies leave for cities around the world. To the thousands of Brazilians who come here looking for work, the city promises large rewards to the ambitious and industrious. But it is also a city of *favelas*, shantytowns of cardboard and wood that grow like crooked mushrooms in the canyons of concrete and steel.

While his companions drowsed in the backseat, Snow gazed out of the open window at the passing show. In the wide doorway of a shop, boys in sweat-stained T-shirts twisted hot glass for neon tubing into large letters. A few blocks farther on, two bare-chested boys played on a dirt lot by an old church, performing the half-dance, half-combat of *capoeira*. Laughing and hooting, they slapped the ground, sending tiny clouds of red dust into the air. The car passed parks ringed with tall, thick-trunked palms in whose shade stood stalls displaying paintings in bright, tropical colors and bolts of crimson weavings. On either side of the road, new skyscrapers loomed, while at their curbed feet, well-dressed business people and beggars shared the sidewalks.

The Chevy careened up the drive of the São Paulo Hilton. Snow suspected this was the right place as soon as he spied the journalists milling around the front door. "Oh, my God, look at this," the driver said as soon as the pack rushed toward the car. As microphones snaked through the open windows, the group leapt from the car and bolted for the hotel door, leaving the driver to bring their bags. "Well, fellahs," Snow called to his colleagues as the crowd parted before them, "welcome to the Barnum and Bailey sideshow."

That afternoon the Chevy returned to the hotel to collect the three scientists and take them to the Medico-Legal Institute, where the bones had been taken after the exhumation. The institute was housed in the city morgue, a short drive from the hotel. A drab, postcolonial slab of cement, it sat like a cast-off shoebox next to São Paulo's largest hospital. Clerks waited nervously for the scientists at the institute's entrance. They ushered the scientists into an anteroom where a handsome, bearded man in his late thirties introduced himself as Daniel Muñoz, an anthropologist. "Yes, Doctor Snow, I have read your work," he said with a broad smile. "I look forward to working with you." Muñoz led Snow, Lukash, and Fitzpatrick up a flight of stairs and into a large meeting room.

The Wiesenthal team was the last to arrive. Snow caught sight of Levine and Kerley on the far side of the room, next to a row of bookcases containing musty textbooks and jars of autopsy specimens. They were deep in conversation with three Brazilian scientists who, like Muñoz, wore white lab coats. A round of introductions was made, followed by polite conversation and several cups of inky Brazilian coffee, served in cups barely larger than eggshells and laced with dollops of sugar.

This was all very civilized, Snow thought, but when do we get to see the bones? Something else bothered him as well. It was time to have a word with the Brazilian scientist, Dr. de Mello, the fellow who was present when the police dug up the bones at Embú. With the forensic pathologist from the Justice team, Iranian-born Ali Hameli, Snow circled the room until he found the Brazilian.

"Dr. dah Mella, I'm Clyde Snow," the Texan said, his drawl transforming the Portuguese vowels into a Lone Star slur. "How about you and me having a little talk." Snow reckoned if there was going to be any breast-beating about his comments on *Nightline*, they might as well come now. But de Mello smiled diplomatically, waiting for Snow to speak.

"Doctor, I think it might be a good idea to go back to that grave and have another look around," Snow said. "I've done a few exhumations in my time and, uh . . . I think we might find a thing or two in there that got left, er, may not have shown up before." De Mello nodded but promised nothing, as if he had expected the suggestion. In fact, the day before, the Justice Department team had given him the same piece of advice.

Having delivered his message as politely as he knew how, Snow rejoined his colleagues. The politicking had begun in earnest. In a corner by a curtained window, a U.S. marshal was quietly but intently conferring with a Frankfurt policeman and a short, gray-haired man who turned out to be Menachem Russek, head of Israel's Nazi crime section. Russek was mysterious to the point of furtiveness; he was changing hotel rooms almost daily, presumably to avoid being kidnapped. Only the West German anthropologist, Richard Helmer, stood alone. Shy and unsure of his English, he peered down at his coffee cup or out the window at the traffic speeding by on the street below.

The collegial atmosphere was abruptly broken by the entrance of Romeu Tuma, the stocky, fifty-three-year-old lawyer of Syrian extraction who ruled São Paulo's police force. Tuma radiated confidence, buoyed no doubt by the ever-present entourage of detectives at his side. Tuma was something of a Nazi-hunter himself, having captured Gustav Franz Wagner, the "Hangman" of the Sobibor concentration camp, in 1978. Tuma was known in Brazil as a different kind of policeman. He traveled unarmed and neither smoked nor drank. During the years of military dictatorship Tuma's job was to infiltrate student and labor groups. But while some of his fellow officers abducted and tortured opposition figures, Tuma claimed that he personally rejected such techniques as immoral and unprofessional.

Tuma cleared his throat and asked his guests to take their seats around the large table in the center of the high-ceilinged room. "I feel at ease with all of you experts around me," he said, spreading his arms expansively.[26] Snow suspected otherwise. He knew what Tuma knew: these scientists could very well announce that the police chief had botched the exhumation so badly that they were unable to make an identification.

"According to several witnesses," Tuma continued, "the body exhumed in Embú should be Josef Mengele." But, he quickly added, "It's up to you, as scientists, to make the final determination." All he asked of them was that they refrain from leaking information to the press.

Following Tuma, Dr. Wilmes Roberto Teixeira, seasoned medical examiner and official keeper of the bones in contention, gave a brief account of the preparation of the skeleton. In his mid-fifties, Teixeira was a short, pale man, with straight white hair that he kept neatly combed. He spoke fluent English and, as the American experts would soon learn, enjoyed playing the role of the officious shepherd.

"Our investigation will be the classical European way," he said. "This is considered an autopsy. The Brazilian scientists will sign the final report, but we need your endorsement." He went on to describe what sounded to Snow like a piecemeal approach to the examination of the bones.

"Every morning," Teixeira explained, "we'll begin by studying a different feature on the skeleton: first sex, then race, then stature, and so on. Each team — the Germans, Justice, the Wiesenthal people — will make their own examination and come to a conclusion separately. Then we'll compare notes at the end of the day." With that, he rose abruptly from the table. "That will be all for today, gentlemen."

That's it? Snow thought. What about the skeleton? What are they waiting for? As he and the others filed out of the room, Snow stifled the urge to demand a timetable for examining the skeleton. He'd already bruised enough Brazilian egos on *Nightline*, and decided to keep quiet for the moment. But he didn't like the looks of this.

That night the Wiesenthal team sat in Snow's hotel room, on edge. The Brazilians, they agreed, were acting cagey. Were they holding something back? There was so much at stake here, not least of which was their reputations. They felt the uneasiness that comes with being in a place where one doesn't speak the language. And as leaders in their fields, they were unused to taking directions from strangers, especially people about whom they knew almost nothing.

"If I knew this guy Teixeira," Lukash said, a cigar butt smoldering at the corner of his mouth, "I would say, 'Lay everything out on the table.'"

"I think it's time that we did," Snow replied. Lighting another Camel from a new pack, he chose his words carefully. "We can't be party to any dissembling of information."

"Oh, I know it!" said Lukash.

"If we see any evidence of dissembling here," Snow continued, tapping the marble coffee table for punctuation, "and if the forensic science material is not on the up and up, and this includes whether there is a complete skeleton, then we can just pack our bags and leave Brazil and make them call a press conference. We'll say, 'Unh-unh, we don't want to play this game with these folks,' and we could be out of here tomorrow. You agree with that, Fitz?"

Fitzpatrick, who was nervously watching ashes fall from his friend's cigarette and roll down his trouser leg, looked up and replied, "Right, Clyde, but, uh . . . would you put that damn cigarette out before you set all of us on fire?"

Early the next morning, Sunday, June 16, a car pulled out of the drive at the Medico-Legal Institute and headed out of the city. Inside were José de Mello and a morgue worker. The scientist gave the driver directions to Embú, and then to Our Lady of the Rosary cemetery. When they reached the cemetery, the two men climbed out of the car and made their way up a hill lined with white marble tombstones to an open grave strewn with candles and fresh flowers. The morgue worker eased himself into the grave and offered his hand to de Mello. Once he was in the hole, de Mello took a trowel from his satchel, knelt down, and began turning over the loose soil. He found a tooth. He sifted some more and uncovered several small finger bones. Then he heard voices.

He stood up and looked over the edge of the grave. "Mierda," he said under his breath.

Coming up the hill was a television crew, followed by the two West German scientists. With nothing to do that day, Helmer and Endris had decided to drive out to the cemetery. As for the TV reporters, they had somehow heard about the second exhumation and trailed after the Brazilians to record it.

The gravesite now bustled with activity. The newsmen switched on their cameras and recorded de Mello being helped out of the grave by the two Germans. The Brazilian looked sheepishly away from the camera, handed a small plastic bag with the new finds to his assistant, and trundled down the hill.

While de Mello was performing his hasty second exhumation, Snow and Levine met in Levine's room at the Maksoud Plaza Hotel to go over the documents the two American teams had brought. Kerley, a tall, reserved man in his sixties with a patrician bearing, had joined them there. Levine pulled several manila envelopes from his briefcase and laid them out on a coffee table in front of the two anthropologists. "The Justice Department got a hold of these," he explained. "They're Mengele's SS records from the Berlin Documentation Center."

One document was the record of Mengele's 1938 SS physical examination. Another consisted of a series of questionnaires the young Nazi doctor had answered in his own hand and submitted to the *Rasse- und Siedlungshauptampt*, the Central Office for Race and Resettlement, between 1938 and 1939.[27]

One of the questionnaires concerned a lanky, good-looking blond named Irene Schoenbein. Mengele wanted to marry her before he was sent to the Russian front, but since he was an SS officer the two of them were required to undergo a "racial purity check" first. They submitted the necessary forms and the paperwork wound its way through the bureaucracy without a hitch until a senior SS officer raised doubts about Irene's grandfather, who was thought to be the illegitimate son of a Jew. Although Mengele was unable to prove that there was absolutely no trace of Jewish blood in Irene's family, he did produce glowing character references from Irene's friends, emphasizing her "very Nordic ways."[28] In March 1939 the race and resettlement office declared Irene racially pure. Four months later, Mengele slipped a ring on her finger.

These early SS files were the forensic team's Rosetta stone. They contained the physical description of Mengele that they would have to compare with the Embú skeleton. The medical report described Mengele as a white male, 174 centimeters tall, with a head circumference of 57 centimeters. His dental chart, a drawing of the teeth, showed that twelve of them had fillings. But it failed to note the type of fillings or their exact location on the teeth. The chart also made no mention of Mengele's gap-toothed smile. By forensic standards, Snow thought, it was hardly a gold mine.

Snow leafed through Mengele's genealogy and racial-fitness report until he found the Nazi doctor's early medical history. According to the report, Mengele had undergone an operation to repair a right inguinal hernia at the age of thirteen. He had also suffered from nephritis, an inflammation of the kidneys, between 1926 and 1927, and he withdrew from the *Sturmabteilung*, or the Brownshirts, Hitler's bullyboy storm troopers, in 1934 because of the ailment.

The hernia operation and the vague diagnosis of renal disease were tantalizing clues but of little help now, as they left no signature on bone. What caught Snow's attention was an entry on the next page: Mengele had contracted a rare inflammatory bone disease known as septic osteomyelitis when he was fifteen years old.

Snow marked his spot with a finger and looked up at Levine, who was rummaging in his briefcase again. Levine pulled out a memorandum he had received earlier in the week from David Marwell, an historian with the Justice Department's Office of Special Investigations, and handed it to Snow, who read it aloud:

> We received news this morning that might be helpful in identifying the recently located remains in São Paulo. A former medical school colleague of Mengele's related the following: He was dining with Mengele in a Munich restaurant before the war, and Mengele commented on his vegetarian diet. . . .
>
> According to this source, Mengele had an osteomyelitis in his leg. Associated with this osteomyelitis was a sequestrum,

which is apparently a piece of bone that has broken away from the site of the infection in the bone. An operation (sequestration) was performed to remove the sequestrum, a procedure designed to aid the healing of the bone. According to medical authorities whom I consulted this morning, the osteomyelitis and the resultant sequestration would leave evidence on the skeletal remains. According to the source, the osteomyelitis was on the tibia and probably resulted in an asymmetry of the legs. It is not clear whether this asymmetry would have led to a limp. The source was not clear on which leg the osteomyelitis occurred, but pointed to his own right leg when explaining the condition. . . . The best evidence for locating and evaluating the possible evidence of the osteomyelitis would be X-rays of the bones in question.[29]

Snow exchanged a knowing glance with Kerley, who, as a fellow anthropologist, was aware of exactly how valuable this lead could be.

By definition, osteomyelitis is an infection of the bone cortex and marrow that may stimulate excessive growth in the affected bone.[30] *Staphylococcus aureus*, a pyogenic, or pus-producing, microorganism is by far the most common cause and can reach the bone via fractures or surgical wounds to the skeleton. Other routes include infected soft tissue adjacent to the bone and blood-borne bacteria distributed throughout the body that can settle in the bone. Once bacteria reaches the marrow an abscess forms and then expands, compressing the surrounding bone. Eventually the blood in the vessels adjacent to the bone coagulates and the bone dies. The dead bone, or sequestrum, is resorbed and replaced or surrounded by new bone. Today doctors treat osteomyelitis by surgically removing the dead or infected bone and treating the infection with antibiotics. If left untreated the infection can recur repeatedly over a lifetime.

Snow and Kerley rarely encountered modern skeletons with signs of osteomyelitis. Before the availability of antibiotics in the 1940s, however, the ailment was common, particularly among children and adolescents who contracted diseases such as typhoid, tuberculosis, syphilis, or sickle-cell anemia. In the middle-aged it was often associated with urinary bladder infection. Osteomyelitis also infected soldiers wounded in battle. Kerley had found evidence of the disease in many of the more than three thousand bone specimens he examined during his nine years at the Armed Forces Institute of Pathology in Washington.[31]

The scientists weighed the merits of the osteomyelitis evidence. Anecdotal reports suggested that some sign of the disease, especially if it had been chronic, should appear on the bones. Then again, they had no X rays or detailed clinical descriptions of the location and severity of the disease to guide them in their examination of the Embú remains. Also, how reliable was Mengele's own recollection of the disease? The fact that he was a physican was not particularly significant, as the condition had reportedly occurred long before he had any medical training. Even assuming he had had osteomyelitis, how likely was it that its marks would remain on a sixty-nine-year-old skeleton? Bones, unlike teeth, are dynamic tissues, capable of remodeling themselves over time. If the osteomyelitis that supposedly struck Mengele at age fifteen had been mild, and if Mengele had stayed relatively healthy during his life, there was a good possibility that time had eroded its intaglio from the bone.

On Monday morning, June 17, the foreign experts gathered again in the meeting room at the Medico-Legal Institute. Morgue workers served them coffee as they milled about swapping stories of past cases and speculating on the delay in seeing the bones. Snow looked at his watch once again. It was already ten o'clock and there was still no sign of Teixeira, although several of his compatriots had trickled in and were mingling with their foreign colleagues.

Finally Teixeira arrived. The room fell silent in nervous expectation.

"Good morning, gentlemen," the Brazilian said. He was far sunnier in disposition than he'd been the day before. Snow suspected they were going to get an exercise in Latin hospitality for the rest of the morning. His American companions, he could see, sat somewhat grim-faced, determined not to allow the morning escape without getting what they wanted: the bones.

"Now," Teixeira said, "if you'll follow me, we'll have a look at the skeleton."

He led the scientists up a flight of stairs. They trooped silently down a corridor past several small laboratory rooms, each marked with the name of the team assigned to it. Teixeira stopped at the door at the end of the hall and reached in his pocket for the key.

"Onde esta a chave?" he asked a colleague.

"Eu, não sei," the man replied, his palms uplifted. Feet shuffled, eyes focused on the floor. The Brazilians checked their pockets. One of them finally found the key and handed it to Teixeira, the sunniness now absent from his face. He hurriedly unlocked the door and stood back as the scientists went in.

The room was bare except for a sofa and two tables. Sheer white curtains billowed inward from the tall, open windows. The morning sunshine cast a soft yellow light on the set of human bones laid out, in rough anatomical order, on the larger of the two tables.

The scientists crowded around the table, hesitant at first to touch anything. The anthropologists moved first, edging their way around the table as they counted the tawny specimens. Snow and Kerley discretely moved phalanges — finger and toe bones — into their proper places without mentioning that the Brazilians had positioned them incorrectly.

The skull, perhaps the most critical piece of evidence, lay in pieces. Helmer shook his head when he saw its wretched condition. He lifted the cranium from the table and turned it gently in his hands. At least that piece had escaped the gravedigger's spade. Setting it down, he picked up several brittle pieces of nasal bone, some crushed to the size of pumpkin seeds, and cradled them in his palm. It was a mess.

Lukash and Hameli, the two pathologists, stood on either side of Helmer staring at the fragments in his hand as if they were reading tea leaves. "Dr. Helmer," Lukash finally asked, "do you think you can reconstruct it?"

"It?"

"The skull."

"Oh . . . certainly. Yes, I can do it."

He could, but it would be like assembling a holographic jigsaw puzzle.

9

———

NO BONE UNTURNED

FINALLY at work, the scientists lost track of time, pausing only occasionally to sip coffee and compare notes. Outside, trucks sounded their horns and ground their gears as they sped past on the city's main thoroughfare. Every half hour or so an ambulance pulled through the institute's front gate and honked for attention. Morgue workers appeared, shouting greetings as they opened the ambulance's back doors, pulled a gurney onto the drive, and pushed it into the dimly lit morgue. By midday, the building's dead outnumbered its living.

In the examining room above the morgue, most of the foreign experts and their Brazilian colleagues had already scotched Teixeira's soccer-team approach to the investigation and divided themselves up by discipline. Only the West Germans stayed together.

Helmer commandeered the room next door. He then descended to the main entrance, where a large plastic crate, festooned with Lufthansa stickers, had been delivered earlier in the morning. With the help of a morgue worker, he lugged it up the stairs to his room and closed the door behind him.

Meanwhile, the other anthropologists — Snow, Kerley, and the Brazilian Daniel Muñoz — took the cranium, pelvic bones, and two of the long bones from the table to the room assigned to the Wiesenthal team. They sat on rickety wooden stools and spread the bones out on a white Formica counter. Snow snubbed out a cigarette on the

176

tiled floor and picked up the cranium. He turned it so the others could see the mastoid processes, the two protrusions of the temporal bones that can be felt directly behind the ear. "I'd say they're big enough to be a male's," Snow said. Kerley leaned forward, pushing his glasses back to the bridge of his nose. "I agree," he replied. Muñoz nodded. Snow tilted the skull back slightly to look at the nucal crest, the ridge at the nape of the neck. "That's too well-developed to be female," he said. Kerley noted the finding on the worksheet. Snow turned to the skull's face. The supraorbital, or brow ridge, was large and prominent, another masculine feature.

They moved on to the two innominate, or hip, bones. These, along with the sacrum and coccyx, make up the pelvis. During puberty, the shape of the pelvis begins to take on distinctly male or female features. To the trained eye these traits provide the most reliable clues for morphologically, or visually, sexing a skeleton. For example, the mature male pelvis is usually more robust, with well-marked muscular impressions. The female's pubic opening is broader, while the bone may feel noticeably lighter. When normally aligned, the hip bones look something like the wings of a swallowtail butterfly that have bowed inward and joined at the bottom tips. At the point where the two bones meet lies the small, cork-shaped pubic symphysis, which separates the ends of the two bones. The lower end of this joint is narrower in males than it is in females.

The overall shape of the innominates and the pubic symphysis looked like a male's. Turning one of the hip bones over, Muñoz followed the contour of the edge of the bone to find the sciatic notch, about as wide as a twenty-five-cent piece. It was comparatively narrow and deep, again a distinctly male trait. He also examined the acetabulum, the socket in the hip bone that receives the head of the femur. Its diameter was wide and its borders well developed. Again, male traits.

Another, though less consistent, method for sexing a skeleton involves measuring the vertical diameter of the heads of the humerus and femur. The pioneering forensic scientist Thomas Dwight (introduced in Chapter 2) discovered this sexual dimorphism after examining four hundred male and female skeletons in the early 1900s.[1] Dwight found that femoral heads exceeding forty-five millimeters in diameter usually belong to adult males, while those less than forty-two millimeters usually come from females. (Those in between may belong to either sex.)

Kerley applied the calipers to the femoral head. "Fifty-five millimeters," he dictated to Snow. Repeating the process on the humerus, he measured fifty-two millimeters. Both values, Snow noted on the worksheet, were well above Dwight's upper limits for white females.

The anthropologists, in less than an hour's time, were certain that the skeleton belonged to a male. And he had been right-handed: the long bones on the right side were markedly longer than those on the left.

After sex and handedness came race. The intact part of the skull was narrow and small-browed, strongly suggesting that the bones belonged to a Caucasoid. To verify this the anthropologists would have to wait until Helmer patched the facial bones back together. Then they could measure several points on the skull to confirm what their experienced eyes already suspected.

The next task was to determine if the remains of this white, right-handed male could be those of Wolfgang Gerhard, the man who the Bosserts first told Brazilian authorities they had buried in 1979.

The anthropologists knew of two characteristics that would distinguish Mengele from Gerhard — age and stature. Judging from the bone loss around the teeth and the abrasion on them, this skeleton appeared to belong to a man between sixty and seventy years old. Though the range was broad, it seemed to rule out Gerhard, who in 1979 would have been in his fifties. Stature, however, gave the scientists their first strong clue that maybe this time the discovery of Josef Mengele was not a hoax. The Bosserts had called Gerhard "Langer," the equivalent of the American nickname "Stretch." In fact, he was nearly fifteen centimeters taller than Mengele.

Snow and Kerley set about measuring the femur and tibia of the skeleton. Snow placed the femur on an osteometric board and slid the block against the end of the bone. "Forty-nine point one centimeters," he said. Snow repeated the process with the humerus, which measured 35.7 centimeters. Kerley added the measurements and applied them to a regression equation.

"Clyde, check in my notebook to see what Gerhard's stature is," he said.

178

Snow flicked to a page marked "Wolfgang Gerhard" and ran his finger down it until he found a figure circled in red ink. "One hundred and eighty-eight centimeters," he said.

"Now, turn the page over. What does it give for Mengele?"

"One hundred and seventy-four centimeters."

Kerley, his dark eyebrows rising, looked at Snow and Muñoz. "Well, at least we're on the right track. This man here was roughly one hundred and seventy-three point five centimeters tall. That rules out Gerhard for sure. And it keeps Mengele in the running."

Two doors down from the anthropologists, in a room fitted with an X-ray viewing screen, Levine switched off the overhead light and pulled up a stool next to Carlos Valerio, a Brazilian dentist in his early fifties with a broad forehead and graying temples. Radiologist John Fitzpatrick and the institute's chief radiologist, Luis Donato, a large, bespectacled man in his late thirties, stood behind them with their arms folded. Valerio switched on the X-ray panel, bathing the room and the men's faces in a phosphorescent glow.

Valerio and Levine had examined the ten teeth found in the grave with the skull and compared them to Mengele's 1938 SS dental chart. Nothing, as far as they could find, was inconsistent. Valerio slipped an X ray of the skeleton's upper jaw onto the screen and asked the Americans what they thought. Levine stroked his bushy black mustache and chuckled. "Okay, Fitz, this one's for you. Tell us what you see. What's odd in this X ray?"

Fitzpatrick drew a pencil from the pocket of his white shirt and leaned across Donato's shoulder. Holding the pencil tip a hairbreadth away from the screen, he traced the white line that bisected the image of the skull's palate. "Well, that's the incisor canal joining the two halves of the upper palate, and it's awfully wide. . . ."

"Which means?"

"Which means . . . this guy must have had a gap-toothed smile."

Levine was already searching at his feet for his briefcase. He pulled it up onto his knees and snapped open the latches. "And here, gentlemen," he said as he laid a large eight-by-ten-inch glossy photograph on the countertop, "is a portrait of Mengele taken when he was twenty-seven years old. Luckily for us, he's smiling. And there's the gap between his front incisors." It was a diastema, an inherited trait in which the left and right halves of the upper palate of the mouth do not come together completely. It is found in 11 percent of the world's population.

That evening the Wiesenthal team found Ralph Blumenthal waiting for them in the bar at the São Paulo Hilton. The reporter introduced himself to Snow and his colleagues and invited them to sit at his table. The encounter began awkwardly. Lukash told Blumenthal that if he wanted details about the investigation, they'd have to set some ground rules first. Snow, meanwhile, ordered a round of *caipirinhas*, a potent mixture of lime and *cachaca*, or sugarcane rum.

He and his colleagues, Lukash said, would answer questions only on the condition that whatever they said could not be published until after the results of the investigation had been announced. Blumenthal agreed and wasted no time getting down to basics. "When would that be?" he asked as he slipped a spiral notebook from his jacket pocket.

"Hard to say," Lukash replied. "For all we know we could be here another month. As Clyde can tell you, the skeleton's a male and its stature, age, handedness, and race are consistent with Mengele's SS records. But that's not enough to go on."

"So it isn't Wolfgang Gerhard?" Blumenthal asked.

"Definitely not. Age and stature rule him out. . . ."

"Besides," Snow interjected, "the Austrian government turned up Gerhard's death certificate. He died of a cerebral hemorrhage in Austria in 1978."

Blumenthal looked up from his notebook. "Look, as I'm sure you know, there are a lot of people who have serious doubts about the Bosserts' story. I spent the day with Tuma and he brought in a Brazilian dentist by the name of María Elena Viera de Castro. She claims she treated Mengele in her clinic in March or April 1979, a month or two after the Bosserts say he died. Also, Tuma says the Mossad now claims it has a 1980 photo of Mengele driving a Mercedes in Asúncion."

Up until then Fitzpatrick had listened without comment. He normally ignored the "background noise" — the speculative give-and-take — that accompanies most criminal investigations. He was the original I-won't-believe-it-until-you-show-me type. Like most radiologists who take up forensic work, he rarely visited crime scenes or interviewed relatives of the deceased. His stock-in-trade was hard evidence — the unmistakable images of X rays.

Fitzpatrick tossed back his drink and broke into the conversation. "You know, in the end, we might be able to exclude or identify this skeleton as Mengele within a given range of certainty. But there's one thing that could sure cut this whole thing short and that's an antemortem X ray. If you ask me, everybody ought to spend less time speculating and more effort trying to track one down."

No one could disagree. In the world of forensic anthropology the antemortem X ray is like a fingerprint. Instead of whorls and grooves, the skeleton's uniqueness manifests itself in the anatomical shape and structural components of each bone. Injuries, such as an old wrist fracture, or even the curve in the root of a single tooth, can solve a case as soon as the X ray is mounted on a viewing screen.

"Now somewhere in this city," Fitzpatrick continued, "there should be a set of X rays or at least a dental cast of this guy's teeth. He's got partial dentures, right? And they're fairly new. The bones aren't going to tell us where they are. So Tuma has to get the Bosserts or some of this guy's other associates to fess up."

"Well, I'm not so sure we should just leave this in Tuma's hands," Snow said as the group rose to go to dinner. "I wouldn't mind a crack at the Bosserts myself."

Early the following morning, Tuesday, Teixeira gathered the scientists together in the meeting room at the institute. He had bad news: the West Germans had failed to find any X rays in Mengele's SS records. But, he added optimistically, Tuma would send out an Interpol request for any of Mengele's medical records that might be held by the governments of Argentina or Paraguay.

Fitzpatrick and Donato returned to their X rays of the bones. They had found several healed fractures and signs of arthritis, as might be expected on an aged skeleton. Now they searched the glowing black-and-white montage for signs of osteomyelitis. If Mengele had had the disease, and if it had been chronic, the X rays of the femurs should reveal a thickened cortex and small cavities within the bone. They found nothing.

One of the fractures, however, came with a story. The day before,

Snow and the other anthropologists had discovered a healed break on the right acetabulum that extended well into the pelvis. X rays of the fracture line revealed that it had been caused by an upward thrust of the thigh bone into the socket. And the right femur measured one centimeter shorter than the left one. Exactly how old the fracture was they couldn't say, but they could see that the bone had remodeled itself sufficiently to indicate that the injury had taken place years, and possibly decades, before death.

Was there evidence somewhere suggesting that Mengele had broken a hip?

Several documents in Mengele's SS files pointed to such a conclusion. One stated that during the German invasion of the Ukraine in 1942 Mengele, then a young medical officer, was seriously injured and later decorated with the Black Badge for the Wounded. Unfortunately, the document did not describe the injury.

A German-police court report said Mengele had been "injured" in a traffic accident near Auschwitz. "On 21 June 1943 around 1600 hours," the report read, "[Mengele] drove with the motorcycle SS 16314 from the hospital barracks of the concentration camp Auschwitz, by way of the Officers' residence and the community camp, to the prisoner of war camp in Birkenau." As Mengele turned a corner at the camp entrance, he collided with a tractor and "was thrown onto the railway track at the right side of the road."[2]

Had the motorcycle accident broken the hip? Possibly. But that was as far as the scientists were willing to go. The police report contained neither X rays nor a clinical description of the injury. It didn't even mention the location of the injury and whether Mengele had required treatment. Also, since the accident had taken place in 1943, thirty-six years before his alleged death, sufficient time had passed for Mengele to have suffered other injuries that could be linked to the same fracture. In the end, the scientists concluded that the hip fracture on the skeleton was at least "consistent" with the assumption that Mengele was injured in the motorcycle accident. But it fell far short of actually proving that the Embú skeleton was Josef Mengele.

Another puzzle materialized that morning, one that was to divide anthropologist Snow and odontologist Levine. The point of contention was a pea-sized hole on the left zygoma, or cheekbone. It looked

182

as if a tiny volcano had erupted on the bone and left behind a rust-colored crater.

Levine told the group the hole looked like a fistulous tract, or duct, caused by a tooth infection. He had seen similar ones on patients when he practiced dentistry in New York City. The infection couldn't drain through the tooth, so it channeled its way through the bone to a point where it finally broke out into the adjoining soft tissue.

Snow wasn't convinced. "It's postmortem artefact," he argued. The X rays of the circular rust pattern around the hole, he said, matched X rays of rust-colored stains on the clothing recovered from the grave. Since the body had been buried for six years, water had probably seeped in by corroding the nails and other hardware on the casket. Rusty droplets of water had dripped onto and through any clothing and exposed bone. "Sort of like Chinese water torture," Snow suggested.

It wasn't the first time Levine and Snow had disagreed. They were both confident of their skills and more than a bit headstrong. The origin of the bony defect remained a point of contention. "You see," Levine said later of the disagreement, "I have a big advantage over anthropologists when you talk about disease processes. Because they're only used to looking at bones, they don't really have an understanding of what goes on in life. . . . Those of them that treated living patients thought it was real and those that were anthropologists went to the artifact."[3]

Though the simple identification work — sex, race, and stature determination — had fallen into place easily enough, the scientists weren't much closer to identifying the skeleton. They needed harder, more specific information. They got it from Kerley. Kerley had forged a name for himself twenty years earlier by discovering a method for estimating a skeleton's biological age, or age at death, from various microscopic changes in the cortex of the long bones.[4] Prior to Kerley's technique, age estimates of skeletons over fifty years old at death were based on such criteria as arthritic lipping, the texture and weight of the bones, or the closure of the cranial sutures. Kerley's method took time and a careful eye, but anthropologists considered it to be the most accurate means of aging older skeletons.

Earlier that day, Kerley had taken the skeleton's left femur to the

University of São Paulo's training hospital. In a room set aside for him, he fastened the femur with C-clamps to a counter top. Like a carpenter slicing a dowel into thin wafers, he delicately sawed three cross sections from the bone. Using two different grades of sandpaper, he ground each wafer down to the thickness of one tenth of a millimeter and then placed them on separate slides. He examined two of the cross sections under a microscope, saving the third for study in his laboratory back at the University of Maryland.

Through the lens, he could clearly see blood-carrying canals, or osteons, in the bone's cortex. Magnified one hundred times, the osteons and lamellae, or concentric layers of bone, that surround them look much like the age rings of a tree. The longer a person lives, the more numerous and fragmented the canals. In old age, virtually every complete osteon is surrounded by the fragments of several older ones. Kerley counted the osteons and osteon fragments and applied them to his equation for calculating age. This person, he decided, had lived to be between sixty-four and seventy-four years of age. Splitting the difference, he calculated that the man had died in his late sixties, within a 5 percent margin of error.

If the Bosserts had told the truth, Mengele was a month shy of his sixty-eighth birthday when he drowned in 1979.

At precisely ten o'clock on Wednesday, June 19, Tuma marched into the meeting room at the institute where the scientists had assembled to await him. He motioned to a detective, who carried an open box to the conference table and tipped it over. A jumble of objects spilled onto the lacquered surface: brass buttons, a worn spectacle case, a small piece of green felt, two .45-caliber bullets, a broken picture frame, a teak pencil box, a billfold, and an assortment of pill bottles.

"These, gentlemen," he said, "my men and I discovered in the attic of the house where Mengele lived."

Teixeira, the medical examiner, turned over the boxes and bottles with a pencil, to avoid leaving fingerprints. He translated the labels for his foreign colleagues. "Those are aspirins. And that there is some kind of . . . how do you call it? Heat rubbing for sore muscles."

"Any prescription labels, Doctor Teixeira?" Lukash asked.

"No, none that I can see."

"Well, the man certainly was a pack rat," Lukash observed. "Some of these medicines look as if they've been around for decades."

Snow leaned across the table and pointed to a small black box with gold lettering. Helmer stood next to him, his normally pale cheeks flushed pink.

"Hey, Doctor Helmer, tell 'em what it says on this one," Snow laughed. Helmer looked uncomfortable as all eyes turned toward him. "Well, it's in German," he mumbled. "They're what I think you call . . . condoms."

Teixeira gently pried open a tin box with his pencil and found it filled with barbiturates, some morphine, hemorrhoid suppositories, a syringe, a rusted needle, and a small vial of unidentifed powder. Evidence of a lingering, or at least imagined, virility notwithstanding, the personal effects suggested that the last years of this man's life were burdened with chronic pain.

Tuma announced that he would bring the Bosserts and another witness to the institute for questioning later in the day. Then, with his usual abruptness, he wheeled out the door, leaving a detective behind to collect the dead man's paraphernalia.

It was just after three o'clock when the scientists returned to their seats in the meeting room for the interrogation. Tuma ushered in Gitta Stammer, a petite, hazel-eyed woman in her sixties, followed by a younger woman who, Tuma said, was to be their interpreter. Gitta's hands, bedecked with rings, shook slightly as she fumbled with the latch on her purse. She drew out a cigarette, lit it, and blew a long ribbon of smoke toward the ceiling.

Tuma explained that in the first week of the investigation in São Paulo, he and his detectives interrogated nearly a dozen of Mengele's associates in the area. Besides the Bosserts, the other key witness to emerge was Mrs. Stammer.

According to the history compiled by the Brazilian and German police, Mengele had lived in Argentina and Paraguay before coming to Brazil. Apparently, Mengele had made little attempt to hide his identity after he arrived in Buenos Aires in 1949. He even had a telephone listed in his own name. In 1954 he divorced his wife, Irene, who was still in Germany. Four years later, still using his own name, he married his older brother's widow in Uruguay. Shortly thereafter, Mengele left her and, in 1959, moved to Paraguay, taking shelter with Nazi sympathizers.

In 1960, after Israeli agents in Buenos Aires kidnapped Adolph Eichmann, Mengele suddenly went underground. His pursuers presumed that he was being protected by a Nazi organization such as Odessa or Kameradenwerk. But if Tuma's sources proved correct, anonymity may have been Mengele's best camouflage when he slipped across the border to Brazil in 1961. He soon made the acquaintance of Senhora Stammer and her husband, Geta.[5]

"Senhora Stammer, you may begin," the police chief instructed his charge.

Gitta stubbed out her cigarette, folded her hands in her lap, and began her story. She and Geta first met Mengele in 1961 when her husband's friend, Wolfgang Gerhard, introduced them. Mengele then called himself Peter Hochbichler, claiming he was a Swiss. Gerhard, a former Nazi corporal, told the couple that his friend was looking for temporary work. The Stammers agreed to let Peter manage their small farm in the Austrian and German colony of Nova Europa in Araraquara, about three hundred kilometers northwest of São Paulo. In 1962 the Stammers moved to another farm at Serra Negra, about 160 kilometers closer to the city, and Peter followed.

It was there, Gitta said, that she began to suspect that Peter wasn't the Swiss laborer he claimed to be. She noticed, for instance, that although he never gave an indication that he was a physician, he skillfully treated sick and injured farm animals. And his tastes were unusually sophisticated for a farm laborer — he read philosophy and history and in the evenings enjoyed listening to classical music.

One day Gitta opened the *Folha de São Paulo* newspaper and saw a photograph of Mengele at Auschwitz. The picture showed a young man in his late twenties. The Nazi's face looked familiar. She noticed his smile and the gap between his two front teeth. "He still had his front teeth then," she told her listeners.

Gitta showed her employee the picture and kidded him about the resemblance. "It made him pale," she said, and he fled the room. Later that evening he confessed: "I have been with you for two years, and you have a right to know," he told her. "I am Doctor Mengele."

When the couple confronted Gerhard with Peter's real identity, he told them they were lucky. "You used to be nobodies, unknown," he said. "Now a great thing has happened in your lives."

Mengele remained under the Stammers' protection for the next twelve years. He shunned most personal contacts, making an exception for sex. According to Gitta, Mengele had several affairs with housemaids and local farm girls during those years. "Men are men, you know, even in Hell," she had once told a reporter. "He could not get involved with women of his own station, for fear of detection."

The scientists, who were anxious to obtain medical information, asked Gitta about the gap between Mengele's teeth.

"Yes," Gitta responded, "he had a space on his upper teeth."

"Did he complain of toothaches?" Levine queried.

"Yes, a couple of times, but when he was with us he never went to a dentist."

"Did you ever notice any gold caps on the bottom of his teeth?"

"Yes, in the back but I don't remember which side."

"Did you ever observe a swelling on Mr. Hochbichler's left cheek?" Levine asked as he looked waggishly in Snow's direction.

"Yes, I did. I thought it was a toothache."

"Did it come and go?"

Gitta thought for a moment and replied: "If you mean the swelling, yes, it appeared maybe two or three times in all those years."

Seeing that he was about to be trumped by his friend, Snow broke in and asked if Hochbichler had ever treated the swelling.

"If I remember correctly," Gitta said, "he would take a hot towel and place it over his cheek."

"That's the fistulous tract on the cheekbone. The pus drains in the direction of heat," Levine whispered to Hameli.

"Was there a scar on his face? Even a small one?" Snow asked.

No, she didn't remember that sort of thing.

"Okay. Did he have any scars anywhere else on his body?"

"There was something on his back," she replied, beginning to relax a bit as she realized that the scientists valued her knowledge. She turned in her chair and pointed to the small of her back on the right side. "It was not very big. . . . He said it was something that happened a long, long time ago, in his childhood."

"How do you know he had this scar? Did you see it?" Snow continued.

Gitta blushed when the question was translated. The Brazilian newspapers had already hinted that Gitta and Mengele may have been secret lovers. She had tearfully denied the charge to foreign reporters, despite the discovery of several love poems from Mengele dedicated to the "beautiful" Gitta.

Gitta's voice quavered as she answered. "The only reason I know it is that my son fell down one day and in order to console him [Peter] told him he, too, had fallen and that he had hurt himself. Then he showed the scar. *That's* how I learned about it."

"Mrs. Stammer," Lukash asked politely, "did the man you knew as Mr. Peter Hochbichler ever see a medical doctor when you knew him?"

"Yes, there was one time when he had some trouble. . . ." She stopped and made a comment to the interpreter, who explained, "Uh, she doesn't want to say the area, but it was behind."

Gitta continued, "He did go into a hospital and the doctor made a small incision and removed a little clot or a ball. . . . He said he had swallowed a lot of hairs from his mustache. As I recall, it was the only time he saw a doctor. He had trouble evacuating. He said it was the ball that had caused it."

"Christ," Snow whispered, elbowing Fitzpatrick, "the guy had a hairball, like one of my damn cats in Norman."

"Do you remember which hospital he went to? And when he went?" Lukash asked the woman.

"I didn't go with him. No, I don't know which hospital. I don't remember when exactly. But it must have been one or two years before he left us."

That was the extent of Gitta's recollections. The scientists thanked her and she was led away, to be replaced by Lisolette and Wolfram Bossert.

Brazilian detectives, over the course of the week, had already grilled the couple for more than six hours. Foreign journalists, late off the starting block, were still descending in droves on their suburban home. The strain now showed on the couple's faces. The roughest assault, however, had taken place early that morning. Tuma learned that the Bosserts had sold several of Mengele's notebooks, ones that the police had overlooked, to the German magazine *Stern*. The police chief was furious. He cabled the West German authorities, demanding that they impound the papers, and dispatched his detectives to search the Bosserts' house. Among the items they found there was a reel-to-reel tape of a speech by Adolf Hitler, a Burberry raincoat, and a hat that the couple said had belonged to Mengele.

Lisolette spoke first. Sometime in 1970, Wolfgang Gerhard, an old friend of theirs, introduced them to Peter Hochbichler. The Bosserts became Peter's confidants, sharing his greatest secret. Wolfram even went so far as to help his new friend commit forgery in 1971. That year Gerhard had decided to return to his native Austria. Before his departure he gave Mengele a precious gift — his Brazilian identity card. Wolfram, an amateur photographer, took several passport-size photographs of Mengele, then sliced open the laminated I.D. card and slipped Mengele's photograph over Gerhard's. Meanwhile, Gerhard paid a visit to Our Lady of the Rosary Cemetery, eighteen kilometers west of São Paulo, where he secured a burial plot next to his mother's. He then left for Austria.

Mengele finally left the Stammers' farm in Caieiras in 1975 and eventually moved into a small bungalow, a yellow stucco building the Stammers owned on Alvarenga Road in Eldorado, a suburb of São Paulo. The Alvarenga house was cold comfort to a man whose spirit was withering from loneliness and paranoia. He had developed a host of aches and pains that often kept him in bed. In May 1976 he suffered a stroke and spent several days at the Santa Marta Hospital in nearby Santo Amaro. (When the police searched the hospital's files for medical records and X rays in 1985, however, all they found was an admitting card under the alias Wolfgang Gerhard, the length of stay, the sickness, and the name of the doctor responsible for his treatment.)

In 1976, shortly before the forged identity card's expiration date, Gerhard returned to Brazil, at Mengele's expense, to manufacture a new card. During his stay he visited the cemetery again and told the director, Gino Carita, to prepare for the arrival of a "sickly older relative." Gerhard returned to Austria where he died two years later.

By the mid-1970s relations between the Stammers and Mengele had begun to deteriorate. Mengele had grown crotchety and more authoritarian. He complained about the way the Stammers were raising their children and urged them to be more strict. "He also became moody, and even quick-tempered with our children, whom he adored," Lisolette told the scientists. He occasionally fired farmhands without consulting the Stammers, which infuriated Geta. On one of his cash runs to Brazil, Mengele's old friend Hans Sedlmeier tried to patch things up between them. But diplomacy failed; Geta even bought an apartment in the city just to get away from the old man.

A neighbor on Alvarenga Road told the police that the man he knew as Señor Pedro had a Mauser that he kept by day in a locked box in his bedroom and at night by his bed. He and others said that Mr. Pedro had fallen in love with a former housemaid, Elsa Gulpian de Oliveira, but that she refused to marry him. When she married someone else in 1978, the old man became annoyed and depressed.

Realizing that the story was drifting away from Mengele's medical history, Levine broke in. "Mr. Bossert, did Peter Hochbichler ever mention if he'd been seriously ill in his childhood?"

"Well, yes, he did," Wolfram replied, sitting up in his chair. He was a thin man whose long, spindly arms poked out from his starched white shirt like twigs in a snowbank. "He told our children that he had a lot of illnesses and diseases when he was a child. That was why he missed out of school a lot and had to make up for it by working very hard in order not to be left behind by his younger brothers."

"Did he ever mention having any dental work done?"

"Yes, he often complained about his teeth. He told me that somewhere in Paraguay he had some work done to hide the gap in his teeth. But it was very badly done."

"Did you or your wife ever see any gold teeth in his mouth?"

"Yes, on the lower left-hand side there was a gold crown or some sort of gold work," Lisolette replied.

"Did he ever say where he got it?"

"No, but it was not here. It was a long time before he came to Brazil."

"Do you know where he had the dentures made?"

The couple conferred and Wolfram replied, "He had a dentist . . . during the last three years of his life. There was no dentist in the area where he lived. So he must have gone to some other part of São Paulo. He never mentioned the name of the dentist, however."

Lisolette chimed in. "He would have looked for a relatively cheap dentist. I am certain he would not have gone to a German dentist or a dentist with predominantly German clientele because he would not want to be recognized or say anything that might lead to his identification."

Snow added a question: "Was he right- or left-handed?"

"He was right-handed," Wolfram replied. "You see, I'm left-handed, and we certainly would have talked about it if he had been as well."

The Bosserts described the final turn in the downward spiral of Mengele's life. The end, they said, came on a beach just south of São Paulo on February 7, 1979. "We invited him to join us at a house we had rented for the weekend at Beritoga," Wolfram explained. Mengele arrived by bus, as he had neither a car nor a driver's license. At about five o'clock in the afternoon, Mengele rose from his chair, next to where the Bosserts and their children were sitting on the beach, and dove into the breakers. Stroking vigorously, he broke through the surf to calmer water and began swimming parallel to the beach. Moments later, Lisolette noticed that he had stopped swimming and seemed to be thrashing about with one arm. She cried out to her husband, who immediately ran into the water and swam toward Mengele. Throwing an arm around the drowning man's chest, Wolfram pulled him toward shore as the waves crashed over them.

At this juncture in the story, Wolfram leapt to his feet, wheeling his arms in the air and puffing up his cheeks, to illustrate the scene. The interpreter struggled to keep up as his words tumbled out.

"I was growing exhausted. But then I thought, why not use the waves? So I dove under and held him up. . . . Then he stopped moving and I felt his head droop against my shoulder." Several bathers ran into the water and pulled the men to the beach. Wolfram collapsed next to Peter. "He was lying there in the sand and I sort of instinctively picked his head up and put it on my arm. . . . I was breathing heavily. . . . I remember foam coming out of his mouth."

The police took the body to the local coroner, Dr. Jaime Edson Andrade Mendonca, who cursorily prodded the corpse and pronounced the cause of death as drowning. He issued a death certificate in the name of Wolfgang Gerhard. Meanwhile, Lisolette rushed her vomiting husband to the hospital; he himself had nearly drowned in the rescue attempt.

The following morning Lisolette hired a hearse and driver and set out for Embú with the body. During the night a tropical storm had swept down the coast and left deep gullies in the dirt road leading out of town. As the hearse slid between the ruts, she watched nervously as the casket slid from side to side, its lid chattering open and shut. Suddenly the car lurched and skidded off the road and a rear tire sank into the mud. It took her and the driver two hours to dig it free.

Lisolette was vaguely aware of sunlight breaking through the clouds when the hearse finally approached the outskirts of São Paulo. The driver, now confident they would reach their destination without further delay, leaned back in his seat and recounted misadventures he'd experienced in the funeral trade. Lisolette half-listened, her tired eyes fixed on the road ahead of them. Having nothing to say but feeling the need to be polite, she asked the driver his name. "It's María Elena," he replied. Momentarily perplexed, Lisolette turned to study this man with a woman's name. Sensing her confusion, the driver explained, "It's my Christian name. I had a sex change several years ago. Perhaps it's strange, but everybody still calls me María Elena. So why change it?"

Lisolette was in a dreadful state when she arrived at Our Lady of the Rosary cemetery in Embú. Her hands trembled as she handed the death certificate to the funeral director, Gino Carita. When he saw Wolfgang Gerhard's name and the cause of death, he remembered the tall Austrian who, two years before, had asked him to prepare a grave for an old relative. "Well, well, so this is how the world goes," he said. Death had chosen Gerhard instead. He asked Lisolette if he could open the casket. "No, I don't want to, I can't," she blurted hysterically. "My husband is ill and I don't know how he is, and I am all alone here and I want to get the whole thing over with as quickly as possible." Carita bridled his curiosity and gave in to her wishes. He told his secretary to send workers up the hill to prepare the grave.

Two mourners stood that afternoon by Wolfgang Gerhard's open tomb as the gravediggers slipped ropes around the casket and lowered it into the earth. Lisolette cringed as the coffin jerked and scraped against the sides of the hole. Hat in hand, María Elena, the transsexual hearse driver, bowed his head.

Later that day Lisolette called Gitta Stammer. "The old man's dead," she said.

"Which old man?" her friend asked.

"Peter. It's Peter, he's dead."

"Well, thank God it's over," Gitta sighed.

With those words Lisolette Bossert ended her deposition. "There's nothing more I can say," she said as her shoulders slumped and her hands dropped into her lap. Wolfram, his gaze anchored to a crack in the tiled floor in front of him, looked like a marionette that someone had left draped over a chair.

Just before dawn on Thursday, June 20, Richard Helmer left his hotel, hailed one of the few taxis cruising São Paulo's gray streets at that early hour, and directed the driver to the Medico-Legal Institute.

At the institute a light shone in one of the laboratories. The diligent Daniel Muñoz was, as usual, the first to arrive. He sat hunched over an examining table, the turned-up collar of his lab coat giving him the look of some sort of television detective. Not one to chat, especially when he had a job to do, Helmer offered a brief hello and went into his lab.

The hub of the investigation sat balanced on a cork ring on a bench to one side of the room. Helmer picked up the skull and inspected his craftsmanship like a sculptor worrying over the details of a marble bust. It had taken hours of work with tweezers and glue to return the paper-thin bone around the eye sockets and the nasal opening to their original cast. Now it was time to give the skull back its grin.

With a small hand drill, Helmer bored holes in both sides of the mandible, then two more in the parietal bone of the cranium, just above the temples. He fixed springs to the mandible, looped them under the zygomatic arches that curve back from the cheekbones toward the ear, and secured them to the cranium with small screws. One more detail remained. Helmer slipped the dentures recovered from the grave between the upper and lower jaw, locking them into place next to the ten natural teeth.

Hamlet once held aloft a skull and wondered if he could discern its owner's identity. Helmer now asked himself the same question. But he had at his disposal a technique that Hamlet could not have imagined.

By the late 1970s Helmer had perfected a video-imaging process called skull-face superimposition, in which a video image of a photograph is placed over a video image of a skull to determine whether the two are the same person.[6] Snow had used a simplified version of Helmer's technique by 1975, and then applied it to identify the cowboy mummy of Elmer McCurdy in 1977 and one of Custer's soldiers in 1985. Since then, Helmer had taken much of the guesswork out of the technique. In his laboratory at the University of Kiel, he had studied the topography of hundreds of skulls, much as an engineer might measure the vaults and arches of a cathedral, and reduced them to geometrical formulas. The result was a procedure for positively identifying unknown persons that had become admissible as evidence in the West German courts.

The core of Helmer's technique lay in the fact that the contours of a skull vary greatly from one person to the next. The skull may be broad or narrow at the forehead, long or short from forehead to chin, or it may have high cheekbones or protruding eyebrow ridges. The eye sockets vary in size and placement. Nasal apertures may be wide or narrow. Diseases or injuries can also influence the features of the skull during life. All of these variabilities make each of us unique — in life and in death.

If the man who was buried at Embú was Josef Mengele, the skull should match his photographs. Helmer had two sets of prints of Mengele. One consisted of two SS portraits taken of Mengele in 1938, when he was twenty-seven. The other was the collection of portraits shot by Wolfram Bossert, the aspiring photographer, two years before the drowning.

Not satisfied with roughly laying the image of the living person over the image of a skull and simply eyeballing the closeness of a match, Helmer insisted on lining the two up to the closest millimeter. To do this, he had devised an ingenious if bizarre-looking method. First, he consulted his tables of facial-skin thicknesses, just as the facial reconstructionist Betty Pat Gatliff would do before sculpting a face over a skull. He got measurements for thirty points on the face. These measurements had to be appropriate for a Caucasoid male in his twenties; thicknesses for a female, a black or Mongoloid, or a young child would be different. He took the standard measurements: supraglabella, at the midline of the forehead; nasion, just above the bridge of the nose; mid-philtrum, the especially fleshy midpoint between the bottom of the nose and the top lip; three points on each cheekbone; the mental eminence, the lowest point on the chin before it starts to curve back toward the neck; and others he had compiled.

Helmer took thirty pins; each was to be secured with a dab of clay at one of the thirty points on the skull. First, however, he slipped a white marker down the shaft of each pin and secured it at the point where the skin of the face would have extended out from the skull in life. On the pin destined for the mid-philtrum, for example, the marker sat eleven and a half millimeters from the skull end of the pin. At the nasion, the distance was five millimeters; for the mental eminence, ten and a half millimeters.

Once the pins were anchored to the skull, Helmer took the skull to a small, windowless room normally used as the institute's photo lab. The room was hot and stuffy, and the air stung his nose with the odor of developing fluids. Pinned to the room's pale green, peeling walls were dozens of faded photographs of crime scenes, bullet cartridges, and fingerprints. Helmer mounted the skull on an aluminum post. It looked like a novelty item you might find in a tacky souvenir shop, somebody's idea of a funny pin cushion. He attached the 1938 SS photo on another aluminum post next to the skull.

The scientist had already set up two high-resolution video cameras in the room, mounted on tracks so that they could slide forward and backward. The video images were relayed to an image processor and thence to a television monitor. Helmer, now scientist turned cameraman, squinted into the viewfinder of one camera, bringing the skull into focus. He moved to the next camera and did the same for the photograph. He shuttled between the two, sliding them back and forth along their tracks until the two images of skull and face on the monitor were the same size. With the image processor, he superimposed the images over each other, lining up the flesh of the face at each pinpoint with the white marker. If this were Mengele, then skin and marker had to match, point by point. If they didn't. . . . Well then, someone else had been buried at that grave at Embú.

At noon Helmer emerged from the photo lab. He took a deep breath of fresh air and hurried down the corridor, searching for his colleague Rolf Endris, the dentist on the German team. When he found him, the usually unflappable anthropologist sputtered excitedly, "Rolf, it's finished. Come. And bring everyone with you."

Minutes later the scientists crowded into Helmer's lab. The German flicked on the cameras. The pin-cushion skull came into focus on the television monitor with the photo superimposed onto it. The sight was unnerving. It took a moment for the eye and brain to process the peculiar image. They were seeing a human as no one in life could, as if the skin were a ghostly film. The contours of the face in the photo — the angles of the jaw, the slope of the forehead, the placement of the nose over the aperture — perfectly matched the shape of the skull. They scanned the face pinpoint to pinpoint. At each spot, the white marker lay at the skin line.

"Now you see that this isn't fantasy," Helmer told his hushed audience. "This is Josef Mengele."

That evening, the American scientists gathered at the U.S. consulate across the city. A large room had been made ready for them. A coffeepot sputtered on a hot plate and an oversized air conditioner rattled at full throttle in the window. A large oval conference table sat heavily in the middle of an expanse of wall-to-wall carpeting, its surface as glossy as the consul-general's limousine. Old Glory hung stiffly in one corner.

Police chief Tuma, anxious to close the investigation, had announced at a press conference that afternoon that he believed all the circumstantial evidence pointed to only one conclusion. The remains exhumed at Embú were those of Josef Mengele.[7] At the consulate, Lukash opened the discussion by noting that Tuma was certainly entitled to his opinion. But it was up to the scientists to decide, based on their own analysis of the *physical* evidence, if indeed the skeleton belonged to Mengele. "Or," Lukash said, "we can decide that there simply isn't enough physical evidence to say one way or another. Remember, this isn't an ordinary case and the public, and especially the skeptics, aren't going to accept just ordinary evidence."

Levine searched Lukash's face for some sign of why he was raising doubts at the eleventh hour. Levine had half-expected that Lukash would cause some sort of fuss about the wording in the report, maybe just to bully him for having turned him down in favor of joining the

Justice Department's team. But no, he realized, there was more to this than just wounded pride.

"Okay, Leslie, you've seen all the evidence," Levine said. "So what's bothering you?"

"Well, to begin with, why aren't the Germans here?"

"Because the German government told them to hold off from making any public statements until they'd written their own report. Anyway, they've agreed to be at the press conference tomorrow. You saw Helmer's work. He's convinced it's Mengele."

"Sure I did, and I was impressed. But it's not my technique and I'm the one signing the report."

"What about the diastema? The gold crown?" Levine asked, growing more incredulous by the second.

"Consistencies, but without dental X rays it's not conclusive proof. You know that, Lowell."

"Age, sex, stature, handedness, and race?"

"Consistencies."

"The motorcycle accident and the pelvis fracture?"

"A possible consistency, but mostly circumstantial."

Lukash stood, rammed his hands into his pockets, and began to pace. "Look," he said, his voice rising a notch. "My problem is we're dealing with the Bosserts and Stammers and they're Nazis of the first order. If one can conspire to hide an individual, one could conspire to do a lot of things. Understand, we don't have any records. The only thing we have is a certificate of death of Wolfgang Gerhard. There are no medical records, no dental records. There is a tremendous amount of circumstantial evidence. Okay, when you put together the anthropological evidence and matching the skull in the pictorial techniques and even the dental to a limited degree, you can come to a conclusion that it is reasonably Joseph Mengele. But the absolute is missing."[8]

Lukash reached into his shirt pocket and withdrew a telex he and his team had received from Rabbi Marvin Hier of the Wiesenthal Center earlier in the day. He read it aloud. Hier asked the scientists to hold a press conference to demand more medical records from Mengele's family in Germany, records the family had promised but never delivered. Only after seeing these records, Hier said, should the scientists come to any conclusion. Otherwise, the Mengele family could simply echo whatever they read in the press about the scientist's physical examination.[9]

Lukash pulled off his bifocals and stared at Levine. "Now, Lowell, is that an *unreasonable* request?" he demanded.

"Politics, Leslie, pure politics," Levine replied.

Snow watched as the debate continued. Things obviously were turning sour. Only a week ago the scientists had arrived in São Paulo as enthusiastic as schoolboys readying for a treasure hunt. The only tension that showed through the veneer of collegiality came from the competitiveness common to any group of equals trying to solve an important mystery. But these were men whose hard-won reputations were on the line.

Snow realized that Lukash had a point: this was no ordinary case. But he also had to accept that not one piece of physical evidence suggested that the skeleton was *not* Mengele's. When you weighed that against the striking number of consistencies between the skeleton and what was known about Mengele, there seemed to be no reason not to go all the way.

"Look," Snow said as he glanced at the clock at the far end of the room, "I'd like to suggest that we approach the writing of this report as follows. First, let's go, step by step, to see if there is even one inconsistency. Next, we'll review each of our findings against Mengele's SS records."

The American scientists agreed, and for the next five hours they haggled over the merits of each piece of evidence. Besides their own findings, they had been given a report written from a team of West German experts who had compared photos of Mengele recovered from the Bosserts house with Mengele's 1938 SS photo and found twenty-four matching physical traits.[10]

The only piece of conflicting evidence was the lack of any sign of osteomyelitis.

Fitzpatrick argued that there simply had been a misdiagnosis. Kerley and Snow agreed but said that they would prefer to leave it open-ended, as it was highly likely the infected bone had remodeled itself over the years.

The night dragged on. Snow asked a secretary if she could arrange for some food to be brought in. When she returned and plunked two large paper bags on the table, Lukash looked disdainfully at the clown dancing under the golden arches on one of the bags. "You mean to tell me we're in Brazil on the most important forensic case in history and all the U.S. government serves us are McDonald's hamburgers?"

At 1:00 A.M. the group agreed to end the debate and settle the thing on paper. To avoid disagreements, they decided that everyone should leave the room except Snow and Kerley, who would draft the report. Snow took out his Hewlett Packard laptop computer and, as Kerley read over his shoulder, began to write:

Based on our examination of the remains exhumed at Nossa Señhora do Rosario Cemetery, Embú, Brazil on 6 June 1985, we conclude that these remains are that of a white male who was of medium build and between 64 and 74 years of age at the time of death. From the length of the leg bones, we calculated that his stature before death was approximately 174 centimeters. Studies of the bones of the upper extremity indicate that he was right-handed.

Pathological and radiological studies reveal an old, healed fracture of the right hip, a healed fracture at the base of the right thumb, a healing fracture of the right shoulder blade (scapula), and an old, healed injury of the collar bone. There are arthritic changes throughout the skeleton. In addition, there is a bony defect of the left cheekbone.

Examination of the upper jaw reveals the presence of three molars containing silver amalgam filling. The lower jaw contains seven teeth, two of which have gold veneer crowns. All missing teeth, except third molars, have been replaced with removable, partial dentures made of what appears to be chrome alloy and acrylic. In addition, there is skeletal evidence indicating that the upper central incisors were widely spaced prior to their removal.

We have reviewed medical, dental, investigative, and other biographical information on Josef Mengele provided by several governmental and private institutions and compared this data with our findings. We have also reviewed the photographic skull-face superimposition analysis and photographic comparison studies of West German forensic scientists. In addition, we have received the report of handwriting analysis of Questioned Document Examiners.

Based on the above, it is the opinion of the undersigned that the exhumed remains are definitely not those of Wolfgang Gerhard. It is further our opinion that this skeleton is that of Josef Mengele within a reasonable scientific certainty.

A more detailed report will be issued at a later date.[11]

Lukash protested that "reasonable probability" rather than "reasonable scientific certainty" should have been used, but he signed the document. One by one, the others added their names, picked up their papers, and filed out of the room, too exhausted to revel in the success of their mission. Snow was the last to go. The clock on the wall read 3:00 A.M. as he closed the door behind him.

10

THE NAIL IN THE
COFFIN

ON Friday morning, June 21, the camera crews arrived at
the federal police headquarters. In a third-floor meeting
room, technicians spent two hours unloading their shiny
aluminum cases, raising tripods for cameras, arranging telescoping
stands for lights, taping cables to the floor, and checking sound levels
on their microphones. The pencil press, among them Ralph Blumenthal, arrived shortly thereafter and immediately complained to the
TV crews that they and their cameras were blocking their view of the
table up front where the scientists were to speak. Words escalated to
shouts, then to angry gestures, until one reporter finally pushed a
member of the TV crew, who promptly punched him back. The two
managed to knock over a chair but, being journalists, realized that
they might actually get hurt and lowered their fists. Just as things
were settling into an uneasy truce, the police's public relations man
walked in and told everyone to move to the other side of the room.
Technicians swept up their equipment and raced to the new location.
Those unburdened by electronic gear got there first. More shoving
matches ensued until a new order was established.

On the floor below the scientists were filing into Tuma's office.
The long week had begun to show in bluish pouches under their eyes.
Fitzpatrick was the only member of the Wiesenthal team to show up;

Snow and Lukash had decided to skip the dog-and-pony show to catch up on some sleep.

Levine distributed copies of the report to the West German and Brazilian scientists. When they expressed satisfaction with it, Tuma, smartly attired in a light gray suit, his jet black hair and mustache neatly trimmed for the occasion, stood and addressed the group.

"Gentlemen, this is like what they say at a wedding," he said. "Speak now or forever hold your peace."

No one said a word.

"All right. Let's go upstairs and meet the press."

Tuma led the group up to the third floor and into the mobbed meeting room. "Shit," Levine thought, "this is a zoo."[1] Tuma assembled the scientists around the speaker's table.

Blumenthal had managed to wedge himself into a spot near the front. He found himself standing next to the Brazilian anthropologist Muñoz, who held a large box under one arm.

"Hey, what have you got there," the New Yorker joked, "the bones?"

"Some of them," came the deadpan reply.

"You're kidding."

"No. Here, look for yourself." Muñoz slipped the top off the box just enough to let Blumenthal peek inside. Sure enough, there was the skull.

The fog of reporters closed around the speakers' table. Tuma spoke first. He said that the scientists had confirmed that the skeleton at Embú was that of Josef Mengele. Then several of the scientists added their observations, which, like paving stones laid end to end, led to what they said was an inevitable conclusion.

"It is almost impossible from a mathematical point of view that this could be another person," said Teixeira.

"The odds are astronomical that this could be anyone else," Levine added, holding up a copy of the report.

How sure are you? he was asked.

"Within a reasonable scientific certainty." Realizing the ambiguity of this scientific term, he added, "That represents a very, very, very high degree of probability. Scientists never say anything is one hundred percent."

Blumenthal sidled up to a man in the audience he had not yet met but to whom he very much wanted to talk. Menachem Russek, the graying Nazi-hunter from Israel, stood watching the proceedings with scorn written on his brow. "Well, what do you think?" Blumenthal asked Russek.

"No comment," Russek replied, barely turning to answer.

"What do you mean, no comment?" Blumenthal blurted. "Here's the skeleton. Do you disagree with it?"

"I don't want to say anything," Russek insisted.

Blumenthal's face flushed with anger. This was the time, damn it, that the Israelis had to say something. They couldn't stonewall now. He tried to bait the Israeli.

"Isn't this what you've been waiting for? Are you casting doubt on the Brazilians? Do you disbelieve them?" But Russek wouldn't budge, saying simply that reporters should address their questions to the Brazilians.

At the front table, the scientists were completing a show-and-tell with photographs of their methods. Muñoz, still wearing his white lab coat and ignored until then, brought forth his box. He slid off the top and reached in gingerly, as if he were removing rare pottery. Out came the skull. The dentures, still in place, froze the mouth in a bizarre grimace. Muñoz turned its face forward toward the cameras. Several thousand frames of film were instantaneously exposed, then the head went back into the box. There, in a locked storeroom in São Paulo, alongside the rest of Josef Mengele, the skull remains.

Back in their respective countries, the forensic scientists had barely unpacked their bags before the doubters emerged to challenge their findings. Survivors of Auschwitz understandably felt robbed that Mengele had not been captured alive. To many of his victims, Mengele had become an almost mythical character, a Jungian creature shaped by their collective nightmares and kept alive by their loathing. They wanted Mengele to face his accusers and suffer the consequences. Now, in less than a week, scientists had turned him into a set of measurements and statistics, denying them not only justice but the opportunity to purge their anguish.

Politically, however, ending the chase for the number one Nazi in hiding seemed less certain. On June 23, in Tel Aviv, the Israeli government, whose vaunted intelligence machine had failed over decades to track Mengele down, stated that while it did not doubt the expertise of the three teams of scientists, its own forensic experts would have to examine all the forensic and material evidence before it would close the case.[2] Meanwhile, the U.S. government was prepared to accept the experts' report, its attorney general, Edwin Meese, calling it the "final chapter in a tragic and horrible part of world history."[3] So, too, did Hier of the Simon Wiesenthal Center, although with some disappointment that Mengele cheated fate.[4]

Several staff members at the Office of Special Investigations (OSI) at Justice, however, had begun to complain privately about the scientists' inability to confirm or disprove Mengele's reputed case of osteomyelitis, which various acquaintances of his had noted over the years.[5]

To allay its lingering doubts, OSI turned to Donald Ortner, a physical anthropologist at the Smithsonian Institution in Washington, D.C. Ortner had occasionally helped the FBI investigate bones recovered in criminal cases. In 1981, he had coauthored a leading text on diseases of the bone, *Identification of Pathological Conditions in Human Skeletal Remains*, and was considered among the best osteopathologists in the country. The OSI believed he could be trusted to judge the bones in Brazil with a cold and calculating eye.

In January 1986, Ortner flew to São Paulo. He had already been skeptical of one part of the first investigation, Helmer's skull-face superimposition, which had so swayed the forensic team. To Ortner, the technique hadn't been exhaustively tested for reliability. At the Medico-Legal Institute he examined all the bones except the skull, which was in the hands of a Brazilian facial reconstructionist, as well as photos and the X rays taken of the bones. What he saw disturbed him. The X rays, for example, showed that someone had sectioned the fistula in the left cheekbone, unnecessarily, he thought, and possibly destroying evidence. He found the healed lesion on the right hip bone and the bony spur, a projection about one centimeter in diameter and three to four centimeters in length in the area of the origin of the rectus femoris muscle.[6] The lesion on the hip bone *could* have been evidence of an injury serious enough to result in osteomyelitis, Ortner thought, but it certainly wasn't clear-cut. As for the bony spur, it had also been sectioned.

Ortner returned to Washington with a report that no clear sign of osteomyelitis could be found on the bones. But something serious had happened to the man dug up from Embú when he was younger. The bony spur on the hip had to have come about from an injury. From the X rays in São Paulo, Ortner could see that the tendon and muscle fibers in the spur lay in an opposite direction from those in the surrounding bone. After a traumatic injury, muscle and tendon can often ossify. The muscle tissue provides cells that contribute to the formation of a callous around the site of the fracture. As with bone, the trauma to muscle tends to produce hematoma. With time the hematoma usually dissolves, but occasionally the muscle tissue will respond to the trauma by producing bone in the muscle itself, often in association with the hematoma. The excessive formation of bone by muscle can be entirely separate from the bone or it can become part of existing bone tissue. This condition is known as traumatic myositis ossificans and is usually associated with injuries in adolescents and young adults. The outward signs, Ortner suggested, could have been mistaken for osteomyelitis, which would corroborate the diagnosis of the disease in Mengele's 1938 SS records.[7] Ortner advised the Justice Department to look into any school records of the young Mengele to see if he had been out of school with an injury for a period of months.

Meanwhile, German investigators had found a tantalizing new clue in Mengele's diaries, a link the scientists had sought in Brazil but failed to find: a dentist. A notation recorded two visits, on December 5 and 11, 1978 — two months before Mengele's death — to an unnamed dentist. The dentist had examined his patient's teeth and concluded that he needed a root canal, which he couldn't perform. Recorded in the diary was the name of the root canal specialist: "Dr. Gama" in the town of Sama.[8]

Pay dirt, thought the Justice investigators. Where there is a dentist, there are X rays. If they could find Gama and an X ray of his patient's teeth, they could compare them to images of the Embú skull. A match would sweep away any clinging doubts, even if questions about Mengele's supposed osteomyelitis were never resolved.

Back in Brazil, an oral pathologist turned diplomat, Stephen Dachi, began the search for the mysterious Dr. Gama. Dachi was the fifty-five-year-old U.S. consul general in São Paulo. Born in Hungary and raised in Rumania, Dachi had been captured by Russian soldiers at the age of eleven during World War II, but had escaped and taken refuge in a synagogue. After the war Dachi made his way to Canada and then to America, where he earned a medical degree and subsequently taught dentistry.[9]

Dachi mulled over the key entry in the diary. For starters, the town Mengele had called Sama didn't exist. As for Gama, it was a common name. The only description of Gama in the diary was that he was bald and round-faced. The Brazilians had interviewed several Gamas and come up empty-handed. Perhaps something more lay between the lines. Could the entry be in code? Dachi wondered. In fact, Mengele's protectors, the Bosserts and Stammers, had said that Mengele did all sorts of odd things to disguise himself and his whereabouts. He would wear a hat, for example, even in the sweltering tropical heat, because he thought it would make him less recognizable. Other parts of the diary, Dachi knew, had been written in code.

Dachi initiated his own investigation.[10] The American read through lists of members of dental societies and customers of dental-supply companies. Of the seven dentists named Gama he found, one had died, four had graduated from medical school since 1979, and one had never practiced dentistry. He interviewed the last suspect and ruled him out; he didn't do root canals.

Riding back from his interview with the last Dr. Gama, Dachi pondered the name Sama. Could it be an acronym? Or an abbreviation of some kind?

Could it be Santa Amaro?

Back at the consulate, Dachi and his vice-consul, Fred Kaplan, rifled through files and bookshelves until Dachi found an old copy of the yellow pages phone book. It was the sort of thing they normally wouldn't have checked, because so few people in this country of on-again, off-again telephone systems bothered with the official telephone book. Dachi paged through it looking for listings for the suburb of Santa Amaro. Yes, he almost shouted, here's a Gama. . . . Hercy Gonzaga Gama Angelo.

Dachi asked his Brazilian secretary, Stella, to call Gama — he didn't want to raise suspicion with a non-Brazilian accent. The dentist's secretary said that Dr. Gama only did root canals. That's fine, Dachi nodded to Stella, that's just fine. Stella continued, telling the dental assistant that a friend had recommended Dr. Gama to her, but she wanted to be sure she had the right one. Was the doctor bald and kind of round-faced? Oh yes, the secretary replied, that's my boss. Stella made an appointment for Friday, March 21.

On the appointed day, Dachi, Kaplan, and a plainclothes police officer drove to the suburb of Santa Amaro. Gama's office wasn't listed on the building directory, but they found it eventually. Gama was surprised by a visit from three men who clearly hadn't come to get root canals. When shown a photo of Mengele, he recognized it from having followed the news accounts the previous June of the investigation. But he couldn't recall ever having treated this man. He sent his secretary back to his files to check. She returned about thirty seconds later shaking her head.

"I've got a patient waiting," Gama told his visitors. "Perhaps you will come back some other time."

"No," the policeman said. "Not later. Bring the records out now."

Gama, droplets of sweat forming on his hairless pate, complied and then returned to his patient. The three men divvied up the piles of folders and checked the dates, looking for those from late 1978. Within forty-five minutes, they found a chart dated December 5 and 11. It described root-canal and upper molar work. It showed that the patient had paid two thousand and one thousand cruzeiros for the work, just as it had said in Mengele's diary. Dachi flipped the chart over. It read: Pedro Hochbichler, 5555 Estrada Alvarenga.

Gama looked stunned. "Wait'll I tell my wife," he said, shaking his head in amazement. But he swore he had no X rays of this patient. As was his custom, he had sent them to the dentist who had first treated Hochbichler. Who was that dentist? Dachi asked. Dr. Kasumasa Tutiya, Gama replied.

"By then I was hyperventilating," Dachi remembers. "Mengele had told Mrs. Bossert that he went to a Japanese dentist because, he said, just as all Japanese looked alike to Europeans, all Europeans must look the same to Japanese. But he never told Mrs. Bossert the name of the dentist."

Tutiya worked in an office just down the street. The three investigators practically ran the two blocks. They found the building, a seedy block of concrete that housed a secondhand clothing store, climbed the darkened staircase to the second floor, and followed the room numbers down a gray corridor to suite number two. They stood in the waiting room as the receptionist fetched the dentist. Dachi noticed that the latest issue of *Veja*, Brazil's version of *Time*, lay on a corner table, a photo of the triumphant face of Romeu Tuma on its cover.

Tutiya took them into his office. He was a careful record keeper. Within seconds, he located Hochbichler's file. In it were dental charts for the period 1976 to 1978 describing work he had done on Hochbichler and the amount paid for each visit.

An exhilarated Dachi tried to remain calm. "You wouldn't happen to have any X rays, would you?" he asked.

"Wait a minute," Tutiya said. He left the room for what seemed to Dachi an hour. He returned with an envelope and opened it over his desk. Out slid eight negatives. Dachi felt as if he had just won the lottery.

Before the group left Tutiya's office, they showed the dentist a series of photographs of men in their late sixties, including a portrait of Mengele taken by Wolfram Bossert for his fake identification card. "Can you identify your patient?" asked Dachi.

"Certainly," Tutiya said with a broad smile, "I recognize him. He's the one with the hat."

A week later, OSI sent Levine back to São Paulo to check Tutiya's X rays against those taken of the skull from Embú. When Levine compared the two sets of X rays, everything matched: the widely spaced upper incisors, the wide diastema, the shapes of the fillings and the floor of the antrum, and the unusual bend in the root of the lower-left canine. There was no question about it, Levine told OSI. Tutiya's patient and the man buried in Embú were the same person.

But as of the middle of 1990, a final report on the Mengele investigation has not been released. According to an official involved in the Justice Department's investigation, the U.S. government has completed an official account that confirms that the bones from Embú are Josef Mengele's. But the Justice Department won't release it until the Israelis act. The West German authorities also have completed their report, but are waiting as well for word from Israel.

According to Dachi and the Justice official, an Israeli pathologist has looked over the remains and the forensic data and is convinced that Mengele has been found. "When he came," says Dachi, "he said, 'You really did correct work here and I really can't say this isn't Mengele. But the problem is the osteomyelitis. I can't find any sign of it.' " But Dachi and others involved in the investigation believe that some politicians in Israel prefer to leave the verdict hanging. Says Dachi: "The Israelis are just flat-out wrong. . . . The Israelis have never looked at this scientifically. They are looking at it politically or emotionally." Dachi says an Israeli investigator told him in São Paulo that it was possible Mengele had found another man in Brazil who looked just like him — "right down to the bones," Dachi says incredulously — and followed his trips to Tutiya and Gama, marking down each in his diary as if he had made the visits. Then he killed the man and buried his body in Embú and made sure the diary was found. Besides being far-fetched on its face, says Dachi, such a tale doesn't make sense. He told the Israeli, "Why would Mengele go to all that trouble when in seventeen years you [the Israeli authorities] never got near him?"

The American government wants to conclude the case with an official report, not least because it wants to show that taxpayers' dollars have been well spent in the effort. The West German Prosecutor's Office wants to retire the arrest warrants for Mengele. However, says the Justice source, the Israelis "have nothing to gain by closing the investigation." So an official OSI report on the Mengele investigation sits in a classified file at the agency's office on Fourteenth Street in Washington, D.C. Everyone must wait, he notes, because "if the Americans and Germans release a report without the Israelis, the doubters will say it is a coverup. . . ."

In a last-ditch attempt to end the episode, Hans Klein, the West German prosecutor in charge of the investigation, turned to a British scientist, Alec Jeffreys, in September 1989. Klein had heard about an extraordinary new technique recently applied to questions of paternity or maternity and used in criminal investigations: DNA fingerprinting. Deoxyribonucleic acid is the chromosomal material that carries genes, the blueprints of every organism. Within the three billion chemical units of a person's entire set of chromosomes lie features unique to each individual. By the same token, some of these features are common only to members of the same family, and are handed down generation by generation.

In forensics, DNA is extracted from fluids or tissue found at a crime scene, often sperm or seminal fluid from the bodies or clothing of rape victims, or blood found at the scene of a violent crime. The molecular features that vary among individuals are located and reproduced in a laboratory on an autoradiograph, a print much like an X ray. These variable "polymorphisms" show up as a row of blotches irregularly spaced in a vertical lane. These "bands" look something like a bar code used to mark goods in a supermarket. If a suspect in a crime had been collared, a similar autoradiograph can be made from his or her DNA, and the two prints compared. If the bands match, the DNA at the crime scene belongs to the suspect.

The method, while not infallible, is highly reliable. But it has never been conclusively applied to bone alone. A company in Maryland, Cellmark Diagnostics, attempted to extract DNA from bones buried for over ten years in Argentina but failed to get enough intact DNA for a high-quality autoradiograph. Bacterial DNA could have contaminated the bones' DNA, according to Cellmark's technician, Karen Markowicz, or the action of some unknown inhibitor could have sliced the DNA into unworkable fragments.

A scientist in Oxford, England, Erika Hagelberg, has applied a more refined technique, called polymerase chain reaction, to extract and amplify DNA from bones from some of Oliver Cromwell's soldiers buried in a seventeenth-century graveyard. But the quality of the amplification is not appropriate for use as forensic evidence. The most thorough attempt to get DNA images from buried bones has been undertaken at the laboratory of Henry Lee, chief of forensic sciences for the Connecticut State Police. Lee has buried a set of bones and at regular intervals recovers a sample to extract DNA to see if it is still intact.

Lee's experiment had not been completed when Klein called on Jeffreys, at the University of Leicester, to look at several of Mengele's bones brought up from Brazil by Romeu Tuma. Jeffreys was a logical candidate to try the technique on Mengele — he invented DNA fingerprinting. At the time he agreed to help Klein, however, he was unsure whether bone would give a good DNA print. A print by itself, of course, wouldn't prove anything. It would have to be compared to a living relative of Mengele's. Two such people were alive: Rolf, Mengele's son, and Dieter Mengele, his nephew, and Klein had not yet won agreement from them to cooperate.

It remains to be seen whether DNA fingerprinting will work with bone. If it does, it will revolutionize forensic anthropology as it already has forensic pathology. But DNA or no DNA, the last word on Mengele probably will belong with those he tried to exterminate.

PART

———

11

A SOUTHERN
EXPOSURE

C LYDE SNOW drew a deep breath, preparing to bring his presentation to a close. For over an hour the anthropologist had held his audience spellbound as he spoke for the deceased. He talked of the two little Oklahoma girls, the fallen soldiers at the Battle of the Little Bighorn, the victims of fiery plane crashes and of serial murderers. In each case, with the aid of slides, Snow had shaped a story to illustrate the techniques he and other forensic anthropologists use to breathe life into bone. ("Bones," he said once, "just have a way of fascinating people.")

The occasion was the annual meeting of the American Association for the Advancement of Science (AAAS), held in May 1984 at the Hilton Hotel in New York City. Snow had come to talk about the role forensic scientists could play in the investigation of human rights abuses. Several months before the meeting, he had received a phone call from the symposium's organizer, Cristián Orrego, inviting him to participate on the panel. Orrego had introduced himself as a Chilean molecular biologist living in Boston and a member of the Association's Committee on Scientific Freedom and Responsibility. Orrego asked Snow if he'd heard about the thousands of people who had disappeared in Argentina. Yes, Snow replied, he'd read about them. Orrego said it was almost certain that military and police squads had killed most of the disappeared and buried them in unmarked graves.

Now, with the return of civilian rule, many of the families of the missing wanted the graves opened and the remains of their loved ones identified. They had turned to the AAAS for scientific expertise. Would Snow, Orrego asked, be willing to help out?

As the last slide flickered off the screen, Snow turned and looked down the line of scientists assembled at the speaker's table. "Time permitting," he said, pausing long enough to see Orrego nod, "I'd like to end my presentation by reading the first verse of a poem by the Spaniard Federico García Lorca. It's called 'The Ballad of the Civil Guard' and begins with guardsmen descending on a gypsy village."

Snow read:

> Black are the horses.
> The horseshoes are black.
> On the dark capes glisten
> stains of ink and wax.
> Their skulls are leaden,
> which is why they don't weep.
> With their patent-leather souls
> they come down the street.
> Hunchbacked and nocturnal,
> where they go, they command
> silences of dark rubber
> and fears of fine sand.
> They pass where they want,
> and they hide in their skulls
> a vague astronomy of shapeless
> pistols.[1]

Snow set the poem aside and continued. "García Lorca wrote that poem when he was a student in Madrid in the late 1920s. Years later, in July 1936, at the outbreak of the Spanish Civil War, he fled the city. The Francoists had branded him undesirable. Like the gypsies in his poetry, García Lorca's ideas had apparently wandered too freely. Fearing for his life, he fled to the hills of Andalusia, his birthplace. He found refuge there in the house of a friend. Then, late in the evening of August 19, a group of Francoists came to the house and took García Lorca away to an olive grove, where they shot him and buried his body in a hastily dug grave. The grave has never been found. Today we would call García Lorca a *desaparecido*, a disappeared one.[2]

"The way I look at it, García Lorca's death amounted to state murder. Of all the forms of murder, none is more monstrous than that committed by a state against its own citizens. And of all murder victims, those of the state are the most helpless and vulnerable since the very entity to which they have entrusted their lives and safety becomes their killer. When the state murders, the crime is planned by powerful men. They use the same cold rationality and administrative efficiency that they might bring to the decision to wage a campaign to eradicate a particularly obnoxious agricultural pest.

"The homicidal state shares one trait with the solitary killer — like all murderers, it trips on its own egotism and drops a trail of clues which, when properly collected, preserved, and analyzed are as damning as a signed confession left in the grave.

"The great mass murders of our time have accounted for no more than a few hundred victims. In contrast, states that have chosen to murder their own citizens can usually count their victims by the carload lot. As for motive, the state has no peers, for it will kill its victim for a careless word, a fleeting thought, or even a poem."

Snow's voice thickened as he levied a challenge as much to himself as to his forensic colleagues in the audience.

"Maybe it's time for the forensic scientists of the world to heed the old call of our favorite fictional prototype: 'Quick, Watson, the game's afoot!' — and go after the biggest game of all."

As the audience clapped politely, Snow joined Orrego at the speaker's table. "Well now," he said to the Chilean, "when do we go to Argentina?"

Buenos Aires was unseasonably cool on the morning of March 24, 1976. In the city center, a fine mist settled on the jacaranda trees that line the perimeter of the Plaza de Mayo. At the northern end of the two-hectare square, next to the cathedral where the remains of Argentina's national liberator General José de San Martín lie in a crypt, a group of soldiers huddled over a small charcoal stove. Three of the men squatted with their backs pressed against the side of a jeep. Smoking and occasionally fanning their hands over the small fire, they watched their commanding officer lift a small black kettle from the stove and pour a stream of hot water into a pear-shaped gourd. A greenish liquid called *maté* bubbled to the neck and the officer passed it around. The men caressed the hot brown gourd and sucked the bitter drink through a metal straw.

By Latin American standards, the military coup that had toppled President María Estela "Isabel" Martínez de Perón the night before had been chivalrous. At 12:45 that morning, the forty-five-year-old President had boarded a helicopter to travel from the Casa Rosada, the rose-colored presidential palace on the Plaza de Mayo, to the presidential residence on the outskirts of the city. In the air, the pilot had told her that one of the turbines was not functioning properly and that they would have to land at the metropolitan airport. When the helicopter touched down, Perón was met on the tarmac by three military officers. "Señora, you are under arrest," one of them said.[3] He asked her to hand over her purse. He opened it, removed a small revolver, and returned the bag to her. As Isabel Perón sat smoking in a guarded lounge, an army van sped to her residence and returned with several suitcases that had been packed with clothes by her own servants. The officers then placed the deposed President aboard an air force jet and flew her across the pampas to a turreted lodge in the Andean foothills.

Isabel Perón's government was the fifth civilian government overthrown by the armed forces since 1930. In fact, since World War II no freely elected administration had lasted its full term except that of Isabel's husband, army general Juan Domingo Perón, who ruled the country from 1946 to 1955.

At the turn of the century, Argentina — with its fertile pampas, thriving cattle industry, railways, and ports — rivaled the United States as a magnet for Europeans seeking freedom and opportunity. Prosperity accelerated during World War II as war-torn Europe turned to Argentina for grain and cattle. The country started manufacturing many of the products it had previously imported and soon developed an industrial base that complemented Argentina's agricultural bounty. Gold reserves filled the Central Bank, and middle-class Argentines enjoyed a high standard of living.

In 1943 a clique of colonels, Juan Perón among them, seized power. From his posts as vice president and secretary of labor, Perón united the workers, who had been crowding the nation's cities to work in newly created factories where they were ill-paid and denied benefits. Like Benito Mussolini, Perón used his charisma to consolidate power. He soon built such a following that by the time elections were held in 1946, he won with 56 percent of the vote. Five years later, he was reelected by an even larger majority.

Perón ruled Argentina for nine years. He raised the workers' wages, built public schools for their children, and fueled their nationalistic pride by expropriating railroads and utilities built by the British. But if Perón offered himself as the worker's defender, it was his second wife, the fabled Evita, who became their saint.

A young, beautiful movie actress, Evita called herself "the bridge of love" between her husband and the workers — *mis descamisados* ("my shirtless ones"), as she referred to them.[4] Herself the product of poverty, she established a foundation in her name to improve the lives of workers, destitute women, and needy children. Unlike previous Argentine first ladies, Evita led rallies, visited slums, factories, and union headquarters, and went on the radio to urge workers to support her husband's economic policies. Then, in 1952, at the age of thirty-two, she died of cancer. Three years later Juan Perón, having lost control of the military, was ousted by a coup.

Perón had given the workers self-respect, but he had also polarized the country and turned Argentina's democracy into a sham. In the final years of his presidency, he imposed censorship, jailed and exiled political opponents, impeached members of the supreme court, intervened in the universities, and created a secret police.

After his ouster, Perón spent the next eighteen years in exile, first in Paraguay and then in Panama. He met his third wife, Isabel, in a Panama City nightclub, where she worked as a chorus girl. He continued his migration through a string of Latin American countries until 1960, when he finally settled in Spain.

Meanwhile, in Argentina the Peronist movement, although banned by successive military governments, had emerged as the standard-bearer for opposition to the armed forces. By the early 1970s, the various factions within Peronism — the far-left Montonero guerrillas, the conservative old-guard politicians, and the right-wing labor bosses — had put aside their quarrels and agreed to return their leader to power.

When Perón returned to Buenos Aires on June 20, 1973, hundreds of thousands of people thronged to greet him at Ezeiza airport. Drums, the pulse of any Peronist rally, thundered along the highway to the airport. But what should have been a celebration turned into a bloodbath. Right-wing Peronists were determined to control the event and maneuvered to plant their banners near the speakers' stand. When left-wing supporters pushed to get closer to the stand, gunfire erupted, then the sound of automatic weapons. The battle raged until dark, leaving hundreds dead or wounded.

As the mayhem at the airport presaged, Perón, now in his late seventies and increasingly feeble, could not control the Argentina he had called into being thirty years before. Even so, six months after his return the aging patriarch, with his wife as his running mate, was elected president of Argentina for a third time. Barely twelve months later, in July 1974, Perón died and Isabel assumed the presidency.

The Montoneros, having been expelled from the Peronist movement just before Perón died, went underground and declared war on Isabel's government. From their clandestine bases, usually houses and apartments in urban areas, Montonero leaders recruited new members from the university Peronist organizations and trade unions, leaving those activists who rejected violence vulnerable to right-wing death squads. To finance their revolution the guerrillas kidnapped wealthy industrialists for ransom, extorting $60 million in one celebrated case. In carefully executed maneuvers, they placed bombs in the homes of policemen and ambushed their cars, killing hundreds and leaving heaps of scorched metal in the streets as signatures of their handiwork.

In the final six months of her abbreviated term, Isabel Perón approved a gloves-off attack on the Montoneros and another terrorist organization, the Trotskyist *Ejército Revolucionario del Pueblo* (ERP), or People's Revolutionary Army. Though the ERP guerrillas numbered far fewer than the Montoneros, they carried out equally vicious assaults on military and police installations. In an effort to break the back of guerrilla insurgency, the police and right-wing groups organized themselves into private armies. Senior military officers hired bodyguards for their own protection, and also sent them out to abduct and murder leftist leaders and their families. One of Isabel's own ministers, José López Rega, known as El Brujo (The Sorcerer) because of his fascination with the occult, ran the notorious death squads of the Argentine Anti-Communist Alliance, or "Triple-A," from his office in the Ministry of Social Services on the Plaza de Mayo.

Buenos Aires became a city prowled by goons in unmarked cars, usually Ford Falcons with their license plates covered or missing. Inside, men with no fear of governmental reprisal — because, more often than not, they *were* the government — cradled sawed-off shotguns in their laps, their eyes invisible behind dark glasses. They called each other by nicknames: Tiburón (Shark), Víbora (Viper), Panza (Potbelly), Oso (Bear). They issued *"pasajes,"* or "tickets," as they jokingly described them, to their intended victims — one-way passages to the mortuary. By the end of 1975, they had eliminated as many as fifteen hundred people.

Isabel Perón's government could neither control nor salvage an ever more divided and violent country. According to one newspaper, during the last month of Isabel's tenure, there was a bomb attack every three hours and a political killing every five. When the military finally made a move, most of the nation sighed in relief.

The day after the March 1976 coup, a three-man junta placed army general Jorge Rafael Videla in the presidency. They also made it a crime, punishable with up to ten years in jail, for anyone to divulge news, communiqués, or views with the purpose of disrupting, prejudicing, or lessening the prestige of the armed forces. One evening a little less than a month later, Videla went on national television to present the military's program for the permanent restoration of order: "The Process of National Reorganization," or *El Proceso*.

Videla told millions of viewers that night that the junta would save the nation from "sectarianism, factionalism, and personalism." Gone were the days of *caudillos*, that old Argentine malady of strong-minded leaders. There would be no more Perón, no single passion-inspiring demagogue, to poison the country's social order. Instead, the junta would calmly and methodically create a whole new society: Christian, moral, antisubversive, secure, with a restructured economy and an educational system designed "to meet the nation's needs."

Eventually, the junta would leave, Videla declared. And democracy would work.

In the name of El Proceso, the junta dissolved congress, banned political parties and labor unions, suspended the activities of business organizations and professional associations, and replaced the members of the supreme court. It appointed retired and active military officers as university rectors and presidents. The junta liked clean walls, so it had the slogans scrubbed off the concrete walls of the universities.

The junta called its antisubversive campaign the *guerra sucia* ("dirty war"), a genuine if twisted reference to the guerrilla tactics of unannounced bombings and kidnappings. But as it soon became apparent, it was the junta that would bypass all legal channels to "win" a war declared against its own people.

Relying on an extensive intelligence network, military and police death squads, known as *grupos de tareas* (task forces), began to operate out of a labyrinth of 360 secret detention centers.[5] These squads abducted thousands of people suspected of sympathizing with the insurgents. Many were arrested because their names were similar to someone else's or because they happened to appear in a suspect's address book. Others disappeared simply because they were journalists or psychiatrists or social workers in some slum. Lawyers vanished because they filed habeas corpus petitions on behalf of those who were abducted and made to disappear. No one summed up the military's philosophy more succinctly, or chillingly, than President General Videla, who explained to foreign journalists in December 1977 that "a terrorist is not just someone with a gun or a bomb, but someone who spreads ideas that are contrary to Western and Christian civilization."[6]

More than ten thousand people disappeared during the seven years of military rule that ended in 1983. Often blindfolded and spirited away in Ford Falcons, detainees would arrive at a secret detention center, where a guard would assign them a number and lead them to a cell. The task forces called such an operation a *chupada*, literally, to "suck up" or "swallow" people. Most of those taken were tortured — given "intensive therapy" or "softened up," as their torturers liked to call it. Antonio Horacio Miño Retamozo, one of the few who survived "disappearance," later described the torture he suffered in August 1976:

> At the [Federal Security Headquarters] I was taken straight to the *parrilla* (grill). That is, I was tied to the metal frame of a bed, electrodes were attached to my hands and feet, and they

ran an electric prod all over me, with particular savagery and intensity on the genitals. . . . When on the "grill" one jumps, twists, moves about, and tries to avoid contact with the burning, cutting iron bars. The electric prod was handled like a scalpel and the "specialist" would be guided by a doctor who would tell him if I could take any more. . . . The worst was having electrodes on the teeth — it felt as if a thunderbolt was blowing your head to pieces. . . .[7]

Elena Alfaro, a detainee held at the El Vesubio center, was made to watch the torture of her husband. A fellow prisoner, Irma Beatriz Márquez, was forced to witness the torture of her twelve-year-old son, Pablo.[8] "Of all the dramatic situations I witnessed in prison," wrote editor and author Jacobo Timerman of the horrors he suffered and observed in detention from 1977 to 1979, "none can compare with those family groups who were tortured often together, sometimes separately but in view of one another. . . . The entire [world of affection], constructed over the years with utmost difficulty, collapses with a kick in the father's genitals . . . or the sexual violation of a daughter."[9]

Many detainees, particularly the elderly, died under torture. Some were eventually freed or transferred to officially recognized jails or prisons. Most, however, were secretly executed without charge or trial. The task forces disposed of the bodies in ways that, they believed, would conceal the crimes. They dropped some victims from military aircraft over the Atlantic or into the estuary of the River Plate. Survivors at the Navy Mechanics School in Buenos Aires, among the most notorious detention centers, recall that prisoners were often drugged before being removed from the center and thrown into the sea.[10] The joke among the military was that they were dumping "fish food." Sometimes the corpses washed up along the Argentine and Uruguayan coasts. Other victims were incinerated in crematoria or open pits. One police officer later testified that at a secret detention center called El Banco, the police "made what they called 'traps,' which were rectangular pits fifty or sixty centimeters deep and two meters long. I saw these pits, the size of a person. . . . They put human bodies inside these pits, sprinkled them with petrol . . . and burnt them to ashes."[11]

In most cases, however, military or police squads delivered the bodies of their victims to municipal morgues, where the police surgeon gave them a brisk examination. Many morgue workers were well aware of the atrocities committed around them. Army trucks would arrive at morgues late at night, carrying bodies, often mutilated and bearing signs of torture. Officers ordered the morgue workers not to perform autopsies and simply to register the bodies as "N.N.," for "no name." These were usually buried in unmarked graves.

One of the most graphic accounts of the way the military and police disposed of their victims is contained in a plea to improve working conditions sent to President General Videla on June 30, 1980, by the staff of the Judicial Morgue in the city of Córdoba. The seven-page, typed letter contains this passage:

> It is impossible, Mr. President, to give a true picture of what we experienced when we opened the doors of the rooms where the corpses were kept. Some of the bodies had been stored for more than thirty days without any sort of refrigeration. There was a cloud of flies and the floor was covered in a layer about 10.5 centimeters deep in worms and larvae, which we cleared away with buckets and shovels. The only clothes we had were trousers, overalls, boots and gloves, while some people had to do the work in their ordinary clothes. . . . With morgue staff and technical autopsy assistants travelling in the back of the truck beside the corpses and a guard of two Provincial Police cars which had been assigned to the operation, we went to San Vicente cemetery. The sight which met us at the cemetery was horrible. The police cars lit up the common grave where the bodies were deposited, identified by number and using the pillars in a nearby wall as reference points. Behind this and even from the roof tops the neighbors watched the macabre task in progress.[12]

The workers at the Córdoba morgue returned frequently to the mass grave. They would watch as a backhoe, kept permanently at the site, widened the pit. "After the first batches came more of five, eight, seven," recalled Francisco Rubén Bossio, one of the autopsy technicians who had signed the petition.[13] "The bodies had bullet wounds, some with a lot of perforations, sometimes as many as eighty. . . . They all had painted fingers [apparently for fingerprinting purposes] and bore clear marks of torture. They had marks on their hands as if they had been tied with cords."

Bossio and his colleagues apologized in their letter to the president for bothering him but explained that everybody else in the line of command had already been notified about this situation and had failed to respond. The crushing work load had not let up, not for a single weekend in years. Couldn't the president do something? The workers desperately needed help. They wanted more time off — and a raise.

The Córdoba petition bears a stamp — *Presidencia de la Nación* — and scribbled under it, in the "received" box, is the date July 1980. Had one of Videla's assistants failed to show him the letter? Or had the President read it and simply tossed it aside? The morgue workers never heard a word in response.

President General Videla may have ignored the Córdoba complaint, but he couldn't have overlooked the curious event that took place across the street from the presidential palace three years earlier on the afternoon of Saturday, April 13, 1977.

The Casa Rosada sits on the east side of the Plaza de Mayo. From its gray-shuttered windows on the second floor one can see the full length of the square. A cobbled walkway, lined with flower beds and olive green lampposts, stretches from the palace's main entrance to the Cabildo, the old town hall, at the far end of the plaza. A statue of a woman bearing a shield stands atop a narrow obelisk in the center of the square, a monument representing the republic. The circular garden at the base of the pyramid contains soil from the country's twenty-two provinces.

At three o'clock that Saturday afternoon, fourteen middle-aged and elderly women converged on the Plaza de Mayo and filled its wooden benches. When the Cabildo clock tower struck the half hour, the women — all mothers whose children had disappeared — withdrew white kerchiefs from their purses and wrapped them over their heads. Rising from the benches, they silently gathered around the statue and began walking slowly in a circle.

The vigil marked the creation of the *Madres de la Plaza de Mayo* — Mothers of the Plaza de Mayo. Many of the women had first become acquainted in the dark-paneled waiting room at the Interior Ministry or outside the offices of police stations and military barracks, where they had gone to seek information about their missing children.

Within a year hundreds of women began appearing at the weekly demonstration. Among the demonstrators were dozens who protested the disappearance not only of their sons and daughters but of their grandchildren as well. These women eventually formed their own organization, the *Abuelas de Plaza de Mayo* — Grandmothers of the Plaza de Mayo. All told, at least three-hundred children had fallen into the hands of Argentina's warlords. They called them *botín de guerra* — war booty. Many of the children, perhaps most, were born to young women while they were being held in the secret detention centers. Others had been abducted with one or both parents who were later killed. The kidnappers treated the children like the objects — wristwatches, radios, antique vases, televisions, spare change — that they looted during raids. Some children were sold on the black market, while others were given to childless military and police families or abandoned by their kidnappers at the entrances of hospitals and orphanages.

Although the military generally treated the Madres as merely a nuisance, it was not above retaliating when the movement became too visible. In late 1977 the Madres' vice president, Azucena Villaflor de Vicenti, was abducted while leaving her home. Days later, two French nuns, Leonie Renee Duquet and Alice Domon, along with several Madres and their supporters, were kidnapped by men in Ford Falcons at the Santa Cruz church in Buenos Aires. No one taken that night was ever seen again.

Scorned or ignored by much of Argentina, the Madres and Abuelas managed to gain the attention of the foreign press and Amnesty International. Amnesty launched a worldwide campaign, calling on its members to send "politely worded appeals" to the Argentine authorities for an accounting of the disappeared. In response, angry Argentine supporters of the military inundated the organization's London headquarters with postcards supplied by a popular Argentine magazine. Mocking the concept of *derechos humanos*, or human rights, the postcards read: "*Nosotros los Argentinos somos derechos y humanos*" ("We Argentines are upright and humane"). Argentine officials angrily denied that anyone was being held in unofficial custody and charged that the so-called disappeared were all guerrillas or their sympathizers who had broken with their families and gone underground, or else had fled to Europe where they were living it up in Paris or Madrid.

Gradually, as evidence mounted that the government had sanctioned abduction, torture, and execution, its ministers began to talk of "mistakes" and "excesses." On September 12, 1979, the government presented its solution: the Law on Presumption of Death Because of Disappearance. The decree enabled the state (as well as relatives) to declare dead anyone registered as missing between November 6, 1974, and September 12, 1979. Minister of the Interior Albano Jorge Harguindeguy, an army general who was one of the authors of the new legislation, announced that the intention of the law was "to regularize the rights of missing persons," as well as those of their spouses and next of kin.[14] Now widows and widowers of the disappeared, he suggested, could put their estates in order, perhaps remarry, and begin new lives. But behind the law's veneer of practicality skulked its real purpose: to impede any future investigation into the fate of the disappeared.

By 1981 El Proceso had lost its momentum. Even supporters of the military takeover were growing weary of military rule. The government had failed to improve the economy and the world, it seemed, was denouncing Argentina as a monster that ate its own young. In March the junta swore in a second military President, General Roberto Eduardo Viola, former army chief of staff. Months later, a palace coup replaced Viola with Lieutenant General Leopoldo Galtieri, the dipsomaniacal commander of the army. Galtieri made economic reform his first priority by vowing to put a tourniquet on Argentina's hemorrhaging foreign debt, which had risen from $6.4 billion in 1976, when the military took over, to $30 billion in 1981. But his government's austerity measures only fueled more distrust for the military. Argentines, shaking off their lethargy and fear, rose up in a series of strikes and mass protests demanding a better standard of living and a return to civilian rule.

On April 2, 1982, Galtieri landed a thousand troops on the Falkland Islands, or Islas Malvinas, as the Argentines prefer to call them, a cluster of windswept islands that had been the object of a 150-year-old territorial dispute between Argentina and Great Britain. Britain's Prime Minister Margaret Thatcher surprised Galtieri by sending troops to recapture the Falklands. As the battle unfolded on the barren South Atlantic islands three hundred miles off the tip of Patagonia, Argentines united in a brief crescendo of nationalistic euphoria. But Galtieri's inability to predict British resolve and American loyalties, which went with Thatcher, ultimately led to Argentina's humiliating defeat.

On June 16, two days after the last Argentine garrison surrendered, the junta cashiered Galtieri and, shortly thereafter, appointed retired major general Reynaldo Bignone as president. Bignone, faced with violent antimilitary demonstrations, lifted the six-year ban on political activity and promised elections in late 1983. Before leaving office the caretaker president took care to declare an amnesty for all those who might be brought to trial for crimes committed in the "dirty war."

Bignone kept his promise to return Argentina to civilian rule and on October 30, 1983, Argentines went to the polls. To the surprise of almost everyone, Raúl Alfonsín, a fifty-seven-year-old former small-town lawyer, and his Radical party won the election easily, overwhelming the Peronist candidate, Italo Luder.

Alfonsín took office in December 1983. Within the first few weeks of his administration, the new leader retired dozens of generals and, after persuading congress to nullify the military's self-amnesty law, ordered the prosecution of the junta leaders. Alfonsín also created a blue-ribbon panel of prominent Argentines chaired by the novelist Ernesto Sábato to probe the fate of the disappeared.

In his inaugural address to congress on December 10, 1983 — International Human Rights Day — Alfonsín preached an old-fashioned liberal ethic of moderation, decency, and the rule of law. "Today public immorality has ended," he said. "We are going to build a decent government." But the loudest applause came when he called for the "dismantling of the state's repressive machinery."[15] Then, riding with his wife in a 1954 Cadillac convertible that had previously served President Juan Perón, Alfonsín traveled to the Plaza de Mayo and climbed the steps to the Casa Rosada. Once inside the palace, he received the presidential sash from General Bignone. Facing the Plaza de Mayo, from which Perón had stirred the multitudes and the generals had spread terror, Alfonsín addressed a crowd of one hundred thousand people. "It is a happy coincidence," he began, "that this day on which we Argentines are beginning a century of peace, liberty, and democracy should also be Human Rights Day." The crowd roared its approval.

On the morning of June 9, 1984, a young Argentine by the name of Morris Tidball Binz strode through the wide cobblestone streets of the city of La Plata on his way to work. Dressed in jeans and a white woolen sweater, his straight blond bangs falling across blue eyes, he looked more like a ski instructor from Colorado than a third-year medical student from the pampas. Near the city's central plaza, Tidball stopped to read a sign taped to a door. Handwritten in bold black letters, it read:

SEMINAR ON THE FORENSIC SCIENCES
AND THE DISAPPEARED
SPONSORED BY
THE NATIONAL COMMISSION ON DISAPPEARED PERSONS
AND
THE AMERICAN ASSOCIATION FOR THE ADVANCEMENT OF SCIENCE
ALL WELCOME

Curious, Tidball swung open the door and made his way to the auditorium, where he took a seat and quickly surveyed the audience. He recognized Juan Ramos Padilla, the bearded young judge who was helping the Grandmothers locate their disappeared grandchildren. On the stage sat five American scientists. A young woman was interpreting for one of them, a tall aristocratic-looking man whose nameplate on the speakers' table bore the name Luke Tedeschi. The interpreter knew very little English and was struggling to keep up. Suddenly she broke down in tears and said that she couldn't go on. Tidball, whose schooling in English had been seasoned with a year's travel in the United States, offered his services.

Tidball's knowledge of English and medical terms served him well. He finished translating Tedeschi's presentation on the physical consequences of torture and then interpreted for Leslie Lukash, a forensic pathologist from Nassau County, New York. The pathologist spoke about the virtues of the independent medical examiner's system and its ability to safeguard against partiality and official coercion. Next, Tidball translated for Clyde Snow, a Texan, he thought, judging from his accent and cowboy boots. After Snow finished, Tidball relayed questions from the audience. Near the end of the session, a man stood up and asked Snow if scientists could determine whether or not an empty coffin had ever contained the remains of a five-month-old baby. Perplexed, Snow looked at Tidball, who repeated the question. Sure, it might be possible, Snow replied, and then moved on to the next question.

Later, as the auditorium was emptying, the man approached Snow and introduced himself as Juan Miranda.

"Doctor, I know my question confused you," he said as Tidball interpreted. "But if I could just explain. You see, it is very important to us, to me and my wife. The baby I mentioned, she's our grand-daughter. If you have a minute . . ."

The disappearance of Juan Miranda's granddaughter took place on a September night in 1976. Just before midnight, soldiers arrived at the house of his daughter and son-in-law, Roberto Lanuscou, both suspected Montoneros, in San Isidro, a suburb of Buenos Aires. The soldiers opened fire with guns and then stormed the house. Neighbors heard more gunshots inside, then the sound of a baby crying as the soldiers left. The next day, a local newspaper carried photographs of the bullet-riddled house and an official statement saying that the army had killed five "extremists" in a shootout. That puzzled the Lanuscous' neighbors, who knew them as a quiet if reclusive family with two children aged six and four and a five-month-old baby. The newspaper account made no mention of the family's whereabouts.

Years after the incident, the Mirandas and the parents of Roberto Lanuscou went to the office of the Abuelas in downtown Buenos Aires. They brought with them copies of five death certificates that they had recovered, with the assistance of their lawyer, from the Boulogne Cemetery in San Isidro. The certificates were dated September 5, 1976, two days after the raid, and signed by a physician, presumably employed by the cemetery. Each certificate was marked with an "N.N." and contained physical descriptions that matched those of the Lanuscou family. Cause of death for the mother and the three children was "a single gunshot wound to the head," whereas the father died of "multiple wounds." The cemetery's log stated that workers buried the five bodies in separate caskets in a common grave.

With the assistance of the Abuelas, the grandparents of the Lanus-cou children eventually convinced a judge to order the graves opened. On the afternoon of January 25, 1984, gravediggers went down the line of five graves, unearthing casket after casket and piling up the bones on a plastic sheet. When they reached the smallest grave, they raised a tiny wooden coffin. Prying open the lid, they found only a small green blanket, a faded rose-colored baby's jumper, a pacifier, and a pair of little socks.

At this point in his story, Miranda paused and looked at Tidball and then Snow.

"Dr. Snow, is it possible that Matilde's bones had dissolved?" he asked.

"Well," Snow replied, "it's impossible, unless the soil was highly acidic. But I'd have to look at the casket and clothing to be sure."

Miranda smiled and his eyes glistened as Tidball translated Snow's reply.

"Thank you, Dr. Snow. Thank you," Miranda said, rising from his seat and clasping the anthropologist's hand in his own. As he left, Snow turned to his young interpreter.

"Your name's Morris, right?"

"Yes."

"Well, Morris, how would you like a job?"

"A job?"

"Yeah, as my assistant. I'll need help if I go out to look at that baby's coffin."

Tidball eyed the American anthropologist suspiciously, uncertain of how deeply he wanted to get involved in this business.

"Well, think about it," Snow said as he rose to join his colleagues.

Snow and his colleagues had come to Argentina at the request of Alfonsín's human rights commission, the National Commission on the Disappeared (CONADEP), to meet with judges, morgue workers, human rights activists, and relatives of the disappeared. At the end of the trip, the scientists were to formulate recommendations for the commission on the best means of exhuming and identifying the remains of the disappeared. It was a tall order for a ten-day tour.

The Americans learned from their hosts that during military rule families of the disappeared had been virtually helpless in their attempts to determine the fate of their loved ones. In a few cases, morgue officials informed families of the death of a detained relative and provided a grave plot number. Even so, judges were generally unwilling, either out of fear or indifference, to order exhumations for forensic examination. That changed shortly after Alfonsín took power in 1983 and established CONADEP. Its commissioners, along with several judges, ordered hundreds of N.N. graves excavated. Cemetery gravediggers aided by heavy earth-moving equipment performed the exhumations.

The result was disastrous. As bulldozers and workers with spades and shovels heaped mounds of bones next to the opened graves, the callous mishandling of the remains drew angry protests from the families of the disappeared. Human rights lawyers also recognized that little usable forensic evidence would be recovered from these grisly harvests. In early February 1984, representatives of two human rights groups — the Grandmothers of the Plaza de Mayo and the Center for Social and Legal Studies — met with CONADEP and urged them to seek help from the AAAS.

After their first seminar in La Plata, the American scientists traveled to Buenos Aires and then to Córdoba, one of Argentina's largest and most beautiful cities. East of Córdoba lies the open expanse of the pampas. To the north, south, and west, green hills undulate toward the Andes. Hidden among the sierras are vast estates with carefully tended lawns that reach down to small lakes. It was near one of these lakes, Lago San Roque, that the Third Army Corp operated La Perla, a concentration camp sometimes called the Auschwitz of Argentina. Nearly three thousand people passed through the camp between 1976 and 1979. Camp guards executed many of the detainees and buried some of the bodies in a pit a short distance from the camp. Others were sent by truck to the San Vicente Cemetery, on the outskirts of Córdoba.

Late in the morning on the day after their arrival in the city, the Americans visited the cemetery. "We froze our asses off talking to those gravediggers," recalls one member of the scientific delegation, odontologist Lowell Levine. "I'll never forget — they brought out the cemetery superintendent. He was lightly dressed as if he didn't think he was going to be there long, with the cold wind blowing.

Well, we got him talking, and the colder he got, the more forthcoming he became."[16]

The superintendent led the Americans through rows of tombstones to an open area about eighty feet long and sixteen feet wide. It was here, he said, that scores of *desaparecidos* had been buried in the mid- to late 1970s. In 1979, after the last burial, cemetery workers leveled and seeded the surface. It had been all but forgotten until early 1984, when a group of lawyers representing families of the disappeared persuaded a court to investigate the site.

For one of the lawyers, a short, soft-spoken man named Ruben Arroyo, the pit at San Vicente was something of a personal obsesssion. He believed that one of the bodies in the mass grave belonged to Cristina Costanzo, the daughter of an old friend. Arroyo had known her since she was an infant. And if his information was correct, Cristina, along with six of her friends, had been buried there in 1976.

Arroyo intensified his investigation after his appointment as legal counsel to the Córdoba office of CONADEP in January 1984. His new position gave him greater access to cemetery and morgue records, as well as to police files. Gradually he pieced together the fate of Cristina and the others. Their tragic story, he learned, began on October 14, 1976.

Early that morning police agents in the city of Rosario, three hundred miles east of Córdoba, picked up Cristina and several of her friends in separate raids around the city. The reasons for their arrest are unclear, but some of them may have been members of a banned organization, the University Peronist Youth Movement. After detainment at the police station, all but two of them were killed.

One of the survivors, Gustavo Piccolo, later described to a CONADEP investigator what he had witnessed at the station.[17] Shortly after his arrival, he said, he was tortured for hours with the *picana* — the cattle prod — and then led to a cell. It was there that he met his childhood friend, Carlos Pérez Risso. Pérez told Piccolo he had been picked up with Cristina Costanzo, who was in the adjacent cell. Piccolo eventually learned that there were nine detainees, including himself, in the cell block. He gave one of them, who was naked from the waist up, his woolen jacket.

Three days later, in the early morning, guards stormed through the cell block, shouting out names and pulling people to their feet.

"I guess I wasn't taken because my uncle was a federal judge," Piccolo told the commission. Nor was Pérez, who was also well-connected through his father, a police commissioner. Later that afternoon, Piccolo heard a group of men enter the cell block. One of them told a guard that "the operation in Los Surgentes had been carried out without a hitch."

The following day, a police patrol found seven bullet-riddled bodies in a field near the town of Los Surgentes, at the boundary dividing the provinces of Córdoba and Santa Fé. The police fingerprinted the bodies and sent them to the Córdoba city morgue, where they were registered as N.N.s and transferred to the San Vicente Cemetery.

On March 3, 1984, three months before the arrival of the American scientists, a federal judge arrived at the cemetery and ordered a small part of the mass grave opened. With him was a former cemetery foreman who pointed out the spot where he recalled burying the seven bodies.[18] A backhoe peeled away the rocky soil and cemetery workers picked dozens of skulls and bones from the dirt.

By late afternoon heaps of bones surrounded the site. The judge called the workers out of the pit and ordered them to place the remains into large polyurethane bags. They were then transported to the city morgue.

The Córdoba morgue was not Leslie Lukash's idea of a well-run operation. "To see that foul-smelling place," he recalls, "was disgusting."[19] As Lukash gnashed his teeth, the rest of the American delegation politely questioned the morgue's head pathologist, Dr. Héctor Alfredo Camara, about how he and his staff had managed during the military years. Spreading open the morgue ledger, he showed the Americans page after page of N.N. entries. Many of the entries bore his signature. Yes, he'd signed out the disappeared ones. He'd had no choice, after all.

"I tried to be very nonjudgmental about it," Levine remembers. "I didn't know if Camara and his staff were acting in concert with the murderers or if they were coerced into signing things out. Obviously, they had to know what was going on. Nobody could be that dumb. . . . So, obviously, they were party to the people becoming N.N.s. . . . They told us about the night they brought a truck in there with twenty-seven bodies with blood flowing out of the truck's tailgate. They were told to bury them and the medical examiner was told to sign them out. Well, [the morgue staff] had wives and kids. And if there are twenty-seven bodies in a truck, an extra one wasn't going to make any difference. . . . So the fear was very real . . . and, very candidly, if somebody told me, 'Listen, you've got two sons and we know exactly where they are, and they'll be the next ones in the hole,' I don't know what I'd do. I'd like to think I'd know what I'd do, but damn it, nobody can ever say."[20]

Camara eventually led his visitors to an examining room, where his staff had assembled. Thirty-eight plastic bags, bulging like sacks of potatoes, lined the floor along the tiled walls. Here and there, bones had fallen out and lay, collecting dust, on the grimy floor.

Snow asked Camara if any families had sent in antemortem records. The pathologist motioned to a young man, the morgue's consultant dentist, Gaston Fontaine, who handed Snow a small brown envelope. This was all they'd received, the dentist explained. Snow opened the packet and fished out a dental chart and three dental X rays, each marked with the name Cristina Noemí Costanzo and dated September 1975, a year before her disappearance. On the chart, the girl's dentist had written her birthdate: August 12, 1951. The girl had died just two months after her twenty-fifth birthday.

Snow asked Camara if he and Levine could examine the skulls. Camara nodded and several sacks were set on the examining table. Snow and Levine moved the skulls across the marble slab like chess pieces, grouping them first by sex and then, as best they could, by age. Many bore the executioner's signature — a single gunshot wound in the back of the head.

Eventually they singled out a skull and mandible that roughly fit Costanzo's age range. Several teeth had been lost at the exhumation, making it impossible to match the dental chart with the fillings in the skull's teeth. Luckily, though, enough of the teeth shown in the antemortem X rays were still intact to compare with X rays they could take of the mandible.

"The next problem was where could we X-ray the teeth, as it was getting late in the day," Levine remembers. "Well, Fontaine, the morgue's dentist, who's been watching us with great interest, steps forward and says he's got an X-ray machine in his living room at home. As it turns out, he's been saving his money to open a dental office. It was the first thing he'd bought."

At eleven o'clock that evening, Levine met Fontaine at his apartment and they began X-raying the teeth. The Argentine was nervous. He confessed to Levine that he wanted out of forensic work. The pay was terrible, he said, and at times, the job was downright dangerous. Yes, things were better under the new government, he conceded, but just being associated with the disappeared, even as a scientist, could mark him forever.

Levine returned to his hotel in the early hours of the morning and immediately called Snow's room. "It was her, all right," he told the anthropologist. "The fillings were identical, the root shapes, the bone trabecular pattern. There's no doubt about it, Clyde. Cristina Costanzo was buried in that grave."

That afternoon Levine went to the old stone building that housed CONADEP's offices in Córdoba. "Arroyo was there. So I went through how we had identified Cristina. Then he spoke. He must have talked for an hour as Marita, the interpreter, whispered the translation. He said he had known Cristina since she was born. Her father was an old friend. He talked about attending her confirmation. And that after Cristina disappeared, her father had retained him to find her. He had been looking for her for seven years. His final words were, 'So this, Doctor, closes the circle.' " Levine found his hands trembling as he opened the door. Stepping out onto the cobbled street, he looked up past the rows of whitewashed houses to the hills. Christ, he thought, any one of those kids could have been one of my boys. Moving his hand to his face as if to shade it from the sun, he wept.

When the American scientists returned to Buenos Aires, they found Morris Tidball waiting for them at their hotel. Ramos Padilla, the aggresive young judge handling the Lanuscou case, wanted Snow to examine the family's remains and would send a car for him first thing in the morning. Tidball had even called a friend, a physician, who'd agreed to let Snow use the X-ray facilities at the San Isidro hospital.

The next morning, in a small, dimly lit room of the cemetery morgue in San Isidro, Snow sifted through the Lanuscou remains. Sorting the bones by size and indications of sex and age, he reconstructed the skeletons of Roberto and Barbara Lanuscou and their two eldest children. He failed, however, to find any bones of the five-month-old baby, Matilde, even after X rays were taken of the baby's clothing and the lining of the casket.[21]

"Matilde was never in that coffin," Snow told Ramos Padilla. "It's as simple as that."

What had happened to her?

The commission on the disappeared had at least a partial answer, one suggesting that Matilde was still alive. Its source was a car salesman named Hugo Ciarroca who at the time of Matilde's abduction in 1976 had been supplying the navy with cars for their kidnapping operations.[22] Ciarroca told the commission that in late 1976 — he couldn't remember the exact date — he had delivered a Peugot 504 to the naval dockyard in Buenos Aires. He turned the car over to an officer and a nurse, a tall, redheaded woman called Gabriela. On previous deliveries he had learned that she was in charge of the kidnapped children. As Ciarroca chatted with a guard, Gabriela and the officer loaded three babies into the backseat and drove out of the compound. Later, the guard told Ciarroca that the babies were being taken to the navy hospital for medical attention. After that, they would be adopted by military families. The guard also said that one of the babies was called "Lacanau or Lanascau or something like that" and had been taken during a raid in San Isidro.

The Grandmothers of the Plaza de Mayo were pleased with Snow's findings on the Lanuscou remains. From an assortment of bones the anthropologist had salvaged a glimmer of hope: just possibly, Matilde was now a seven-year-old girl.

Hope had turned these women into detectives. Over the years, they had examined thousands of pages of public documents, conducted stakeouts, and gone undercover in their search for clues. In one case, a grandmother had even worked as a maid in the home of a military couple whom she believed had adopted her grandchild. By June 1984, the Abuelas had located twenty-five missing children.

Sleuthing was easy compared to convincing the courts that the children were biologically related to the grandparents who claimed them. As Chicha Chorbik de Mariani, the president of the Abuelas, recalls:

The quandary we faced had been born in the uncertainty of how we would identify the first two little girls we located in 1980. We had photos and other evidence, but that wasn't enough. The judge wanted more. It had been three years since their kidnapping and they were taller and of course they had aged. And so we asked ourselves, "What are we going to do with children who were born in detention?" In some cases, we didn't know their sex, or even to whom they belonged. Well, we thought of everything possible. For instance, I had cut locks of hair from my granddaughter before she was kidnapped. I sent them to Amnesty International to see if they could be used to identify her. I received a reply saying it would be difficult, particularly because the hair had been cut many years before and because it didn't contain follicles. Other grandmothers asked, "I have a baby's tooth which I've kept of my grandchild, could it be used in identifying him or her?" Then one day in 1981 I read an article in *El Diario del Día*, a newspaper in La Plata, that said scientists had found a way of identifying a person through analysis of the blood. Well, I didn't understand all the scientific terms but the gist of it was that there was an element in the blood that repeated itself only within the same family. I cut it out. And when I traveled abroad I'd take it with me. I asked scientists and doctors and scientific institutes if this new discovery would help us identify our missing grandchildren.[23]

In October 1983, during a visit to Washington, D.C., Mariani posed the question to the American Association for the Advancement of Science, which relayed it to Mary-Claire King, a geneticist from the University of California at Berkeley. As the Grandmothers had hoped, King replied that thanks to numerous and highly specific "genetic markers" — including human leukocyte antigens (HLA), blood groups, red-cell enzymes, plasma proteins, and variations of sequences in DNA — grandpaternity, like paternity, could be determined with a high degree of certainty.[24]

The biological basis of the approach is that whereas a child's clothes, name, and hair color can be altered, the genes never change. Thus the evidence for relationship of a child to his family remains with that child and his relatives forever.

The procedure for determining that relationship is straightforward. Small blood samples are taken from the individuals who might be related. The cells of the adults and the child are tested for matching genetic markers. When certain markers match, scientists can say how likely it is that the adults and the child are related. The most reliable system for this analysis uses HLA proteins, which are found in white blood cells.

Mary-Claire King traveled to Argentina with the AAAS delegation in June 1984 and met with the Grandmothers of the Plaza de Mayo. They introduced her to Ana María Di Lonardo, an immunologist at the Durand Hospital in Buenos Aires. Together, the two women developed an HLA-based test for grandpaternity. A judge, meanwhile, agreed that the scientists could apply the test in the case of a suspected kidnap victim.

The case involved an eight-year-old girl named Paula Eva Logares, who was living with a former police chief, Rubén Lavallén, and his Uruguayan girlfriend. In court the couple claimed that Paula was their biological daughter. To prove it, they produced a birth certificate signed by a police surgeon. A fellow policeman testified that he was the owner of the house where the birth had taken place.

The Abuelas argued that the couple and their cohorts were lying and that the certificate was bogus. The true story, they argued, began on the afternoon of May 18, 1978. On that day, heavily armed men kidnapped Paula, then twenty-three months old, and her parents, Claudio and Monica Logares, who were never seen again. The first sign of Paula came in April 1980 when the Grandmothers received an unmarked packet. In it were photos of a small girl bearing a remarkable resemblance to Paula. An address included with the photos indicated that she was living in the home of Rubén Lavallén. Paula's maternal grandmother, Elsa Pavón, was certain that the girl in the photos was her granddaughter.

Anxious to see Paula, Pavón would stand for hours outside the Lavalléns' apartment building near the botanical gardens in Buenos

Aires. One day she caught sight of the child walking through the park with a woman in her early forties. She followed them until they slipped out of sight. When she returned weeks later, a For Rent sign had been posted on the apartment door.

In late 1983 the Abuelas, emboldened by the military's defeat in the Malvinas, launched a campaign to find Paula. Photographs of the little girl appeared in newspapers and on posters tacked to telephone poles. Then one day Pavón received an anonymous phone call from someone who lived in the same building as Paula. The caller gave Pavón the address of a ground-floor apartment near the Chacarita Cemetery.

Pavón resumed her vigil, but she feared now that if the Lavalléns were aware of the search they might leave the country. Two days after Alfonsín took office, Pavón, having learned that the couple planned to spend the Christmas holiday in Uruguay, turned to the courts. The Federal Criminal Court issued an order prohibiting Paula's departure from the country.

Besides Paula, three of her putative grandparents, including Elsa Pavón, were alive in 1984. Pavón's husband had died years earlier, but his HLA could be reconstructed from two of their children. The Lavalléns refused to be tested, a right guaranteed them under Argentine law. As Rubén Lavallén later told a reporter, "I was unfamiliar with this kind of analysis, [and] when it became clear that it was a humiliation for us and our own daughter, I decided I wouldn't go through with it. I won't allow anybody, anybody, to question my fatherhood, especially since I've seen this child leave my wife's womb. No way will I submit to such tests."[25]

King and Di Lonardo established a 99.9 percent certainty on the basis of HLA testing and blood groups that Paula was a descendant of the grandparents who claimed her. Six months later, she was legally removed from the Lavalléns' home and returned to Elsa Pavón.

W. H. Auden once wrote: "Through art, we are able to break bread with the dead, and without communion with the dead a fully human life is impossible." Had Auden been a forensic scientist and not a poet he might have chosen the word "science" instead of "art." Either way, Auden's notion that the living have a responsibility to learn from the dead is shared by both the arts and sciences. And though the dead may speak softly, only failure to listen and interpret the evidence can dishonor their final testament. It was this message that Snow and his colleagues wished to leave with their Argentine hosts.

On June 16, the day before their departure, the Americans held a press conference. They called on the Argentine government to declare a moratorium on all exhumations and to establish a national forensic center dedicated to the scientific investigation of the disappeared. One grave excavated using archaeological techniques, they argued, would yield more evidence than several hundred demolished by bulldozers.

Argentina's search for the disappeared was locked in a race against time. Many medical and dental records had already been discarded. Most others were incomplete: more than half of the disappeared were between twenty and thirty years old, an age group that generally receives little medical care and thus leaves few antemortem records. Moreover, most of the disappeared had been buried eight years earlier, and hair and clothing were decomposing, erasing vital clues. Such evidence was critical to the conviction of those responsible for these deaths.

Why dig them up? From a humanitarian perspective, the scientists said, families would finally know the fate of their lost ones and be able to give them a proper burial. In addition, through forensic documentation and subsequent litigation, the knowledge that governments can be held accountable for their actions may deter such practices in the future, both in Argentina and elsewhere.

Snow, however, doubted if Argentine forensic scientists, most of whom were police surgeons, were really ready to start exhuming graves and conducting scientifically sound investigations. As far as Snow could tell, the country's medicolegal system had changed little since the nineteenth century and was as rickety as an old buckboard. Besides, the mishandling of the exhumations had already cast a pall over the country's forensic community, leaving the families of the disappeared leery of its motives. Even special techniques such as facial reconstruction or video superimposition would be of little use. Facial reconstructions would mostly look the same: Caucasoids, primarily males, in their early twenties. The sheer number of disappeared, perhaps as many as fifteen thousand, guaranteed that even a single reconstruction displayed in a newspaper would attract hundreds of mothers claiming that this was the face of their son or daughter.

Still, Snow's misgivings didn't prevent him from signing up for one last assignment before he left Argentina. Several days before the delegation's departure, Ramos Padilla, impressed by Snow's work on the Lanuscou case, approached him again. During their visit, the Americans had given their hosts an earful about how not to exhume graves. Now Ramos Padilla was asking Snow what any good Texan would: put your money where your mouth is and show us how you would do it.

Ramos Padilla presented Snow with the case of a thirty-three-year-old woman named Rosa Rufina Betti de Casagrande, who had been abducted on November 13, 1976. If the judge's information was correct, she had been buried in the Boulogne cemetery as an N.N. in early 1977. Snow agreed to exhume the grave. But, he said, they would need archaeologists to plan the dig; he was a bone man first, an excavator only by default.

Several days of telephoning produced nothing. None of the archaeologists at the universities had time, it seemed. Some simply acknowledged that they didn't want to get involved. As the week wore on, it looked as if the chance of exhuming a *desaparecido* would dissolve like a desert mirage.

Morris Tidball suggested that he might be able to round up some anthropology students from the University of Buenos Aires, and maybe an archaeology student as well. Snow, however, was skeptical, both of the wisdom of employing inexperienced students and of his puckish interpreter, who had assumed the role of procurer and man Friday a little too quickly for his taste. Tidball politely if insistently reassured him.

Late in the afternoon of Friday, June 22, four days before Snow's departure, tens of thousands of demonstrators gathered along the city's main avenue, Nuevo de Julio, to protest what they saw as the International Monetary Fund's bullying influence over Argentina's economy. As men and women with arm bands and megaphones shouted slogans over the heads of the demonstrators, a short, sandy-haired anthropology student wandered through the crowd looking for a group of friends. Although he was Argentine, Douglas Cairns's bloodline was Scottish. Cairns, as his ancestors would have said, was as drunk as a newt. Nonetheless, he had a job to do, an important mission for his friend Morris Tidball.

Eventually Cairns found one of his quarry. "Mimi," he yelled over the din. A slender, dark-haired woman turned to face him, "Dougie Cairns, como te va?" Cairns kissed her cheeks in greeting but skipped the usual pleasantries. A scientist, he said, a gringo who was some kind of forensic expert, was looking for anthropologists and archaeologists to exhume bodies of the disappeared. Would she volunteer?

Mercedes Doretti, a twenty-five-year-old student at the University of Buenos Aires, didn't know Cairns very well. Clearly he was *borracho* and probably making up all this nonsense about digging up bodies. Anyhow, she said, she studied cultural anthropology and knew nothing about bones. But Cairns wouldn't hear of it and insisted that she was just the kind of person for the job. Then with a quick good-bye he reeled off into the crowd.

That evening Mimi ran into her friend Patricia, an archaeology student at the university, at a café near the university. Patricia Bernardi was a year older than Mimi and was not prone to excitability; her heavy lids and syrupy-slow speech gave her a Madonna-like peacefulness. Today, however, Pato smoked nervously and deep vertical creases split her brow. Doug Cairns had asked her to meet this American scientist, she said. She didn't know what to do. She asked Mimi to come with her. Mimi said she had seen Cairns as well. Perhaps they could just go to talk, they agreed. Luis Fondebrider, Pato's friend at the anthropology department, would come as well.[26]

By eight o'clock that night, Cairns had managed to find his way to the Continental Hotel. Inside, Tidball paced the lobby. When Cairns rolled into the hotel, Tidball imagined his well-laid plans dribbling away like spilled beer. But he couldn't turn back now. He called up to Snow's room. Cairns was here, he said, to report on his recruiting efforts.

Tidball maneuvered his friend out into the street, hoping his state of inebriation wouldn't be quite so obvious there. Cairns positioned himself under a lamppost and held onto it as if it were a reluctant dance partner. When Snow ambled out in his cowboy boots, a cigarette between his fingers and a hesitant smile on his face, Cairns introduced himself.

"Hey, gringo, welcome to Argentina," he shouted in English, grinning like a sailor on shore leave. Tidball's stomach sank. "So, what's this forensic anthropology?" Cairns bellowed. "Human rights in Argentina? What's that?"

Snow had to smile at this fellow. Knee-walking drunk, he assumed, but not incoherent, at least. Snow asked him how a family of Scots had come to live in Argentina. Soon they got into a discussion of the qualities of scotch whiskey.

A few minutes later, Mimi, Pato, and her friend Luis showed up, along with an archaeology student, a hulking but quick-witted fellow named Sergio Aleksandrovic. They chatted at the hotel bar about what Judge Ramos Padilla had cooked up. Snow tried to keep the pace nice and slow. He suggested dinner at a nearby restaurant, the Maipú, a typical Argentine grill with mirrors and wainscoting of darkly stained wood, starched white tablecloths, and a bevy of attentive waiters in tightly fitting white jackets.[27]

What Snow saw around the table was a group of scared kids. Mimi protested that she had no archaeological skills. Snow reassured her that the work was fairly straightforward. She could screen dirt or take photographs. Would there be flesh on the bones? Would it be depressing? Would the police be there? Yes, he replied to the last question, it was to be an official exhumation. That seemed to worry them. Their concern made an impression on Snow. What must it be like, he thought, to live in a country where the officials are the ones to be feared?

After dinner Snow returned to his hotel while the students met at Pato's apartment. The American had made the work sound fairly easy. His credentials were impressive. He wasn't stuffy or condescending like other scientists they had known at the university. He'd even offered to help pay for the tools they would need: wooden stakes, buckets, string, trowels if they could find them, spoons and knives, and scrapers. An exhumation would be ghoulish, perhaps even dangerous. But part of their country's history lay buried in that cemetery. Could they turn their backs on it?[28]

June 26, a Tuesday, started as drearily as an Argentine winter morning can. Strong winds, as bitter as when they first gathered in Patagonia, had swept rain northward across the pampas, whose utter flatness offered no brake before the weather broke across Buenos

Aires. It had been raining for days and the streets of the city were beginning to flood with water backed up from the antiquated sewage system. The students — Mimi, Patricia, Morris, Doug, and Sergio — made their separate ways through the torrent to the Continental Hotel, shook off their raincoats and parkas, and met Snow in the lobby.

At 8:00 A.M., the group piled into two cars and drove an hour out of Buenos Aires to the Boulogne Cemetery, in the Buenos Aires suburb of San Isidro. By the time they arrived the skies had cleared but a damp chill remained in the air. Although Snow had prepped them the day before in some techniques of forensic exhumation, they were as skittish as caged cats. Snow realized they had good reason to be when they arrived at the cemetery. He recalls the scene:

> The local judge was out there. And his secretaries, a couple of male lawyers. And the relatives of the deceased. That shocked me. We don't let relations within five miles of an exhumation in the States. And there were high-level policemen, three guys in navy blue suits, I think they were majors or colonels. And there were spectators. And gravediggers.
>
> So here come these five frightened kids. We're trying to figure out what to do. The kids are scared to death because the police are out there. I'm scared to death because I don't know what I'm doing.
>
> We've got out our tools. But none of them had dug before, except maybe Sergio. We're sitting there with our trowels, stakes, and string. And here's the judge, the policemen, the secretaries, the onlookers, the kinfolk. And a police surgeon in a camel hair coat. I'll always remember his camel hair coat.
>
> Finally I walked up to Ramos Padilla with Morris. I explained to him that since this was a crime scene, good police procedure called for a 'scene supervisor,' who would be me, and who would establish a perimeter that no one could enter without permission of the supervisor. I took out this horrible badge from the Illinois Coroners Association. "Dr. Clyde Collins Snow, Forensic Anthropologist, Illinois Coroners Association," it said. You gotta remember, whoever has the biggest badge wins.
>
> Well, they went for it. So I told the judge he could come

and go as he wished, but the police, the relatives, and the others would have to stand outside the perimeter. The police officers went into a big huff. But the judge in Argentina is all-powerful. It was a matter of courtesy, I said. If they came within the perimeter, I made them sign a paper. In return, I promised to show them anything that we found that was interesting.

The grave's marker bore the letters "N.N." Using a standard archaeological technique, Snow showed the students how to dig a test probe at the foot of the grave to determine the level of the burial. With this established, he called in gravediggers with picks and shovels to remove dirt to a level of ten centimeters above the skeleton. The students, hands in pockets and shoulders hunched against the blustering southerly, and casting furtive glances at the policemen standing outside the perimeter, listened as Snow gave out assignments for the next phase.

After the overburden, as the surface soil is called, was removed, Snow had the students place wooden planks across the open hole. Stretching across the boards, they reached into the grave and gently scraped away the earth with trowels and spoons. Within an hour they hit bone.

A false alarm, Snow told them; it belonged to an animal. The cemetery had at one time been a dump and the bones of cows and domesticated animals littered the ground beneath the surface soil.

As the team dug, two forensic doctors from the local constabulary occasionally entered the perimeter to observe their progress. The crew, somewhat emboldened by the fact that Snow had kept the police at bay, grew indignant at these encroachments and schemed to play a practical joke on the doctors. Morris, as practiced with displays of humility as with moral outrage, took a couple of cow bones over to the doctors and asked, "What kind of human bones are these?" They puzzled over them for a few moments, then replied stiffly that this sort of thing was not easy to determine and would require more thorough study. The team's spirits rose.

Their mood shifted by late morning, however, when they removed pieces of a disintegrating coffin and, digging still further, uncovered a human skull. Snow stopped their work, leaned over the lip of the grave, and delicately brushed dirt from the skull. The gracile brow ridge and smallish mastoid process indicated a woman. "And there was a bullet hole right up over the eye," Snow remembers. "There was an earthworm right next to it. This was the first *desaparecido* that the kids had ever seen. I didn't know what they were going to do."

The students grew quite still. Looking over Snow's shoulder as he whisked the earth away from the skull, they saw that its jaw hung open, as if in mid-scream. They didn't know that as the muscle and ligaments that hold the jaw together decompose, gravity pulls the mandible down until the chin rests on the clavicles of the upper chest, giving the skull its gape.

Pato dropped her trowel, stepped from the grave, and walked away. Snow reckoned they had lost her, then and there, and maybe the rest as well. But Morris, accustomed as a medical student to seeing skeletons and corpses, kept digging with his spoon at the soil around the remains. The others, though reluctantly, followed suit.

Ten minutes passed in silence. Then Pato reappeared at the side of the grave, her eyes red but her composure regained, and picked up her trowel.

"Morris," Mimi said, "give me your spoon."

He looked up, perplexed. "Why?" he asked.

"Because," Mimi replied, "it's time for coffee."

By six o'clock, Snow and his assistants had uncovered the entire skeleton. They photographed the remains in situ and carefully removed and catalogued each bone. As dusk lengthened the shadows of the tombstones across the soggy ground, the crew carefully placed the bones in small plastic bags.

A starless night had fallen by the time the team drove up to the morgue. Besides Snow, only Morris had ever been inside one. Its dark corridors and unfamiliar smells spooked them, and they grew quiet as they fell in behind Snow.

After he had laid out the bones on the autopsy table in the examining room, Snow took measurements to reassure himself by metric sexing that they indeed had belonged to a woman. Filling in the rough outlines — sex, approximate age, stature — posed no difficulty. Manner of death, however, turned out to be tricky. Certainly, the bullet hole in the skull testified that this young woman had been shot. But was it the kind of wound one would expect from an execution?

The police surgeons, obviously ignorant of forensic anthropology, insisted that the hole bore the marks of a long-range gunshot wound, a finding that would affirm the standard story attached to every *desaparecido*: the victim, a terrorist, had been killed in a shootout with the security forces.

But Snow saw it differently. People shot in gunfights usually get hit in all sorts of places. In this case, he explained, there weren't any other signs of gunshot trauma on the bones. "According to my experience," he said, "it looks like an execution-style wound." Still, since the wound was caused by a bullet, which usually leaves the same diameter hole no matter what range it is shot from, he couldn't be sure whether the hole indicated a short- or long-range wound. The police surgeons insisted that they had found another hole in the skull that surely suggested that the woman had been shot twice. Snow had already seen the hole, about the size of a dime, and knew its source. Here was a chance for a touch of drama. He retrieved a small, roundish shard of bone from the examining table that he had set aside earlier. Holding the skull up for all to see, he pointed to the hole the surgeons had spotted. This was no bullet hole, he explained. It was made when a small island of bone within a cranial suture, called an ossicle, simply dropped out, a common occurrence as buried skulls age. He showed them the bone shard and gently slipped it into the hole. It fit perfectly.

Midnight had come and gone. Ramos Padilla, lighting one cigarette after another as he paced in and out of the examining room, was impressed by the operation. But the most painful task remained. Outside the examining room, Rosa Betti's parents waited to hear whether the remains were indeed those of their disappeared daughter. Snow had no antemortem X rays or dental records to compare with the skeleton. It was strictly a case of comparing descriptions of the young woman against the bones on the examining table. But he had seen enough to make up his mind.

With the team in tow, Snow walked out to meet the Betti family. They had waited for hours with the quiet patience of people who had already waited six years for news, any news, of their daughter. No, Snow said, the remains were not those of their daughter. He explained that the height and age of the skeleton did not match her description. The mother started to cry, whether from grief, catharsis, or a rejuvenated hope that her daughter might still be alive, Snow had no idea. The team stood by, some of them crying as well, feeling lost and useless but unable to tear themselves away. They were at that moment realizing something about forensic work: that the digging had really been the easiest part.

It was past two in the morning when they started back for Buenos Aires. Underneath the fatigue, the students felt a closeness to this strange American scientist. They didn't need translations to understand the gestures and the tone of voice that had coaxed them from the streets of Buenos Aires, calmed their fears, and comforted them at the grave. He had molded them, however briefly, into a sort of family. They began to realize as they drowsed in the darkened car that in a single day they had accomplished more for human rights than they had as faceless participants in countless demonstrations. And how odd that it was an American who had come to their country to search for the disappeared.

Digging up graves . . . Exciting, satisfying in a way, and wrenching too. A once-in-a-lifetime experience.

Or so they thought.

12

LILIANA'S STORY

COCHE PEREYRA sat up in bed and listened. The knock on the door was insistent. Wrapping a dressing gown around her bare shoulders, she groped from the bedroom to the front of the apartment. As she drew near the door, a woman's voice called quietly.

"Coche, hurry. The telephone. You have a call from Mar de Plata."

The Pereyras didn't own a telephone, and Coche sometimes got calls through her neighbor. It was an amicable arrangement, but the hour was late and she hated to abuse the privilege. She padded down the corridor to her neighbor's apartment, apologizing as she went.

"Sí," she said into the receiver.

"Señora," a man's voice whispered. "Your daughter, Liliana . . . I'm the owner of the rooming house where she stays."

Fear rose like a fist in Coche's throat.

"May I speak with her? Is she all right?"

"I'm sorry, Señora. She's not here. We must talk. But please not now. . . . You have the address?"

"Yes, b-but . . ."

The phone clicked.

"Is anything wrong?" Coche's neighbor asked.

"I'm not sure. He hung up. Something's happened to Liliana."

The next day, Coche and her husband drove from La Plata to Mar del Plata, a seaside resort town about three hundred kilometers to the

250

south, where Liliana lived. Coche had slept little the night before. She was not a political person, but she knew well enough that young people who got involved in left-wing politics were disappearing, never to be seen again. She gazed out the windows, thinking only of her daughter as the flat terrain of the eastern pampas sped by.

Liliana was Coche's first child, born September 1, 1956. She was a pretty girl from a middle-class family who did well in school and made friends easily. She went to the Colegio Misericordia, an all-girls school within walking distance of her family's apartment. In 1974, at the age of eighteen, Liliana entered the University of La Plata to study law. She joined the university's Peronist Youth Movement at a time when many of its members were being gunned down by death squads belonging to the AAA, the Argentine Anti-Communist Alliance.

In 1977 Liliana abandoned her studies and went to live with her grandmother in Mar del Plata. She found work in a fish-packing plant, where she eventually met and fell in love with Eduardo Cagnola, an erstwhile law student like herself. Liliana stayed two months in her grandmother's house. The two women argued constantly. Liliana demanded more freedom, while her grandmother discouraged her granddaughter's involvement with Eduardo. One morning Liliana packed her bags and left. She met Eduardo at a prearranged location and soon they rented a room in a pension on the two thousand block of Catamarca Street, across from a tree-lined park.

Coche and her husband were met at the pension by the owner, Andre Barbe. He apologized for being so evasive on the phone and invited them inside, sat them down in the front parlor, and broke the news. Their daughter had been taken, he said. A few days before, on October 5, as Liliana and Eduardo were returning to the rooming house, men in naval fatigues had emerged from the park and wrestled them into waiting cars. He was in the pension when it happened.

Barbe led Coche to her daughter's room. She wept when she saw the bare walls and the broken furniture. A mattress lay on the floor, its bedsheets rumpled in a corner. Next to the mattress Coche discovered something extraordinary. There, on the floor, lay a pair of booties and a tiny sweater. Coche gasped as she picked them up. She knew instantly what anyone but a mother might not have guessed. Liliana had been pregnant when she was abducted.

251

Back in La Plata, the Pereyras frantically sought information about their daughter. They got the same blank response from the police that so many other parents of the disappeared had encountered. Coche withdrew to the apartment for days, sitting alone and distant in Liliana's bedroom. Then, in July 1978, nine months after the kidnapping, she received an unexpected notice from the police in Mar del Plata. It was brutally brief: "Cadaver No. 50.524, N.N. Female. Victim of a shootout with the combined forces in Mar del Plata, July 15, 1978. Identified: PEREYRA, Liliana Carmen."

Coche wrote back immediately. How could her daughter have been in a shootout in July 1978 if she was abducted by navy agents in October 1977? And where was the body? But she recieved no reply.

In 1979 Coche joined the Grandmothers of the Plaza de Mayo; whether Liliana lived or not, Coche suspected she herself may well be a grandmother. By then, the Grandmothers had learned from two former prisoners, Sara Solarz de Osatinsky and Ana María Martí, that doctors at the naval hospital in Buenos Aires kept a list of married couples in the navy who could not have children of their own and who were prepared to adopt a child from among the pregnant detainees held in a special section at the Navy Mechanics School.[1] During their imprisonment at the Navy Mechanics School, Solarz de Osatinsky and Martí were assigned to care for the pregnant women. The two women recalled that Liliana Pereyra had been brought to the center from Mar del Plata in November 1977.[2] She had been about six months pregnant. Solarz de Osatinsky said that during one of her visits to Liliana's cell the girl told her that she had been tortured in front of her boyfriend. It was the last time Liliana had seen him. That Christmas eve, Liliana and her cellmates gave Solarz de Osatinsky a card that they had made from a piece of cardboard. One of them had drawn a teddy bear with its arms stretched out. In a circle of tiny flowers over the bear's head, they signed their names. Osatinsky still had the card.

According to the woman, Liliana gave birth in the center's clinic to a healthy baby boy in early February. Solarz de Osatinsky had assisted a naval doctor, Jorge Magnasco, in the delivery. Liliana then was transferred back to Mar del Plata without her baby. Shortly afterward, two members of naval intelligence, Hector Favre and a man who went by the pseudonym of "Pedro Bolita" took the baby away.

This story was the last shred of information about Liliana's fate that Coche recovered until December 1983, when the military ceded power to the civilian government. With the assistance of a lawyer, she began checking burial records at the Cementerio Parque on the outskirts of Mar del Plata. They discovered two N.N. entries, dated July 13, 1978, that gave physical descriptions similar to Liliana's.

Coche knew that she could never be satisfied with an anonymous entry in a cemetery logbook. In early 1984, she approached Judge Pedro Hooft in Mar del Plata, who agreed to open a formal investigation. It would last over a year. Along the way it would introduce Coche to an extraordinary team of scientists and, ultimately, would inscribe Liliana's last testament into her country's history books.

In mid-February 1985 Clyde Snow returned to Argentina to direct a five-week training workshop in identifying skeletal remains. He was to be joined by odontologist Lowell Levine, radiologist John Fitzpatrick, and forensic pathologist Robert Kirschner. Together, the four scientists were to train a team of Argentines to begin the process of exhuming and identifying the remains of the disappeared.

Much had happened in Argentina since Snow left the muddy, windswept graveyard at San Isidro seven months before. On September 20, 1984, the National Commission on the Disappeared (CONADEP) delivered its report on government-sanctioned atrocities committed under the military dictatorship to President Alfonsín. In his introduction to the report, CONADEP chairman Ernesto Sábato, a novelist, wrote: "The vast majority of the [disappeared] were innocent not only of any acts of terrorism, but even of belonging to the fighting units of the guerrilla organizations: these latter chose to fight it out, and either died in shoot-outs or committed suicide before they could be captured. Few of them were alive by the time they were in the hands of the repressive forces." In all, at least 8,960 people had disappeared into the smoke screen of the military's self-proclaimed dirty war. Sábato cautioned, however, that the true figure of the disappeared was likely to be much higher, as many families were still afraid to report a disappearance for fear of reprisals.

On the day Sábato delivered CONADEP's report to Alfonsín, a throng of demonstrators gathered on the Plaza de Mayo. Hebe de Bonafini, one of the leaders of the march, stood under a huge banner that read, "Aparición con Vida!" — "Let Them Appear Alive!" Bonafini, who had lost two sons and a daughter-in-law to police raids, led a contingent of the Madres de Plaza de Mayo. A hefty woman with iron gray hair and a steely will, she had helped to turn the Madres into a household name in Argentina and was an inspiration to similar groups throughout Latin America.

Bonafini and her followers were angry that Alfonsín had continued to promote military officers despite evidence of their complicity in past atrocities and failed to dismiss judges whom the Madres believed were whitewashing the military's culpability for the disappearances. They also didn't want exhumations. "We, the mothers of the disappeared, will not be converted into the mothers of the dead," Bonafini once declared, ignoring mounting evidence that the disappeared had indeed been executed.[3]

Snow had little inkling of the political maneuverings over the disappeared, but he definitely sensed something was amiss as he sat in a comfortable office in Buenos Aires and listened to the urbane Eduardo Rabossi. By then, Alfonsín had dissolved CONADEP and replaced it with the *Subsecretaría de Derechos Humanos*, the Undersecretariat of Human Rights. Rabossi, a university professor of philosophy, had been named to run it. One of Rabossi's tasks was to develop a nationwide system for excavating graves of the *desaparecidos*. He had personally written to the American Association for the Advancement of Science for help. The AAAS had turned again to Snow.

Snow had sent several letters to Rabossi in advance of his arrival, advising him that in order to run a training workshop, they needed students who had at least some understanding of the forensic sciences. Now, as Snow sat watching Rabossi light and relight his pipe in his office on the second floor of the Teatro de San Martín in Buenos Aires, he grew suspicious. He sensed condescension in this preening, stuffy little man. Exasperated, Snow asked bluntly for a list of the workshop participants that Rabossi was supposed to have drawn up.

Rabossi sucked air through his dead pipe. "Well," he replied, "you must realize that exhumations have become a divisive issue among the human rights organizations." Bonafini and her group were demanding that their children be returned alive. It was irrational, of course, they were no doubt dead. Even so, he explained, his government had to move cautiously.

Snow soon realized that the workshop had been reshuffled to the bottom of Rabossi's deck of priorities. "Doctor Rabossi," he growled, "I've arranged to have three forensic scientists come down here. No one's paying me or any of them for this. Now, are you trying to tell me nothing's been done to get this thing moving?" Rabossi, taken aback by the American's anger, assured Snow that things would be put in order.

When Snow returned to the undersecretariat the following day, he found that Rabossi had assigned two of his staff, Marita Vera and María Julia Bihurriet, to help him salvage the workshop. They proved able beyond Snow's expectations. Vera, a tall, big-boned woman in her mid-thirties, was the daughter of a prosperous wine merchant from Mendoza. She had studied at Argentina's best schools, where she gained a fluency in English and a cosmopolitan charm that proved invaluable in winning concessions from the most reluctant of Argentine officials. Bihurriet, in contrast, was country, a twenty-four-year-old former village schoolteacher with close-cropped, thick dark hair and delicate features. Like Evita Perón, she had been born in Los Toldos, a small farming community to the west, and shared the former first lady's stubborn determination.

Vera and Bihurriet tracked down medical deans, anthropology professors, and directors of forensic laboratories and told them to send their best and brightest. Responses began to trickle in. Snow was impressed. In little over a week Vera and Bihurriet had managed to enroll about twenty students in the workshop and locate two judges, one just outside of Buenos Aires and the other in Mar del Plata, who wanted several N.N. graves opened. Now they would have actual graves and cases to work on. That meant he would need some more experienced help doing excavations. He knew just the group to do it.

Mimi and Pato were reluctant. But Morris and Sergio convinced the two women to join them in helping Snow exhume a set of graves at the Isidro Casanova Cemetery in the western suburbs of Buenos Aires. Pato's friend Luis, who provided not only a strong pair of hands but a wry sense of humor that kept the group at ease, also volunteered his time.

Their first visit to Isidro Casanova, at the behest of a judge investigating eight *desaparecidos* who had vanished in 1976, was anything but reassuring. Indeed, the party that met them at the overgrown cemetery, its tombstones half hidden in waist-high weeds, was more frightening than the one they'd confronted at their first exhumation. Fifty policemen, armed with automatic weapons and equipped with riot helmets, ringed the cemetery. They were there to protect them. But from whom? Snow reassured his suspicious assistants. "Remember," he said, "we control this dig."

Over the next two weeks, under the hottest sun that Snow could remember since Arizona, the group opened eight graves. The heat took care of the police; after the first week, only four remained, and they repaired to the shade of a grove of plane trees, where they stretched out next to a pile of broken tombstones to play cards and sip maté.

Besides human bones, thirty-two bullets and dozens of bullet fragments were removed from the graves. The team packed up the lot and sent it in a police car to the medical school in Buenos Aires. The exhumations had been good practice for Snow's team. But soon they got a new assignment, one that would stand as the high point of their young careers as forensic scientists.

Coche Pereyra had heard of their work through the Abuelas. She asked Judge Hooft if he would arrange to have the team open the grave she believed to be her daughter's in the Parque Cemetery. Hooft called Bihurriet at the undersecretariat and said he wanted the American and his team to exhume three graves at the cemetery. Morgue records suggested that one of the graves contained the remains of Néstor Fonseca, a twenty-eight-year-old man who had disappeared in May 1978. Found dead by the side of a road, the police had signed him out as a "suicide" and ordered his body buried as an N.N. The American anthropologist, the judge said, would have two osteological clues to work with: Fonseca had been left-handed, and he had accidentally shot himself in the right hand on a hunting trip the year before his disappearance.

The other two cases weren't as clear cut, the judge explained. Two young women with almost identical physical characteristics had been buried in unmarked graves. Both had been in their early twenties when they disappeared and had been about the same stature and weight, with the same eye and hair color. One of the bodies was thought to be that of a woman named Ana María Torti. The other, Hooft believed, was Liliana Pereyra.

"There's one thing you should know," Hooft said before he hung up. "Torti's mother is a member of the Madres de Plaza de Mayo, and she's refused to have anything to do with the investigation."

On a Saturday morning, a van carrying Snow and the team rolled through the iron gates of the Parque Cemetery and wound through its maze of gravel paths. It was a barren place, a gray and forbidding public-housing project for the dead and quite unlike the grandiose necropolises of Buenos Aires. The only consolation was the fresh, salty breeze from the nearby Atlantic.

They broke into two groups. Morris, Pato, and Luis dug one grave, while Mimi and Sergio, with the assistance of María Julia and Marita, excavated another. As they worked through the day, a small crowd of onlookers, some with blankets and picnic baskets, gathered on the other side of the rope the police had strung around the graves to keep them out of the way. A television crew also showed up, but police shooed them away, leaving the team to work relatively undisturbed.

Mimi was the first to notice a young blond woman in a beige jacket and blue jeans standing at the edge of the perimeter. The woman motioned for Mimi, who set down her bucket and walked over to her. They talked briefly. Mimi returned to the grave and stretched out alongside Snow as he reached in to brush the dirt from the emerging skeleton.

"A male," Snow said. "Looks left-handed as well." He gingerly lifted several finger bones for closer scrutiny. "He's got several old, healed fractures on the right hand. We'll have to X-ray them for metal fragments. But I'd say this is Néstor Fonseca."

"Are you sure?" Mimi asked.

"Why?" Snow responded.

"That woman standing over there is Fonseca's wife. She wants to see the remains."

Unsure of what to do next, they fell silent. Then Sergio spoke.

"Look at it this way. When did Fonseca disappear? In 1978? That means for seven years now she's been denied the right to know. The military, the police, the courts, they all denied her the truth. Now she has the right to decide for herself. We can't deny her that."

Mimi rose, walked to the woman, and led her to the grave. She introduced her as Fonseca's wife. As the woman knelt by the edge of the opening, Mimi noted with relief that someone had thoughtfully closed the skull's gaping mandible.

"How can you tell if it is him?" Fonseca asked.

Mimi pointed out the left arm bone and explained how they determined handedness. She lifted several finger bones from the soil and, holding them in her palm, showed her the tiny deformities in the bones. The chance that another of the disappeared shared these characteristics, she explained, was extremely unlikely.

Fonseca rose to her feet. Mimi wrapped an arm around her shoulders as they returned to the perimeter. The woman stopped, struggling to speak. "Thank you," she whispered, holding Mimi's hands in her own. "What you are doing, it's wonderful."

By the end of the day, the skeletons of two people had been removed from the soil at Parque: Néstor Fonseca and a woman whose identification would have to wait for a more thorough examination at the morgue in Buenos Aires. The third grave was left partly opened, to be finished the next day.

Sunday morning at daybreak, María Julia and Marita left their hotel for the cemetery ahead of the others. They had expected a peaceful beginning to their final day of digging. They were wrong.

"As we entered," María Julia recalls,

we could see a large group of people standing around the partially open grave. There must have been about fifteen of them, mostly women. We stopped first at a small shed. We heard shouts. But we couldn't make out what they were saying. I asked where the judge was. No one knew. Maybe he was on his way. A policeman came up and told us the people at the grave were members of the Madres. They wouldn't let anyone near the graves that we had dug. He said when he and his men approached, they hurled stones at at them, so they backed off.

Well, I decided if they were Madres, I could talk to them. The policeman warned me not to go, but I did anyway. When I got about thirty meters away, I recognized Hebe de Bonafini. But before I could say anything, they began shouting insults.

"Assassins, *milicos*, sons of bitches . . ." Then the policeman grabbed me and pulled me back. So Marita and I decided we'd better find the judge. Luckily, we intercepted the team on the road.[4]

On the way to the judge's office, María Julia described the scene at the gravesite. The team was stunned. Since Bonafini was running the show, there would surely be lots of publicity. "Mierda, que lío!," Morris swore. Inside the courthouse, María Julia told the judge what had happened. Much to everyone's relief, he suspended the last exhumation. It was agreed that María Julia and Marita would escort the bones they had exhumed the previous day to Buenos Aires.

Mimi, Pato, Luis, and Sergio spent the rest of the day at the beach. "We felt so strange," Mimi recalls, "all these people on vacation around us, and there we were, so white, so completely white. We just sat there, looking at the sun and the sea. Pato was really upset. We all were. It was so terrible having the Madres against our work."[5]

At five o'clock that afternoon María Julia and Marita left Mar del Plata in a police car with the remains. "By then," says María Julia,

> I was very nervous and most of all tired. I was also confused about what had happened that day. About thirty minutes out on the highway, another police car caught up with us. It flashed its lights and we pulled over. We were told to get out of the car and get into the other one. I had no idea what was happening. I was so frightened and tired, I almost panicked. For all I knew, they could have been kidnapping us.
>
> So we continued in the new car. Then another police car overtook us and we went through the same change. I thought again, could this be a kidnapping? The police wouldn't speak to us. And I was so scared I didn't dare ask what was going on. Finally, the men began talking among themselves and it became clear that they didn't know who we were or what we were carrying. So it dawned on me that this changing car business was some sort of police procedure for transporting highly confidential material.
>
> Besides Marita and me, there were always three policemen in the car. Two in front, one guy driving and one guy operating the radio, and another in the back seat with the two of us.

Marita slept. I couldn't. I was too frightened. We were traveling so fast, I thought for sure we'd have an accident. Finally, I mustered up my nerve and told the driver, "Look, you don't know who I am or where I'm coming from or where I'm going. But I know who you are, and I'm going to tell you just one thing. If I see that speedometer pass the one hundred kilometer mark again, I'm going to start screaming into that radio." So he replied, "A thousand pardons, miss. I didn't realize it bothered you."

We must have changed cars seven times that night. At about eleven o'clock we arrived at the Puente La Noria, or at least that's what I thought it was, because it was dark and I don't know the geography of Buenos Aires that well. Anyway, the bridge marks the point where the federal police of Buenos Aires take over from the provincial police. We stopped at a guard post. The guy in charge, a federal police officer, stuck his head in the window and told us he'd been instructed to deliver us and whatever we were carrying to the medical school. But, he said, he first wanted to know who we were and what we were transporting. This caused a problem for me, as I had been instructed by the judge not to tell anyone what I was carrying. But the guy insisted. "Okay," I said, "they're human remains." And I told him who I was and where I worked. "But *whose* remains are they?" he asked. "How would I know?" I said. "They're N.N. remains." With that, he broke into a big smile and showed us into a police car, and several policemen took us into the city.[6]

Waiting at the University of Buenos Aires morgue for the arrival of the mysterious cargo was José Conesa, an anatomist who had been named the liaison between the school and the undersecretariat. He was one of the more eccentric members of the faculty. With his thinning hair, pale face, and soiled, oversized lab coat whose hem swept to the floor, he looked as if he'd been grown in a cellar under fluorescent light. His laboratory, located in a forgotten corner of the medical school, overflowed with tropical plants, caged birds, and dusty jars filled with every human organ imaginable. The smell of the place was potent, a mixture of formaldehyde and neglected kitty litter. Five cats of varying sizes and pedigree prowled the shelves and napped on the windowsills. Conesa's favorite, an old cross-eyed tom, wore a postcard-sized blackboard around its neck, on which Conesa would leave messages for his colleagues.

Conesa stood on the morgue's loading platform, a cat nestled under his lab coat, when the flashing police car shot through the university's side gate. The cat bolted, making a dash back into the building, while Conesa stood frozen in the car's headlights, wide-eyed. Police officers stepped out of the car, their pistols drawn. The last to disembark were María Julia and a sleepy-eyed Marita. Wearily, the two women lifted two crates of bones from the car's trunk, climbed the steps to the platform, and disappeared into the building, leaving Conesa to deal with the gun-toting cops.

It was early in the afternoon of March 28, two weeks after the dash with the bones from Parque Cemetery to the university's morgue. Sunlight yellowed the still air in a sixth-floor lecture hall at the medical school, catching spirals of dust like lazy little cyclones in its rays. Pato stood at a table with Luis and Morris. Luis cradled a plastic bag full of bones in his arms; Morris held the skull, swaddled in a cotton towel, against his chest. Behind them, on a blackboard, was a drawing of a foot, its plantar arteries marked with spidery red chalk lines.

"You'd better erase the board, don't you think?" Pato said. She pulled a new white tablecloth from a bag and spread it across the table. She smoothed out its rigid creases as best she could. That done, she left the room.

Luis and Morris looked at each other uncertainly. In a matter of minutes, the mother of the woman whose bones they held in their arms was due. Morris set the skull on the table. "How do we do this?" he asked Luis. Luis raised his eyebrows and shrugged.

Over the past two weeks, Luis, Morris, Mimi, Sergio, and Pato had worked over these bones, while the other workshop participants had studied the other remains the team had exhumed from Isidro Casanova. Snow had shown them how to determine the skeleton's sex, race, stature, and age at death. Levine, the New York dentist with the bushy mustache and self-assured manner, had taught the team how to read dental charts and spot anomalies in the teeth. Kirschner, the energetic Chicago pathologist and one of the world's authorities on gunshot wounds, had shown them how to tell that the beveled hole they had found in the skull came from a single gunshot blast. In the end, however, it was Fitzpatrick, the radiologist, who had clinched the identification. Working alone in the medical school's radiology laboratory, he had taken X rays of the reconstructed thorax and rib cage and compared them to a chest X ray they had acquired from the family of the supposed victim. Waving the radiographs in the air, his hair and clothes in their usual disarray, he had burst into the morgue shouting, "It's a match! It's a match! There's no doubt about it!"

But no one had taught the Argentines how to present the bones to Liliana's mother.

"We could lay them out in anatomical order," Luis said, trying to sound convincing. But displaying the reconstructed skeleton seemed too scientific, too cold, like a classroom exhibit. "On the other hand, we could arrange them in groups. You know, put the finger and toe bones to one side, the long bones to another, the ribs, and so on." Grouping them, he suggested, might soften the spectacle, make it less shocking, if that was possible. They agreed to arrange the bones in several separate piles.

Just as they finished, Snow rapped on the door and stuck his head in the room. "They're coming," he said. Morris stuffed the plastic bag and cotton wadding into a drawer and the two joined Snow outside. Moments later, the visitors arrived on the landing. Chicha Maríani, the president of the Abuelas, entered first. Coche Pereyra followed with her son and daughter, both teenagers.

"When I saw Coche's face," Luis recalls, "it said it all. It was then that I realized I was doing something important. I knew my contribution was no more than a grain of sand really, but I also knew no matter how minor my role was, it meant something to the family, and I had to continue."[7]

Coche hugged her two children to her side as she looked down at the bones of Liliana. The memory still moves her to tears.

Deep inside I didn't want the remains to be Liliana's, but when Dr. Snow stood with us at the table and explained how he and his colleagues had identified them, I had no doubt. I remember he said he had found pieces of handkerchief with her remains. He described the color. Well, this puzzled me. But later I learned from Ana María Martí, the girl who had been detained with Liliana at ESMA, that my daughter had used a handkerchief to tie back her hair. As we stood there beside Liliana's remains, there were so many questions I wanted to ask Dr. Snow. I remember there was a mark on the skull, and I thought, what is that? But the pain was so great, I just couldn't speak. I was so afraid to know the truth.[8]

On April 22, 1985, the Federal Appeals Court of Buenos Aires opened the trial against the nine generals and admirals who had made up the three successive juntas that ruled Argentina after the 1976 coup. Hebe de Bonafini had been proved right in her mistrust of military justice. In September 1984 the military court charged by the president to try these nine men declared that they had failed to find them guilty of anything illegal. In response, the civilian court empowered to review the military tribunal's deliberations took charge of the case. The government's most seasoned prosecutor, Julio C. Strassera, led the prosecution.

For Argentines who had lived through an almost impenetrable secrecy during the seven years of military rule, the trial was high drama. Of the nine defendants, three were former presidents — Jorge Rafael Videla, Roberto Eduardo Viola, and Leopoldo Galtieri. Never before in Latin America had a civilian government tried military leaders for past human rights abuses. A television camera was installed in the paneled courtroom to record every argument, plea, and gesture of the attorneys and judges, who were to propose and pass judgment on a decade of political chaos. A newspaper was even created just for the trial. *El Diario del Juicio* appeared in newsstands around the country and for the duration of the five-month trial it became the country's best-selling publication.

For most of the proceedings, the defendants chose not to appear in court, sending a bevy of lawyers instead. There could be little doubt of their position, however. Wars have no laws, the defense lawyers insisted. The constitutionally elected government of Isabel Perón had declared a state of siege in 1974, and therefore the military could not be condemned for doing its job. For weeks, the defense bolstered this argument with a parade of witnesses, many of whom were prominent and powerful, who reminded the six judges and the jammed courtroom that the terrorism that had gripped the country during the mid-1970s could only have been defeated with unconventional means.

Strassera led the prosecution with a lugubrious presence; tall and thin with a thick mustache hanging over a pendulous lower lip, his dark hair slicked back like a tango dancer from the 1930s, and vast pouches under his eyes, he looked like a mournful hound. In eloquence he had no peer in that courtroom. When the pace of the proceedings threatened to bog down, he offered epithets and parables. "It is senseless for a man to destroy all the china in his house in order to catch a fly," he lampooned the defense one day, citing the twelfth-century Chinese philosopher Wan Lang. On another day, he asked angrily: "Is it an act of war to occupy houses and keep relatives of those being looked for as hostages? To keep the babies? Are those military objectives? Can you explain the systematic plundering of homes as a necessary measure to seize enemy arms? 'I was robbed of everything, from my wife's underwear to the flint on the kitchen stove,' the witness Hugo Pascual told us. Are we to believe that these are just the unfortunate consequences of war?"[9]

At the prosecutors' table, Strassera's assistant prosecutor, Luis Moreno Ocampo, kept the flow of documents and testimony moving behind Strassera like a stoker on a steamboat. Barely thirty years old, handsome and fashionably dressed, Moreno Ocampo was part of Argentina's new generation. In the 1970s, men and women of his age had formed the ranks of the Montoneros as well as the mid-level positions in the military. Now it was up to his generation to remake Argentina in a civilian mold.

The prosecution had to prove that the nine junta members were directly responsible for the illegal detentions and disappearances. What they needed were signed orders by the accused. But, as Strassera discovered, if there had ever been any, they had already been destroyed. So he decided to demonstrate that the defendants had been well aware of the crimes committed by their subordinates. "It's normal," Strassera explained during the trial, "that when you have a secret organization, the plans are also secret. A Mafia boss doesn't have signed orders on his desk. He doesn't have to. Just because there's a plan doesn't mean you have to have a copy of it. What we know is that the Argentine Armed Forces work on the basis of vertical structure. And only with the existence of a plan at the top could it follow that lower officials had acted in the same manner."[10]

Over eight hundred people testified during the trial. Many were survivors of the secret detention centers. Others were relatives of people who never emerged from the camps. Each one was called before the wide bench to face the judge's impassive but attentive gaze, to give his or her testimony as the audience, crammed into rows of polished wooden pews, strained to hear their echoing, sometimes sobbing, voices. One of those called was Clyde Snow.

Shortly before the opening of the trial, Strassera met an attractive young woman at a cocktail party. She told him about her work with an American scientist who had recently identified the remains of two *desaparecidos* who had been buried in the Parque Cemetery in Mar del Plata. Strassera knew something of it; the protest by the Madres had indeed drawn press coverage, followed by statements of support for the exhumations by other human rights groups. Mimi described the techniques the American scientist had used to identify the skeletons. Strassera was fascinated. And, being a good lawyer, he realized that these curious bone sleuths might help his case.

On the second day of the trial, April 24, Snow arrived at the Café Colon, one of many in the maze of small restaurants and offices of lawyers and bail bondsmen that lined the streets behind the majestic, thick-columned courthouse across from the Plaza de Lavalle. There he met a serious, auburn-haired young woman in a red blouse who was to be his interpreter for the evening. Snow was to testify at about 8:30 P.M. He was uncommonly quiet. Despite a haircut, a fresh white shirt and tie, and his signature tweed jacket, his face betrayed his fatigue. He drank coffee and smoked dark Parisienne cigarettes, the strongest local brand, oblivious to the clatter of dishes and the waiters' banter around him.

At eight o'clock, Snow entered the courthouse with his interpreter. A guard examined their subpoenas and ushered them to a waiting room. An hour later, an officer of the court came and announced that his time to testify had arrived. Snow slung his canvas army-surplus bag full of slides over his shoulder and, with his interpreter, followed the officer down a narrow hallway. They passed through a paneled door into the main chamber. To his left on the dais, in high-backed chairs with black leather upholstery, sat the judges. They were younger than he'd expected, natty in broad ties and tailored suits. Behind them were stained glass panels etched with a tableau of a crucifix and two women in robes carrying swords of justice.

Television lights threw the dias into sharp relief. The gallery vanished into murkiness, lit only by two rows of small lamps, their smoked glass shades formed in the shape of flowers, secured to wainscoted pillars. Below and to the right of the judges was the prosecutors' table. Strassera looked up and nodded as Snow was led to the witness table, directly in front of the bench. Behind him he could hear the rustling of an impatient audience.

After being sworn in, Snow read his qualifications and explained why he was in Argentina. He gave the names of four people whose skeletons he and the team had exhumed and identified. He could see that the judges were tired. He was the twelfth witness to testify that day, and surely their attention had been spent. Snow felt the reassuring pressure of his canvas bag and the plastic carousel of slides against his elbow and knew that he had something that would wake this courtroom up.

Finally, the presiding judge asked him to explain how his scientific methods would be of value to the court. Snow took his slides to a projector set up in front of the bench and aimed it at a large screen on the wall to their left. The first slide, of the Parque Cemetery, appeared on the screen. He explained how a test pit is first dug, and how carefully the overburden must be removed. Slides of María Julia and Sergio sifting dirt through screens followed. Months of fieldwork flashed by. A judge motioned to a secretary to bring him a cigarette and asked Snow to be brief.

Snow cleared his throat and flipped to the next slide. "This is the breastbone, or sternum, of this individual, one of the cases from Isidro Casanova. The circular perforation is a bullet hole caused by a bullet penetrating at the back of the sternum and entering the anterior, or front surface, of the sternum. Even while the bone is still in the grave we can determine this individual was shot in the back."[11] Leather creaked as a judge leaned forward in his chair to get a better look.

"This is the skull of a disappeared we identified as Néstor Fonseca," Snow continued. "And here," he added, showing a slide of an X ray of Fonseca's fingers, "we can see signs of metal fragments embedded in the bone itself, which is consistent with the history of an old gunshot wound."

A new slide clicked into view. "And here," Snow went on, "is a pelvis. From the shape we could determine it was female, and from other features, that she was in her early twenties at the time of death." The audience grew quiet.

The next slide showed a swatch of hair found near the woman's skull. It matched the color and form described by the suspected victim's mother, Snow said. Next came a photograph of the teeth. "The mother said that about one or two months before her daughter was detained, she had had an upper-left canine tooth removed. You will notice a space in there representing the missing tooth."

Snow stopped to move slides around in the carousel. Then, with another click, a full frontal view of the skull appeared on the screen. Several people in the gallery gasped. Snow paused until the hall was quiet. Up in the balcony, Mimi, Morris, and Luis could see that Snow had mesmerized his audience.

Snow continued: "The bones of the skull as we found them were in a very fragmented form. Along with the fragments, we found five — no, excuse me, seven — pellets from a shotgun, badly deformed, the size consistent with the load of buckshot used in shotguns such as the Ithaca that are issued as a standard police and army security weapon in Argentina. We had to reconstruct the skull in order to study the patterns of injuries, about two days' work."

Another slide. "Now, for the right side of the skull . . ." Snow looked up at the bench. Every eye was glued to the screen. "We see a defect there which represents the entry wound of the point where the, uh . . . gunshot entered the skull. Characteristics of the size and shape of this defect led us to conclude that the range at which this shot was fired was perhaps around one meter or perhaps a little less than a meter."

Snow turned to face the judges. "To me an even more significant aspect of this case was the fact that we did not encounter the small bones of a human fetus in the pelvic area of this woman's skeleton. What we did find on the the pelvic bones was a groove in the preauricular sulcus, a small, shallow trench immediately in front of the sacroiliac joint" — Snow reached over to the projecter and pressed the switch to bring up the last slide — ". . . which indicates that this individual had given birth to a term or near-term infant."

A photograph of a pretty young woman filled the screen, her large dark eyes accented with girlish makeup, her pale face framed in long, straight brown hair, the corners of her mouth raised faintly in a suggestion of a smile. In the audience, Coche Pereyra could no longer contain her emotion and broke into sobs.

"We were able to identify her," Snow continued, his voice breaking slightly for the first time, "as Liliana Carmen Pereyra. She disappeared on her way home from work in Mar de Plata on the fifth of October, 1977. She was five months pregnant at the time."

Snow left Liliana's photograph on the screen as he turned to face the judges. "What I would like to point out here," he said, "is that in many ways the skeleton is its own best witness."

13

MERCY TENDERED,
JUSTICE DENIED

AFTER testifying at the trial of the junta leaders, Snow tried to settle down to a normal life back in Norman. He lasted less than a year. In February 1986, before the snow had melted from the cornfields at the end of his suburban street, he was offered his third assignment in Argentina. This time he was to help the government's human rights undersecretariat establish Argentina's own national forensic-science center, whose stated goal was to exhume and identify the disappeared.

Soon after his arrival in Buenos Aires, Snow rented a small apartment on Billinghurst Street, set up his Leading Edge computer, and laid out his Spanish dictionary for easy access. He was glad to be back. The team was blossoming into something more than a bunch of students on a field trip with half-baked notions of archaeology and the names of a few bones on the tips of their tongues. In fact, since Snow's testimony at the junta trial ten months before (at the end of which five of the nine generals were convicted and sentenced for crimes ranging from homicide to robbery), the team had carried out twelve court-ordered exhumations, several of which were to be presented as evidence in the upcoming trial of General Ramón J. Camps, the former chief of the Buenos Aires provincial police. Camps was credited with having overseen the disappearance of five thousand people. The exhumations were a considerable accomplishment for the young scientists, Snow realized. He also sensed that something like a philosophy had begun to crystallize among the Argentine team. It was an attitude he recognized in himself, one that he had embraced as dearly as inductive reasoning and a taste for bourbon. He had acquired it at military school in New Mexico, nurtured it during his years in the air force and again among the paper-pushers at the Federal Aviation Administration, and practiced it in numerous courtrooms as an expert witness. What the team was learning, he saw, was the willingness to question authority. Sometimes even his own.

Snow and his gang of six also realized that they needed to shift their focus away from grand recovery schemes. There were just too many *desaparecido* graves, perhaps as many as eight or nine thousand. To exhume even a few thousand graves, with their limited resources, would be like trying to build the pyramids of Egypt with seven pairs of hands. Also, the powerful effect of Snow's testimony on Liliana Pereyra at the trial of the military leaders, and the value of the physical evidence against Camps that the team had literally brought back from the dead, suggested that they could have the greatest influence with a few carefully chosen cases. Even a handful of exhumations, done the right way, could help put some of the junta's tacticians, some three hundred military men of lower rank now under investigation, in jail.

Although bones were Snow's stock-in-trade, he possessed another tool of the forensic scientist, the cold razor of statistics. He had juggled numbers most of his professional life, not only to confirm evidence from field and laboratory, but sometimes simply to entertain himself. If those who scoffed that the disappeared were really sipping café au lait in Paris bistros didn't believe the stories the bones had to tell, then he would convince them with numbers.

Before Snow left Argentina in 1985, he asked María Julia Bihurriet, his young colleague at the Undersecretariat of Human Rights, to survey all the cemeteries in the province of Buenos Aires, the nation's most populous with some eleven million inhabitants. To strengthen the case against the military, Snow had reasoned, he would have to show with hard numbers that the bodies buried in N.N. graves between 1976 and 1983 belonged to the disappeared and not to society's untouchables — the vagrants, drunks, and abandoned who subsist and, all too often, die unseen under bridges, in alleyways, or in condemned buildings. If the number of anonymous burials and the type of people interred had suddenly changed during the military dictator-ship, the undersecretariat would have the kind of evidence that, along with individual accounts of abductions and murders, could put the military on the defensive. Furthermore, a study of N.N. burials could help the team pinpoint cemeteries where the disappeared had been interred.

Snow had hardly expected Bihurriet to complete the survey by herself. Hence his surprise when he arrived in 1986 to find stacks of records on the floor of her small office at the undersecretariat. Bihur-riet explained to him how she had sent questionnaires to the superin-tendents of the 125 departments that make up the province. All the recipients were asked to provide the date of interment, along with any other recorded information, such as sex, age, or cause of death, of each N.N. buried in cemeteries in their jurisdictions between 1970 and 1984. All but twenty of the superintendents had responded. The result was file after handwritten file, like ledgers from some Dicken-sian counting house, heaped in tottering stacks that surrounded Bi-hurriet's desk.

So much for the raw material. The next step — the careful massag-ing of the data into a statistical comparison of N.N. burials before, during, and after El Proceso — would take months of work. But Snow enjoyed that kind of digging. What others might see only as cemetery records — the dry accounting of death — he regarded as a paper trail into the past.

Snow spent his days tapping the numbers into his computer. At night, he strolled among the throngs of *porteños* who promenaded up and down the noisy streets, past the sidewalk cafés and steak houses and bookshops that stayed open until the early hours of the morning. It was a culture he was learning to love. Buenos Aires buzzed with the enthusiasm of a population emerging from a chrysalis to flap its wings in the fresh air of democracy. Here, the aura of a new beginning made Snow feel young and adventurous. He was even becoming some-thing of a celebrity. At the fashionable Café la Biela near the Recoleta Cemetery, where he often took his morning coffee and cigar in the shade of a the city's biggest ombu tree, patrons occasionally recog-nized the American *profesor* who, the newspapers said, was looking for the bones of the *desaparecidos*. After dinner at Zum Edelweiss or Hispanos he often crossed the Avenida Nueve de Julio to the Grand

Café Tortoni, the elegant 130-year-old landmark on Avenida de Mayo. The city's literati convened there once a week to read their latest poems and sip espressos and brandy under ceilings of stained glass and elaborately pressed tin. At the café he preferred simply to be alone with his thoughts, the silent observer, occasionally playing a game of chess or reading the English-language daily, the *Buenos Aires Herald.* "Yes, I'm an American," he replied more than once to inquisitive patrons sitting around Tortoni's white marble tables. "But I hate the *Yanquis,* too. You see, I'm from Texas."

In Buenos Aires Snow was truly in his element. Here he wrote the rules, organized his own time, set the goals and deadlines, and took the credit or the blame. Here life could be sumptuous, with its lean steaks and sweetbreads, its rich red wine, and its passing parade of exotically beautiful women. And at times it could be backbreaking — bending over an open grave for hours, struggling to understand the language, maneuvering through the political maze of a country that had suddenly been turned on its head. But for the most part, Snow's life in Buenos Aires was uncluttered and straightforward in purpose.

Snow buried himself in Bihurriet's questionnaires. The first task was to establish the historical rate and character of N.N. burials before the 1976 coup. That rate, Snow found, ran at about four or five per one hundred thousand population each year. Most were older men, as would be the case most anywhere.[1]

Next, Snow calculated how many N.N. burials should have taken place during the late 1970s under normal circumstances and compared it with the actual rate. He found that twenty-four departments showed considerable increases in N.N. burials during the period 1976 to 1978, the most intense years of the military's dirty war. He labeled these the "significant" departments. While the number of N.N. burials remained constant at other departments during this three-year period, they doubled or tripled at the significant ones, up to as many as fourteen N.N.s per one hundred thousand people.

The difference between the expected and actual numbers of N.N.s became "excess N.N.s" in Snow's analysis. That number totaled 940 people, 84 percent of whom were buried during 1976 and 1977. Snow also noted that the reports of political disappearances during that same period also skyrocketed.

Snow then looked for the location of "prisoner assessment centers"

(PACs), an Orwellian term the military had used to describe its administrative headquarters, which housed not only offices for its paperwork but holding cells, interrogation rooms, and torture chambers. About ninety such PACs existed at the height of the repression. Survivors and some of the men who had run the PACs had testified that people killed there or at nearby detention centers were usually buried within a few dozen kilometers of the PACs. Snow found, as he had expected, that nine out of ten of the departments he had tagged as "significant" contained a PAC or were located next to one with a PAC. Of the departments where no unusual rise in N.N. burials was found, only 5 percent contained a PAC.

As Snow probed further, he found data that confirmed the largely anecdotal evidence originally compiled by President Alfonsín's commission on the disappeared (CONADEP). Women, for instance, made up about 12 percent of N.N.s before the military took over. But after the 1976 coup, their proportion jumped to 20 percent, a reflection of the fact that many of the disappeared, as the commission had found, were women. Even more striking was the shift downward in age. Among all the departments surveyed, the vast majority of N.N.s before the coup were over thirty-five at death. In 1976, the ages of those buried in anonymous graves immediately started to drop. Whereas previously only 15 percent of them had died between twenty-one and thirty-five years of age (the average age range of most of the desaparecidos), during the military government's first two years that number rose to 56 percent. Meanwhile, in the outlying departments that escaped duty as dumping grounds, the age range of N.N.s did not change.

Finally, Snow combed the questionnaires for the most damning piece of evidence of all, cause of death. Indigents don't often die of gunshot wounds to the head, at least not in Argentina, where death from firearms has traditionally been extremely low by American standards. The numbers were shocking. At the "nonsignificant" departments, the deaths by gunshot wound never rose above the norm of about 4 percent of the total. At the significant departments, however, there was an epidemic of gunshot killings — from $5\frac{1}{2}$ percent of the N.N.s before the coup to over 50 percent during the first two years of El Proceso.

Cold and impersonal, the numbers bore witness for the thousands hidden in the nameless graves. Yet again, they told the same story — lest Argentina forget.

April marks the end of summer in Argentina. It is a month of uneasy transition, when the days grow noticeably shorter and the pale blue skies of summertime give way to a canopy of dull gray clouds. It was on one such day in 1986 that Snow and his team began work on one of the dirty war's most infamous cases, the Fátima massacre.

According to press reports at the time, just before dawn on August 20, 1976, the sound of gunfire woke the town of Fátima, seventy kilometers northeast of Buenos Aires.[2] A series of explosions followed twenty minutes later. A group of laborers on their way to work that morning discovered thirty bodies strewn across a field. One of the men later told a reporter that the bodies, some with their hands tied behind their backs, appeared as if they had been dynamited.

By mid-morning the corpses had been transported to the nearest provincial police station, where a physician, Gregorio Joaquín Ferra, examined the bodies. As Ferra later testified at the trial of the ex-commandants in 1985, a police officer ordered him not to autopsy or photograph them.[3] He did note, however, each victim's approximate stature, weight, eye and skin color, and cause of death. The police, meanwhile, took fingerprints — at least according to their records. The prints, however, were never found.

That evening, as the corpses were being transported for burial in a local cemetery, known as Derqui, the junta, headed by General Jorge Videla, pledged publicly "to use every means possible to investigate the incident and to punish those responsible."[4] Then the government simply forgot about it.

In September 1983, at the instigation of a human rights group, the Center for Legal and Social Studies, a judge ordered seven of the Fátima graves opened.[5] Five sets of remains were identified, mostly based on dental records. The two unidentified bodies were returned to Derqui's soil, where they and the twenty-three others remained until April 1986, when Snow and his team arrived at the cemetery.

It was the biggest job the team had ever undertaken, and during that winter they dug as never before. When they weren't at work at the cemetery, they attended classes at the university or worked at part-time jobs. In the evenings they met in cafés or their apartments to write up their reports and plan for the next day's dig. Some days they had to suspend the work because of rain, returning the following morning to find that water had leaked through the canvas sheets they'd rigged as cover and made bathtubs out of the graves. Other days the frost-shrouded earth was rock-hard and impossible to penetrate.

It took until November of that year to bring up all twenty-five skeletons. They cleaned them and took their basic anthropological measurements. They then began to interview the relatives of eighty-three *desaparecidos* who were believed to have been detained at the Federal Police Headquarters compound in Buenos Aires.[6] According to a guard at the police station, thirty detainees had been taken out of the compound in an army truck on the night of the Fátima executions. These people, he said, were surely the same Fátima victims.

The team's investigation eventually led them to a twenty-two-year-old woman named Marta Alicia Spagnoli de Vera.[7]

Marta and her husband Juan Carlos disappeared on August 3, 1976 — seventeen days before the bodies at Fátima were discovered. Two former prisoners who had been detained at the Federal Police Headquarters told the team they had seen the couple before the Fátima executions but not afterward. Marta's surviving family members described her as being 149 centimeters (about five feet) tall, and nulliparous — she had never borne a child.

These were unremarkable statistics, typical of most of the female *desaparecidas*. Marta had never suffered a fracture or other injury that would have shown up on the bones. The family had no dental or other X rays of their daughter either, although they did remember that she had had fillings in her premolars and molars, especially among the bottom teeth. But something else might prove helpful, they said. Her top-right second incisor tilted toward the back of her mouth and her lower incisors were crowded together and aligned irregularly.

Nine of the skeletons exhumed at Derqui were female. By comparing their statures and ages with Marta's, the team immediately eliminated seven of the candidates. On the pelvic bones of one of the remaining skeletons, they found the telltale pitting and scarring that results from carrying a fetus. That one could not have been Marta.

The skull from the last set of remains rewarded the team's deliberate process of elimination. Ten teeth, five top and five bottom, bore a total of thirteen amalgam fillings, all near the back of the mouth. The fillings were larger on the bottom teeth. And the right maxillary second incisor was pushed inward. The match was close, very close. But the team wanted something stronger. They asked Marta's family one last time if they could locate Marta's dentist. They couldn't, but they found something almost as good — a blurry snapshot of their daughter taken about six months before her disappearance.

Marta had been smiling at the camera. In the photo, the bottom teeth were slightly irregular, just as on the skull. And the twisted upper incisor stood out like a lighthouse in the gloom. The remains were Marta's. Three bullet wounds, evenly spaced, had pierced the back of her skull.

Snow concluded his statistical survey at about the time the team finished its work at Derqui. From a scientific point of view, the past nine months had been a success. Even so, the team's newfound pluck and Snow's statistical "necrography" seemed destined to come to naught.

That winter had seen setbacks for the team. Money, as always, was scarce. Though the Ford Foundation had provided them with a small monthly stipend for part of the year, that source would soon dry up. Meanwhile, relations with the undersecretariat, and especially its director, Eduardo Rabossi, had soured. Rabossi, for the most part, ignored the team. They didn't have professional degrees, after all. In turn, it angered Snow and the team that the government official in charge of human rights wouldn't even take an afternoon to inspect their work. They had tried to convince Snow when he arrived in 1986 that Rabossi's undersecretariat was as inert as the inside of the crypts at the Recoleta cemetery, but Snow counseled them not to break with the undersecretariat completely, as it had resources and authority that they did not. It was the first serious argument between them.

Snow finally came around to the team's way of thinking when he turned over his statistical study of N.N. graves to the undersecretariat. Rabossi buried it, filing it away in what Snow later would call Rabossi's "black hole of Argentina."[8] Snow, however, had the last word. He gave a copy of his report to Luis Moreno Ocampo, the assistant federal prosecutor. Moreno Ocampo leaked the study to the press, who gave it plenty of ink. Rabossi fumed at Snow and his "chicos," and relations between the forensic team and the undersecretariat frosted over permanently. Clearly, the team was not destined to serve on the newly formed technical commission.

The Argentine government may have ignored the *equipo*, but another government in need of help saw value in their unique skills. Corazon Aquino had won the presidency of the Philippines and established a human rights committee to investigate the abuses of her predecessor, Ferdinand Marcos. In November 1986, the committee arranged to fly Morris Tidball, Mimi Doretti, and María Julia Bihurriet, along with Snow, to the Philippines. Waiting for them in Manila were two forensic pathologists, one an American and the other a Dane, and a AAAS staff member. For two weeks they marched thirty-four Filipino physicians and scientists through an intensive training program on how to apply forensic sciences to human rights investigations. At the time, local human rights groups were searching for the graves of over 655 people who had disappeared between 1970 and 1985. Although they were only able to identify one skeleton from the nine graves they opened, the trip boosted the team's prestige as well as their spirits.[9]

On the way back to Argentina, Snow stopped over in Oklahoma for the Christmas holidays. On the day after Christmas, he received a phone call from Morris, who, along with Mimi and María Julia, had arrived back in Argentina only a few days before. Morris's voice, ever the barometer of his mood, betrayed his disappointment. He had bad news. Early that morning the Congress had passed the *Punto Final*, or Full Stop law. It was perhaps the best Christmas present the junta's henchmen ever got.

Law 23.492 set a sixty-day deadline for the formal initiation of new prosecutions of members of the armed services, police, and prison officials accused of past human rights abuses.[10] Afterward, only cases involving the abduction of minors or the falsification of documents could be brought. A third category was also allowed — those in which property was lost. Apparently, lives could evaporate legally, but not possessions.

The Alfonsín government, which had proposed the law, expected that by February 22, 1987, when the sixty days were to expire, only some thirty to forty members of the armed forces and police, mostly in retirement, would still face charges. As it turned out, however, judges around the country rushed to issue summonses against over three hundred officers, including some still in active service.

Although the law had been aimed at appeasing the military, it actually sparked more anger within the armed forces, whose members had actually been hoping for a blanket amnesty. In April, a group of middle-ranking officers took over the Campo de Mayo army base near Buenos Aires. Their message to Alfonsín and the courts was clear: back off or else.

The public poured into the streets in protest against the rebellion, but Alfonsín balked, refusing to roust the officers from their stronghold. Instead, he chose to negotiate (though his government aides bristled at the term) with the rebels, who eventually surrendered.

By then, Snow and the team had reunited in Buenos Aires. They thought the military had exhausted its leverage with the Alfonsín government. But once again, on June 5, the government retreated. It enacted the law of *Obediencia Debido*, or Law of Due Obedience.

The quandary the Alfonsín administration faced was one that had troubled the Allies after World War II, the French after the Algerian War, and the Americans after the My Lai massacre in Vietnam: namely, to what extent are soldiers responsible for their actions while following orders?

Tribunals throughout the world have rendered varying interpretations. The first Nuremberg trial of Nazi leaders resulted in only nineteen convictions, of which twelve were death sentences. Later trials of Nazi and Japanese leaders produced more convictions, but almost all the rulings hung on the question of whether a subordinate knowingly committed a crime. American courts, for their part, were more lenient when judging atrocities committed in Vietnam. In the case of My Lai, where American soldiers killed more than one hundred Vietnamese civilians in 1968, twenty-five American officers and enlisted men were charged, but only one, Lt. William J. Calley, Jr., was convicted. He was paroled after serving three years.

As for Argentina, the Alfonsín government's new law instructed the courts to exempt from prosecution all military and police personnel except those who were chiefs of security areas or security forces. In effect, only thirty to fifty senior officers could still be prosecuted. Only three offenses were exempted from the new leniency: rape, theft, and falsification of civil status, the tactic by which the children of the disappeared were given false identities and delivered to other families. But torture, murder, arbitrary arrest, and misrepresentations to judges could now be overlooked if the alleged perpetrator was able to prove that he was just following orders.[11]

Alfonsín's compromise fell like a hammer on the team's spirits. Alejandro Inchaurregui, a medical student and political activist when he joined the team in 1986, remembers their sentiments: "It upset us a lot. We met, discussed its implications for a few days, and redefined our role from that point on. We decided we had to continue because it doesn't help anyone to feel impotent. . . . The best thing we could have done for the assassins and torturers would have been to stop."[12]

Putting assassins and torturers in jail now looked to be beyond their reach, however. In addition to returning the remains to the families, the team set out a new goal. Just as CONADEP had chronicled the fate of the disappeared through anecdotal evidence, they would now add to that historical record by providing physical evidence, the kind of evidence that doesn't hinge on memory or eyewitness accounts. Says Alejandro:

> The reconstruction of the story [of the disappeared] is extremely important. . . . One of the ways to suppress a people is to alter or destroy their identity. And one of the ways to destroy their identity is to change their history — to make people disappear, to bury them in N.N. graves, to say that this person was never born, to kidnap children, to kill their parents, and then change the childrens' birth certificates and their names and those of their families. This is unforgivable. It is an attempt to erase part of our history, our past. I believe the team's efforts to reconstruct our country's immediate past is not only healthy for our society but also for the generations that will follow us.

On June 20, 1987, a Saturday, Snow threw a party — not an Argentine *asado*, but something Texas-style — in his apartment on Billinghurst Street. In four days' time, he would be back amid the unbroken horizons of the Oklahoma prairie. Guests began to fill Snow's tiny apartment at mid-afternoon. Except for Mimi, who was in France, all the members of the team were there, along with María Julia and one of Argentina's leading investigative journalists, Horacio Verbitsky.

As Snow prepared his chili, cutting strips from a slab of beef and tossing them into a simmering pot of onions and beans, Verbitsky, a balding man in his mid-forties, stood in the kitchen doorway. His recipe, Snow told his interviewer, came from Mark Amspacher, a butcher in Norman who had won considerable renown at chili contests in the southwestern United States. Snow said he had talked Mark into sharing the recipe on the promise that he would use it only in Argentina.

Verbitsky listened patiently, waiting for the opportune moment to steer the anthropologist back to Argentina. "What do you think of the law of Due Obedience, and the fact that the undersecretariat appeared to support it?" he finally asked.[13]

"Look," Snow replied, "I can only talk about what I know. . . . In the undersecretariat's upper echelons there is inertia, a lack of dedication to really upholding human rights. If I had had to depend only on the undersecretariat, I would have wasted a year of my life. That it didn't turn out that way was because of the team. I haven't seen the dedication and the hard work in the undersecretariat that I saw in CONADEP. Maybe this is due to philosophers like Dr. Eduardo Rabossi, who are good at contemplating things but not at actually carrying them out. Is it better that they should have appointed a philosopher than a police detective?

"In the files of the undersecretariat there is documentation on at least 8,961 disappeared. My job is that of a scientific detective. Now when we're dealing with homicides we never close the cases until they are solved because there is no statute of limitations on murder."

Snow stopped his stirring and looked Verbitsky in the eye. "So is my opinion on the matter clear?"

Verbitsky nodded.

"What I *don't* understand," Snow added, "is how they can retroactively legalize murder."

For Snow, this looked like his last trip. Politics had thrust its ugly snout in the way of doing good science, and he wanted none of it. "Sowing dragon's teeth," he said of the two amnesty laws. And although the team was growing accustomed to Snow's north-south oscillations, they thought the latest turn of events in Buenos Aires would put an end to the American's visits.

As the chili bubbled throughout the afternoon, everyone tucked into a large supply of beer and wine. The little apartment grew close with the haze of cigarette smoke and the aroma of beans and beef and peppers. The guests draped themselves over the few sticks of furniture and stretched out on the floor as several conversations competed simultaneously for prominence.

Then Morris got up and asked for everyone's attention. He told Snow that the team had brought him a gift, a woolen poncho typical of northern Argentina. Snow slipped it over his head and pulled it down over his shoulders. There was a round of applause. Morris insisted on snapshots, so Snow, dressed in his straw cowboy hat and new poncho, left his chili pot and posed.

Morris held Snow by the arm and told him there was something more. Everyone fell silent and Morris spoke for the group. He told Snow how just three hours earlier, the father of a disappeared girl had been standing here in his apartment photographing a skull to help another father find his daughter. Events like these, he said, were indicative of Snow's accomplishments in their country. For this, and for so many other things, Morris said, they wanted to give their thanks. He held out a framed piece of paper. It was a hand-stenciled diploma declaring that Clyde Snow was an honorary member of the Equipo Argentina de Antropología Forense. Clyde held it before him, his tough exterior melting, and smiled even as the tears rolled down his cheeks.

"Then we opened a bottle of Bolivian *pisco*," Alejandro recalls. "It nearly did us in. But the chili was so hot, it was the only way we could kill the fire. We went on until two in the morning. But the real conclusion of this dinner came a year later when the owner of the apartment presented us with a bill for one hundred dollars. She had a list of all the things we'd broken. It was amazing! Cigarette burns on the sofa, a torn curtain, I don't know how many broken glasses. . . ."

"Three days after the chili dinner we met Clyde at the airport to say good-bye. It was the same day that we were talking about exhuming a mass grave at the Avellaneda cemetery. So we told him. At first, he didn't say anything. Then, just after he passed through the gate, he turned and said, 'If you take on Avellaneda, I'm coming back!' "[14]

14

TODAVÍA CANTAMOS

ONCE moved, the earth rebels. It does not lie easily in compact strata like the unmoved sod around it. Instead, the earth sits loosely, and is darker in color. If the ground is gently scraped smooth with a trowel, a refilled hole stands out like a knot in a plank of maple.

Cemeteries are full of such scars. They usually mark the orderly interring of the dead, one by one, in the earth. But in Buenos Aires there is a cemetery, in an old neighborhood beyond the slaughterhouses and tanneries of this city of beef and leather, where the turned soil hides a secret from the dirty war. The name of the cemetery is Avellaneda, the *l*s pronounced like a *j* in the local patois. At least two hundred people are buried there in the country's largest mass grave — the *desaparecidos*, enemies of the state, though most of them never knew why.

The cemetery at Avellaneda came into being in 1870. It now sprawls across about six hundred acres, a virtual city of the dead tended by hundreds of workers, most of whom live within walking distance of the necropolis. Like a medieval city, it is encircled by high walls. Avellaneda's are pale pink. Outside the walls, merchants enjoy a brisk trade. Shops sell statuary, bronze plaques, bouquets of freshly cut flowers, icons, and talismans to mourners before they pass through the high-arched gate on Calle Agüero. For the army of gravediggers, cafés provide meals, beer, and ice cream.

Inside the walls an avenue lined with swamp maples leads visitors to narrow paths between the graves, like a river emptying driftwood into a broad delta. The tombs are mostly modest stone crypts sunk into the ground and adorned with flowers, epitaphs carved into the stone, or sun-faded photographs of the long-dead occupants. Mausoleums adorned with spiraling marble statuary testify to a taste for the Gothic. Except for a few islands of dappled shade cast by a smattering of acacia trees, the vista of white stone shimmers under an austral sun.

To the casual observer, Avellaneda looks like many other cemeteries that serve the city's population. In one part of Avellaneda, however, lies sector 134, a walled, grassy rectangle about the size of a tennis court. The ground there sags in places, like a rumpled pillow. The sector is unmarked, and its only access now is a rusty iron gate that bears a crude sign forbidding entry. The west wall separates the sector from the main cemetery, the east from a quiet suburban street.

Just inside the entrance, a few paces to the left, stands an abandoned morgue. Water stains mar the building's crumbling cement exterior, and broken glass lies strewn across its threshold. On the metal door leading into the morgue someone has written in crude red letters: *No cage adentro, estamos en democracia. Gracias.* ("Do not shit in here, we are a democracy. Thank you.")

Inside, the morgue reeks of human excrement. A pallid light seeps through a dozen small, broken windows, too high for anyone to look through. White tiles cover the walls from floor to eye level, their smudged surfaces feathered with cobwebs. An aluminum examining table occupies the middle of the room, its only piece of furniture. A film of dust and grime obscures its top, and a human thighbone pokes out from an opening in its metal base. On one wall, about two feet above the floor, a dull burgundy splotch of old blood disfigures the tile. A spray of droplets spreads from the splotch in a long arc, its shape and pattern suggesting a sudden and explosive separation of blood from body. In a dark corner sits a wooden box labeled, in Spanish, "Selected Argentine Fruit." The box contains a human skull and a jumble of bones.

It is March 1, 1988. Back outside, two women and four men attend to various tasks in the sector, which they are preparing to excavate, slowly, a few centimeters at a time. Mimi, dressed in pale blue shorts and a T-shirt with "University of Oklahoma" written on the front, kneels in a shallow depression, scraping dirt from around a bone embedded in the earth. She concentrates on exposing the bone, using the edge of her trowel and alternating with a small brush. A red barrette fails to hold back her hair, which falls on either side of her face to reveal a sunburned neck and shoulders.

Pato perches crosslegged on the lip of the depression. Her long, veined fingers grip a brightly colored pencil as she sketches the layout of the hole on a pad of drawing paper. It is the first plot of earth the group has opened. She labels it "Cuadrícula D9."

Nearby, Luis, shirtless, hammers a metal stake into the ground with a wooden mallet. He already has driven in several stakes, which stand in neat rows down the length of the courtyard. Luis has placed them to mark off quadrangles exactly two-and-a-half meters square. He punctuates his hammering with off-key and off-color renditions of old songs of Carlos Gardel.

Two other men — Carlos Somigliana, known as Mako, and Alejandro — are stretching a white nylon line from one end of the courtyard to the other. Mako attaches one end of the line to a ringbolt screwed into the south wall. Ale, peering from under a floppy white tennis cap, stretches the other end of the line to pass directly over a row of stakes. His beard and tinted glasses make him look older than his thirty years.

Ale pulls his end of the line tight and ties it to a bolt in the north wall. A small carpenter's level threaded over the line assures him that it is parallel to the ground. He hustles down the row of metal stakes, stopping at each to secure the line by splitting it over a single nail driven into the top of each post.

Each cordoned-off row of squares, or *cuadrículas*, is identifiable by one of five letters, A through E, painted on the south wall, and by a number, from one through nine, painted on the west and east walls. When the team finishes laying out the forty-five squares, the place will look something like a crossword puzzle. As each square in the puzzle is created, it is then subdivided into a smaller square-within-a-square with four short wooden stakes and more string. The smaller squares measure two meters to a side. Digging must remain within the smaller boundary, in order to leave a one-meter wall, or balk, between *cuadrículas*.

Clyde Snow, his thumbs hooked into the belt loops of his chinos, stands in the sun's glare and watches. Sweat dampens his checked shirt where it stretches over a big, hard Texas belly, and his thinning, cornsilk-fine graying hair is damp and matted. He wears dark glasses and cowboy boots that might once have been oxblood but are now scuffed and muddied into an indeterminate neutral shade. The hatching of brown skin underneath his eyes has spread with his four years in the South American sun. A cigarette dangles from his mouth, its ash hanging precariously.

"Remember to keep the earth walls between the *cuadrículas* vertical," he says to no one in particular. "You read the stratigraphy from those balks. It's plain old archaeology."

Continuing with her scraping, Mimi translates Snow's instructions into Spanish for the others while he examines a row of Luis's stakes. "Muy bueno," he says. "But woe to the person who kicks one."

Somewhere on the street beyond the east wall, a loudspeaker crackles into life. "Three australes for a bag of biscuits," a vendor announces in Spanish. "Sweet, fresh, and crisp biscuits. The big bag of biscuits, three australes. And eggs, good fresh eggs. Yes, ladies, believe it, one-and-a-half australes." Variations on the refrain follow, slowly fading into silence again as the biscuit-man draws farther away.

Ready now to join in the work, Snow peels off his shirt, takes a brush from a yellow plastic bucket, and kneels in a *cuadrícula*. Luis drops a cassette into a tape player balanced on a nearby bench that he has constructed from broken gravestones and cinder blocks. The voice of Mercedes Sosa fills the courtyard. "Todavía cantamos," she croons in a husky contralto. "We still sing." Luis picks up a six-foot-long iron rod he has lifted from a nearby construction site and slowly probes the earth around *cuadrícula* E9 for soft spots that might reveal where the earth has been removed and then returned.

Without fanfare, the largest forensic exhumation ever attempted has begun.

Mimi Doretti sits in a folding chair with her legs tucked under her in the one-room office of the Equipo Argentino de Antropología Forense. The room perches like an aviary on the roof of a beaux arts townhouse that serves as the offices of the human rights group Movimiento Ecuménico de Derechos Humanos (MEDH), the Ecumenical

Movement for Human Rights. The hum of downtown Buenos Aires drifts through tall French doors, the only concession to ornament in a Spartan room of whitewashed walls, a plywood board on sawhorses that provides a work surface, and a telephone that functions only when coaxed and when the telephone workers aren't on strike.

It is just past noon on a mid-March day in 1988, and Mimi is reading the transcript of a former detainee at the Banfield police station. With a black felt-tip pen, she circles the names of the people he saw there, people who may have been killed and later buried in the courtyard at Avellaneda. Avellaneda has become the team's obsession. Almost every day now, in small groups or sometimes separately, they board buses and bounce through the potholed streets of western Buenos Aires, across the bridge that spans the Riachuelo River, its current coursing with the runoff from the city's tanneries and meat-packing plants, past the blocks of auto-repair shops and apartment towers, to meet at sector 134.

Like Dante's guided tour through Hell, the team's investigations — the painful, halting interviews with detention-camp survivors, the long nights spent leafing through names and cryptic numbers penciled in police ledgers — have begun to unravel the curtain behind which Avellaneda hid during the years of military rule. Often, the threads began in the western part of the city at the Banfield police station, a solid, stucco building painted yellow and topped by a watchtower.

On a typical night in a courtyard behind the station, plainclothes officers loaded bodies into a van or a Ford Falcon. Sometimes they dragged along living captives, their hands tied behind their backs and hoods over their heads. The prisoners were being "transferred," in the jargon of the Buenos Aires Provincial Police, from the *pozo*, or pit, of Banfield. Usually the order came from Colonel Ramon J. Camps, the chief of the provincial police, or his deputy at Banfield, Amílcar Tarela, more commonly known as Trimarco.

The caravan bumped over the cobblestones and potholes of Calle Siciliano, then past a schoolhouse and the houses of Banfield's well-to-do, each block protected by walls topped with broken glass like the spines of poisonous fishes. The caravan followed the main road, Avenida Hipólito Yrigoyen, named after the revered president of

Argentina during happier days in the 1920s. The hour, as was the norm for such transfers, was late, and the pace slow; they were the police, and no one would inquire into their business.

The cars passed through the barrio of Remedios de Escalada, by places that had become familiar to the drivers: a junkyard on the right; the local Goodyear outlet; the *gomerias*, whose merchandise — used tires — were chained together in stacks on the sidewalk. Next came the Lanus barrio, its tall apartment buildings darkened, the only sign of apparent life the sleepy travelers sitting with their cardboard suitcases on the sidewalk next to the bus depot. The caravan turned right onto Hulgera just after the glass factory and entered a neighborhood of stockyards, whose pungent fumes followed the cars well into the slums, where cement shanties slumped among stands of haggard trees and the rusted wrecks of abandoned cars that ringed Avellaneda.

Finally, the caravan entered Calle Agüelo, which runs along the high pink walls of the Avellaneda cemetery. To the left, the entrances to the cafés and the *bronzeras* that sell plaques for graves were tightly shut behind corrugated metal doors, rolled down over the entrances like lids over a lizard's eyes. The cars made their last turn onto Calle Oyüela and stopped outside an iron gate in a brick wall that led into a courtyard next to a squat cement building. The driver shouted and the gate opened outward. As the cars turned to back in, their lights illuminated the ocher walls and green shutters of a darkened apartment building across the street.

At that moment, some of those who lived in the apartments paused by their windows to peer down at the scene across the street. As they watched, men lit up by the vehicles' headlights like players on a stage carried bodies into the morgue. Sometimes the bodies were simply left there, and the stench would waft up for days until, mercifully, the cemetery workers dug the big pits in the courtyard and buried them. Many of the building's residents had moved away, and those who remained did not tell strangers, or even their friends in the neighborhood, of what they had seen.

The vehicles were quickly lightened of the corpses and the prisoners. The mute witnesses above turned back to their beds, but not yet to sleep. Clocks ticked through the silence and the air hung still. Finally, a sudden burst of gunfire rang out from the courtyard below.

The silence closed in again, and only then did the residents of Calle Oyuela return to their fitful dreams.

Sitting in the cluttered office, Mimi closes the ledger with a sigh. The Banfield story is only one of many that fill the team's notebooks — and that fill their dreams as well.

The team first broke ground at Avellaneda in October 1986. The federal court of the city of Buenos Aires was in the midst of prosecuting Ramón J. Camps. Under Camps's direction, the police ran a number of clandestine detention centers, principally in La Plata and its environs, and in the suburbs of Buenos Aires. The court needed a corpus delicti to bolster its case, and suspected that Avellaneda, which fell within Camps's jurisdiction, would deliver the evidence. The court, to its credit, knew that the undersecretariat couldn't perform an exhumation; it asked the *equipo* to do the job. As for a suspected *desaparecido* to look for in sector 134, the court proferred the name of Rafael Perrota.

Perrota apparently was guilty of nothing more than being particularly flush and, in the opinion of some of the junta's henchmen, of value to its cause. In 1977 Perrota sold his newspaper, *El Cronisto Comercial*, and profited handsomely from the transaction. Much like the leftist Montoneros, the police task forces had adopted kidnapping-for-ransom as a convenient source of cash to keep themselves in Fords and firearms.

Perrota was abducted on June 13, 1977. The same day his kidnappers demanded a large ransom. Although the family delivered the money, they never saw Perrota again.[1]

Survivors of a detention center known as COTI Martínez, including the well-known Argentine author Jacobo Timerman, said they had seen Perrota alive there, though suffering the aftereffects of torture. He also was believed to have passed through Pozo de Banfield, run by the First Army Corps and one of the last stops on the way to the cemetery at Avellaneda. Soldiers who had run the center confirmed in testimony before CONADEP that Perrota had been there.

The team trooped out to Avellaneda. A gravedigger led them to a spot in the walled-in sector near the eastern wall where, he said, they would find bodies. A day's digging uncovered eleven skeletons stacked one atop the other. Some of the skulls contained bullet holes. When the team screened the dirt from the grave through a wire mesh, they found thirteen spent bullets. They found no clothes among the bones, nor were there signs that any of the bodies had been autopsied before being buried. The cemetery records from the period of the dirty war provided the barest of descriptions — the bodies had been listed merely as male or female, sometimes with an approximate age. Any identification would have to be made strictly from the physical characteristics of the bones.

The team measured and sexed the skeletons but none fit the description of Perrota. But they had other prospects. A few families whose relatives had disappeared into Banfield and other nearby detention centers had sent them antemortem records and physical descriptions. They soon matched one of the eleven skeletons with a set of antemortem data. The remains they identified belonged to María Mercedes Hourquebie de Francese. Age, sex, and stature of the skeleton corresponded to the woman's description. Also, a dental prosthesis found with the skull matched antemortem dental records. Hourquebie de Francese had disappeared in 1977 along with her entire family. At the age of seventy-seven, she was the oldest known *desaparecida*.[2]

The team submitted their analysis of Hourquebie de Francese's remains to the federal court, but without a cause of death the information couldn't contribute to the prosecution. The court, as it turned out, didn't need it; Camps was convicted and sentenced in December 1986 to a jail term of twenty-five years.

Nonetheless, the paper trail of documents and testimony convinced the team that other victims of the death squads lay elsewhere in sector 134, perhaps more than two hundred of them. They wrote up the results of this initial probe into the sector and asked the court if they could continue the work there, suggesting that one to two years of archaeologically sound excavation would be needed to finish the entire courtyard. They argued that if they could identify even one person in each pit and trace his or her last days to a detention center and a date, they could follow that lead to identify others in the same pit who might have come from the same center.

But no one seemed very interested anymore in digging up that part of the past. The court declined to take the team up on its offer.

★   ★   ★

A summer passed after the team's first sally into Avellaneda, and the weeds and *cipo* vines and little *pindo* palms quickly grew back over the lone hole dug in the courtyard. The team could do little but wait until a judge traced one of the disappeared to Avellaneda and asked for another exhumation.

Their break finally came in June 1987. A judge in the city of La Plata, Nelky Martínez, gave them permission to start digging again in Avellaneda.[3] The judge believed that somewhere in sector 134 lay the body of María Teresa Cerviño. According to police files, Cerviño, a young woman believed to have been a Montonera, was shot to death in 1976. Police in Buenos Aires found her hooded body hanging from a bridge adorned with a sign that read, "*Soy una Montonera. Sigame.*" ("I am a Montonera. Follow me.")

By the time the team reorganized itself, it was November, the beginning of spring in Argentina, and sector 134 was bursting with weeds. The inside of the morgue, where they planned to set up their own laboratory for examining the bones, had become a toilet for drifters and cemetery workers. For now, the team dropped any pretense of being forensic experts and got down to shoveling broken glass and human feces. That done, they turned to the chest-high undergrowth, slashing at it like jungle guides with machetes and scythes. Eventually the little forest was reduced to something more like the rough on a golf course.[4]

The bones they found in the undergrowth didn't belong to *desaparecidos*, but rather to unfortunates whose families had failed to keep up with the annual payment of a grave tax to the cemetery. Once in arrears, these graves are repossessed. Gravediggers remove the bones and cart them to one of the *osarios*, shafts dug into the earth and topped with cast-iron plates like manhole covers. Into these the bones are ignominiously cast. The *equipo* figured that bones scattered on the surface of sector 134 had fallen off wheelbarrows destined for the *osarios* and that cemetery workers had flipped them over the wall into the courtyard, the one place where they would never be seen.

"The cemetery workers were supposed to help us," Mimi recalls. "Well, we waited, but no one came. I talked to one gravedigger and he said they were afraid of the spirits in the place. It's because of the things that happened there. They were the ones who dug the holes, they called them *vaqueros*, how would you say in English . . . cowholes? Because the pits were big enough for cows. The workers saw what happened. They were afraid to come in. Most of them still don't."

One worker did, however. As the team began its first survey of the sector, he described how the military ran the cemetery as a secret dumping ground. After the vans brought the bodies, the workers dug the *vaqueros*, each about two meters long and two meters deep. They stacked the bodies inside, head to foot to make the most of the space. "We threw them in like sardines," the gravedigger said, "one on top of another. . . . The police would call us over in the mornings after the trucks had come in with the bodies. I remember times when the morgue was overflowing with bodies. They were even in the outside passageway, right under the open sky. It was terrible! A fiesta of worms. The soldiers told us to begin digging holes and then we threw them in."[5]

In late February 1988, Snow, true to his promise to return if Avellaneda was opened, flew to Buenos Aires. Avellaneda, he suspected, was not likely to turn out like any other forensic job he or any other anthropologist had ever seen. It was going to be big, the biggest exhumation ever in forensics, he reckoned. And it would be tough going.

Local officials had made some vague promises to help, but the team's first request, for the removal of the trees and underbrush they'd cut and stacked at the courtyard's entrance, had gone unanswered. The only thing they did get was a lone policeman to stand guard. Paunchy and somnolent, he soon found a shady corner next to a nearby tool shed to make his own, where he sat dozing like a round Buddha, now and then raising his chin from his chest to observe the progress.

In early March, supplies arrived from the States: carpenters' levels for setting lines and Marshal Town trowels. Besides Mimi's camera, the most sophisticated piece of technology on hand was Luis's old radio/tape player, a boom box whose boom had mostly fled and whose aerial was a coat hanger. Luis possessed eclectic taste, so everyone's musical preferences were satisfied at least once in a while. When Snow first arrived on the site, Luis popped in a tape of tunes by Bob Wills and the Texas Playboys, winding it forward to a song particularly appropriate to Snow's arrival: "Big Balls in Cowtown."

In late March rains swept through the cemetery and overwhelmed the hastily constructed plastic shrouds that the team had set up over the holes, turning them into muddy pools. Work on the site slowed. Meanwhile, right-wing terrorists who had backed the military for so many years began to clear their collective throat, voicing their impatience with the course of Alfonsín's civilian government by leaving bombs in movie theaters. As the streets of Buenos Aires flooded and the potholes in the sidewalks turned into invisible traps for the unwary, lovers and drunks were turned out of late-night cinemas as the bomb threats were called in. The climate, literally and figuratively, hardly smiled on the *equipo*.

On a hot afternoon that March, during a respite from the rain, the team was finishing a day's work in sector 134. Outside the courtyard they took turns washing the sweat and clay from their skin in a basin where the cemetery's visitors fill vases for flowers. A pink, heart-shaped soap dish was passed from one brown hand to another. Their hair lay wet and gleaming against their heads.

When the last one had finished, they straggled through the cemetery and crossed the street to the Mathias Bar, a café with a cement floor, fly-specked walls, and the slowest-moving ceiling fan in the Southern Hemisphere. The café had no door, just a wide entryway that was boarded up at night. The proprietor stood behind a counter cutting slices from a hunk of meat impaled on a vertical rod like some sort of beefy barber pole. A foursome of gravediggers sat inside. They were older men, working only part-time now. Their backs were bent and the flesh hung loose and wrinkled around their elbows. They played cards silently, looking up only briefly to acknowledge the young men and women who sat themselves at the lone table on the sidewalk outside the café.

Mimi and Pato ordered Fanta, Luis a beer. Dario Olmo, a serious man in his early thirties who joined the team in 1986, ordered a mineral water and sat silently while the others chatted.

Pato's drooping lids and liquid eyes gave her a sleepy look. Her skin and hair were the same shade of light brown, and her straight nose ended in the shape of a teardrop. She smoked as she talked with an American journalist who asked her what her family and friends thought of her work at the cemetery.

"For me it was a little complicated because of my job. At first, I had to lie. I was working in my uncle's company back then, in 1985, and for him, human rights passed like the traffic. I couldn't tell him I was taking off to exhume graves." She laughed at this, covering her mouth with her hands and smiling with her eyes. "Besides, he has lots of friends who are military men. So I don't know how many exams I invented in that year."

Luis sat next to Pato, one hand wrapped around a lukewarm bottle of Quilmes beer and the other draped over the back of Pato's chair, his fingers touching her hair. He watched her as she spoke, and smiled when she smiled, his dimples barely visible under his usual three days' growth of beard. When she paused, he added:

My situation was a little different. I have four brothers in my family and their political views vary. Some are more militant than others. . . . With my parents and my older brother, there is some worry, but it's okay. With my friends it's different. I have different types of friends — friends from the university, from the neighborhood, friends with whom I play football who aren't really concerned about human rights. I don't talk to them about our work. Sometimes they ask what I do, and, at first anyway, I told them I worked in prehistoric archaeology. Now, my picture is in the papers sometimes. So, when they ask I just don't talk about it much. We all keep an independent life from work. We need to, it should never end up eating your life away. . . .

When I started in this work, in 1985, I had read a lot about politics and what had happened in Argentina, but I hadn't really become involved, say, as an activist. So to jump right into exhumations, well. . . .

His voice drifted off for a moment, as he ran his open hand through his shock of curly hair. "Anyway, it was the right thing to do, to look for the truth. . . . And the important thing now is to be working together, all of us together, that is something I am proud of."

Pato recalled that once she and Ale were going through cemetery records at a court and Ale found that one of his friends, a young woman, was listed as a burial. "I don't know," Pato said with a sigh, "to discover something like that would probably break me." She absentmindedly picked at her cuticles as she considered her words. "I don't have any disappeared in my family and I have never been involved in any political party. But I've always thought if I knew anyone who was disappeared, I don't know what I would do, it would be difficult. But Ale, he just goes on."

"I remember a line of Ale's," Luis said. "We were being interviewed and we were asked how we could exhume graves with bodies that might have been in there for eight years, something like that. And Alejandro replied, 'We're close to death, but we are making a grand act of life.' "

Mimi rejoined the group. She had been inside, talking to one of the gravediggers whose confidence she had won over the past year and a half. Sometimes he suggested where they might dig first. He preferred to talk where they couldn't be easily seen.

Mimi was studying cultural anthropology when she started exhuming *desaparecidos*. She worked on a student magazine and had interviewed some of the government's opponents. She had painted slogans on a wall once. She had never touched a human bone before. At first, she was reluctant to get involved in forensics.

"I knew this was something more, and that after the first exhumation, I'd just be marked," she told the journalist. "It was 1984, democracy was beginning here, and everybody was talking about a new military coup. I was worried that I could be on . . . well, the next list," she said with a wry smile.

"I was also worried about going to a cemetery and getting inside a grave with someone who had died in a violent way. And I was afraid of things that you don't know. We didn't know what could happen to us once we were there."

Over the four years the team had been together, Mimi's fears had subsided but never completely disappeared. She often told Pato of her dreams. Sometimes the skeletons she uncovered in the day came to life at night.

While Pato had become the field leader at the exhumations and Ale and Morris shared the public relations and politicking duties,

Mimi had taken on the task of interviewing the relatives of suspected *desaparecidos* to track down medical records and personal histories that could help in identifying skeletons. She also was the one who usually performed the team's most difficult task: informing families that a set of bones belonged to their lost relative, most often a son or daughter. Mimi recalled one especially trying incident.

"It was in 1986, when we were working on the Fátima case. Thirty bodies had been dumped in a field outside of Buenos Aires in 1976 and later buried as N.N.s. We exhumed twenty-five of the bodies." She paused to ask a waiter for a coffee, then continued:

> We arranged with the lawyers and presumed families to have a meeting every week. And there was a woman who was coming to the meetings, maybe she came three times the whole year. She was looking for her daughter. . . . After we'd exhumed all the bodies, we identified the daughter of this woman. So we arranged a meeting with her to tell her. She was thinking that nobody was ever going to find her daughter. She gave us ante-mortem information but just as a formality, not really believing.
>
> At the meeting, the lawyer said, "Now Mimi is going to describe what is going on." This was the first time I had met her. . . . Well, there was no way to say it in an indirect way. So after five minutes of saying stupid things, I said, "Well, we found your daughter." And this woman started crying. She said it was the most terrible thing to tell her, she would prefer to go on thinking that her daughter had disappeared, that she would reappear someday, and that's the way she wanted things to remain.

Mimi turned her palms skyward and shrugged, more in sadness than exasperation.

The talk turned away from work. Luis and Pato were planning a vacation to the Cataracas de Iguazú, the waterfalls on the Argentine-Brazilian border. Mimi was coaxed into showing some copies of photos she had taken that were to be exhibited the following week at a gallery in the fashionable Florida district. The images were brooding abstracts, all form and texture with few human subjects in the frames.

Ale appeared across the street, passing through the main gate of the cemetery. Short and stocky, his movements were contained and abrupt like a gymnast's despite the suggestion of a nascent paunch. He waited for a funeral procession to pass — a hearse, three ancient Fords and a Peugeot, and finally a pickup truck, its bed filled to the brim with flowers in extravagent arrangements. He strode over to the café, pulled up a chair, and conversed quietly with the team, pulling at his trim black beard as he talked. He had just come from the cemetery director's office. An anonymous caller had telephoned the cemetery the night before and threatened to kill everyone working in sector 134.

The day after the death threat, the team sat around an oval table in a windowless room on the second floor of the MEDH headquarters. The team's computer, marked with the logo of Texas Instruments, hummed on a table in the corner, its well-being the justification for having the only air conditioner in the building turned on. Clyde Snow sat at the keyboard, tinkering with a program he had designed to inventory the remains at Avellaneda.

Alejandro, his elbows planted on the table, leaned forward and explained in Spanish what the director of the Avellaneda Cemetery had told him the day before. "The night guard at the cemetery received several telephone calls threatening him and the police guards at the morgue at Avellaneda," he said. "The caller also said that members of the team would be killed."

Morris, rocking his chair onto its back legs, reminded the group that making death threats was as easy as picking up the telephone. Actually doing something, however, took effort. "We should be surprised if we *didn't* get any," he scoffed.

"The Avellaneda barrio is full of organized crime," Ale added. "People make threats all the time. You don't take them very seriously. This doesn't move even a hair on my head. The way I look at it, if they were really going to harm us, they wouldn't have announced it beforehand. They would have just done it."

Picking up some of the Spanish, Snow turned to the group and said: "Yeah, death threats are so common down here they ought to set up hours of the day when these calls will be taken. You know, the cemetery director gets one and says, 'Sorry, we don't take death threats except between the hours of ten o'clock and two o'clock. You'll have to call back later.' "

Mimi translated and the team laughed, although a little nervously. All had thought long and hard about who might be watching them. Despite the presence of the *cana*, the officer assigned to guard them at the site, the police could hardly be trusted. In 1985, while exhuming a grave in Boulogne Cemetery, Mimi had overheard one policeman say to another, "If we had done the job right in the first place, these people wouldn't have anything to dig up."

They also had to consider the judge, Martínez, who didn't want to draw attention to the dig. Already, word of the team's activities had spread through the community, and in an embarrassing and bizarre way. A commercial company hired by the municipal authorities to haul away the debris cleared by the team had simply dumped it in an overgrown corner of a nearby *villa miseria*, or slum. The residents found human bones in the rubbish and, understandably miffed at having death dumped on their doorsteps, protested to the local government.

The team passed a brown gourd filled with maté around the table as they pondered the danger, real or perceived, of the death threat. "Well, this isn't the first threat we've had," Morris said. "And it won't be the last either." The team had exhumed scores of bodies and encountered plenty of hostility from officials as well as ordinary citizens who wanted to keep the past buried. But the tenor of the times had to be heeded as well. There were those who might be provoked — those who sat quietly smoking in the cafés, or who were counting the passing days in their barracks and fortresslike *estancias* in the countryside, the ones who supported and carried out the dirty war and who wanted to keep its casualties invisible.

After an hour debating the pros and cons of proceeding with the excavation, the team decided to suspend digging for a week. There was plenty of legwork to do chasing down documents and testimony.

Mimi and Snow headed to the narrow staircase that led up to the team's rooftop office. Mimi waited for Snow to go first; the anthropologist's only known concession to physical fitness, besides fieldwork, was his habit of running up flights of stairs, as long as there weren't too many flights. Heavy-footed in his cowboy boots, he made the iron rungs of the staircase ring through the building. Mimi followed cat-like. The rest of the team drifted off into the city, to resume, at least for a few days, something akin to a normal life.

It was on an "office day" that the team received a phone call from Juan Méndez. Méndez was an Argentine lawyer who worked in Washington, D.C., for Americas Watch, a human rights organization. He now used his legal skills and knowledge of Latin-American politics to investigate violations of human rights throughout the region. Méndez knew Snow and the team and had followed their trials and successes for years. On the phone that day, his voice betrayed excitement. He asked for Snow.

"Clyde," he said, "You know about the Suárez Mason case in San Francisco?"

"That's the extradition hearing, right?" Snow replied. Mimi and Morris looked up from their work to listen.

"That's right," Méndez said. "Look, the prosecutor has contacted me. He wants to give the judge as much evidence as he can to show just what kind of things Suárez Mason did. We need the hardest evidence we can get. So I remembered that statistical study you did of the N.N. burials. Do you still have it?"

Snow smiled. "Sure, I've got it."

"Can you write up a condensed version, something the nonscientist, or a judge, will understand?"

"I think we can handle that. When do you need it?" Snow asked. "A week or so? Okay, I'll get it together and send it up, God and the Argentine mail service willing."

Snow hung up and turned to his colleagues. "*All right*, now we got a real case."

The subject of Snow's enthusiasm was a particularly nasty piece of work named Carlos Guillermo Suárez Mason. General Suárez Mason commanded the First Army Corps during the first three years of military rule. He controlled the provinces of Buenos Aires and La Pampa. Within the military, he was known as "Pajarito," or "Little Bird," because of his prominent nose and his tendency to flee the country, as he had done after a failed coup against the government of Juan Perón in the early 1950s. To those in the clandestine centers, however, he had been called "the Lord of Life and Death."

When the military threw in the towel after being humiliated in the

Falklands and vilified on the streets of Buenos Aires, Suárez Mason fled to the United States. Immigration officials finally tracked him down in Foster City, California, in January 1987. He claimed that he had never ordered anyone to be tortured, and that those who might have died at his command were terrorists anyway. Former detainees, including Jacobo Timerman, who described Suárez Mason in his book *Prisoner Without a Name, Cell Without a Number* as the symbol of torture and death, said otherwise. So did the Argentine government, which issued warrants for the general's arrest on forty-three counts of murder and twenty-three of kidnapping. While in jail in San Francisco awaiting his extradition hearing, he coolly argued his innocence. His confident demeanor reportedly broke only once: when a reporter showed him a photograph of a pretty young woman, about the same age as Suárez Mason's daughter, who had been five months pregnant when she was abducted from her home in La Plata. It was a photograph of Liliana Pereyra. "Okay," he told the reporter, "maybe these things happen. In actuality, I knew that people disappeared. Anything is possible. But who did it? You know I'm not a murderer . . . believe me."[6]

Standing in the *equipo*'s office in Buenos Aires, Snow was exultant. Perhaps his months of labor on the statistical survey of N.N. deaths now would find a more useful fate than filling up a file drawer in Rabossi's bureaucratic cul-de-sac at the undersecretariat. He would like to see the philosopher's face when he heard that Argentine and American prosecutors wanted him and the *equipo* to help extradict Suárez Mason with the very scientific evidence that Rabossi had ignored.

Snow had only a few days left in Buenos Aires. He put together a summary of the statistical survey for Méndez, made a few more trips to Avellaneda, and then left the job to his young charges. The team still had some things to learn about archaeology, but they would learn from experience, and they were now as confident in the face of adversity as he'd ever seen them. Who knows? he wondered. Maybe the next chapter in the history of forensic anthropology, and the course it would take hereafter, now lay in the hands of seven young Argentines in a place called Avellaneda.

* * *

It was a sultry January 24, 1989, a day when bands of well-armed soldiers occupied many street corners of downtown Buenos Aires. Left-wing extremism had reappeared like a specter from the 1970s: the day before, a small band of armed civilians had staged a suicide attack on an infantry barracks called La Tablada. Most were killed, and photographs of the carnage on the front pages of the morning newspapers had put a nervous edge on the day.

Clyde Snow had just returned to Argentina after a nine-month absence. He hailed a taxi with a wave of his cowboy hat and directed the driver to Avellaneda. Trucks carrying troops added to the pell-mell of morning traffic. At the cemetery, the cab drove through the front gate and stopped as close to sector 134 as the road went. Here, as usual, nothing indicated the passage of time and travail on the outside. Snow walked the last one hundred yards through the rows of gravestones and tombs to the courtyard. Inside the iron gate, Luis met Snow with a smile and beckoned him inside. "Long time no see," Luis said, practicing a new English idiom.

The scene that greeted Snow was macabre, as if staged by a Hollywood set designer bent on shocking his audience. A trench four feet deep and a dozen yards wide stretched the length of the west side, against the brick wall. Cemetery workers had built a wooden roof over the trench, casting parts of it in contrasting shadow and bright sunlight. Inside the trench stood eight earthen mounds. Scores of skeletons, some fully exposed, some with an arm or leg bone poking out of the dry brown earth, lay in small mesas carved out of the ground. In some places, bones were jumbled together in heaps like a game of pickup sticks. Shreds of clothing, shoes, sandals, a raincoat, belt buckles, nylon stockings, and a scarf adorned some of the bones. Many of the skulls showed single gunshot wounds to the head. In the shadows of the trench, an army of red ants crawled from bone to bone.

"We found a skeleton with its hands and feet cut off," Luis explained as he walked with Snow along the lip of the trench. Snow whistled softly at what he saw. It was just as the gravedigger said: they were thrown in head to foot.

"We found the first bones in *cuadrícula* C9," Pato said, as she joined the two men. "That was last April. Since then we have found about seventy."[7] The team had left each skeleton exactly as excavated to record its position while combing the nearby earth for artifacts that might hold clues to identity or cause of death. They had collected many bullets, which they kept in plastic film containers.

At the edge of one mound, several skulls rested one on top of the other. The team had named it *la cascada*, or the cascade. "This mound is like the Picasso painting," said Mimi, pointing to the next mound. "Like *Guernica*." She turned to yet another mound to point out a skull that had been broken. "This is from our 'terror team,' " she said, referring to Luis and Ale, who had developed a reputation for digging a little too vigorously. "And here, these are tires that were burned. They tried to burn some of the bodies to cover up the stench after they were put in the holes."

Water had been the team's worst enemy. Sometimes after a heavy rain, carefully maintained balk walls and mounds had crumbled, pushing the skeletons out of their original position. Days were lost as the team reconstructed their previous configuration. The ants, whose bites left painful welts, had made life difficult as well. The team had spread ant poison in the trench and varnished some of the exposed bones, a practice common in archaeology, to protect them.

The provincial authorities had finally come through with money. Plumbers were installing water pipes in the morgue, which the team had also painted. In contrast to the support from the community, however, the undersecretariat had dropped any pretense whatsoever of helping the team. The previous July, the newspaper *Página 12* printed a letter from Eduardo Rabossi criticizing them. "It is deplorable," he wrote, "that this painful subject is being used once again by the EAAF for their personal and collective advancement."[8] Snow, however, couldn't let that aspersion go unchallenged, especially since Rabossi had never even observed one of the team's exhumations. The month after Rabossi's complaint, Snow told a *Página 12* reporter that the subsecretariat didn't have the stomach to pursue real human rights cases, and was instead "transforming people into paper."[9]

Morris, shirtless and showing his usual enthusiasm, joined the tour. "This one is totally unusual," he told Snow as they stopped to examine a skeleton with its arms across its chest. "Our hypothesis is that this burial is part of an old cemetery. It's an old person, the arms are folded across the chest, and there's part of a casket. The bones are very fragile, as if they have been there for a long, long time." It was now clear that the sector had once been a part of the main cemetery, probably catering to the poor. Mimi said that cemetery records listed the names and addresses of about sixty people buried here legitimately. That would surely complicate the search for the disappeared among them. Also, in one corner of the sector they had found the skeletons of several infants buried together, without coffins, whose origin remained a mystery.

Snow stood surveying the scene, shaking his head. It was almost more than he could take in all at once. As difficult as the excavation had been, the challenge of sorting out identities loomed even larger. First, Snow supposed, they would have to separate the bones of the "legitimate" burials from those of the *desaparecidos*. Age at death and evidence of bullet wounds would be the first way to discriminate. Already he had seen several bullet wounds and at least one skeleton bearing signs of osteomyelitis. Also, indigents who died anonymously in hospitals usually weren't buried with shoes, which might prove helpful in making distinctions. The team also had discovered the dates, all between 1976 and 1978, when nineteen of the "cowholes" had been dug. But the records don't say which hole was which.

As they left the courtyard, Snow turned to view the scene a last time. The year's work had produced a well-laid-out site. The team had stuck with it, persisting despite the obstacles and the indifference that might have discouraged a less dedicated group. What they still faced would require even more of that kind of diligence. But the work had continued to reward their efforts. The National Academy of Sciences of Argentina had named them *ad honorem* investigators the previous year. The team's sweetest victory had come, however, in May 1988 when, with the help of their report on María Mercedes Hourquebie de Francese, whose skeleton was the first dug from Avellaneda, and Snow's statistical survey of N.N. graves, Suárez Mason was finally extradited from San Francisco to Buenos Aires to stand trial for murder, torture, and kidnapping. And now they were becoming internationally renowned, their unique skills in demand in other countries where families were trying to recover the remains of their disappeared relatives. In a week, the team would be going to Chile to help human rights groups investigate the hundreds of disappearances that took place shortly after the military took power in 1973. And there was interest from the Bolivian government for help investigating reputed executions at prison camps.

They walked through the cemetery gates on their afternoon pilgrimage to the Mathias Café. Morris paused to scrape mud off the sole of his shoe. "This cemetery dirt really sticks to you," he said.

"Yep," replied Snow, "sooner or later it does."

Mimi, Pato, and Luis sit on a grassy bank overlooking a stream in the lush El Tigre delta where the Paraná and Plate rivers meet and eventually flow past Buenos Aires to the Atlantic. At the water's edge, his feet dangling in the stream, Snow is well into a crime novel about a man dressed in a Santa Claus suit who holds up a Texas bank.

The group, faced with three consecutive days of rain, has abandoned its digging in Avellaneda to gather for a brief holiday at a small cottage owned by Morris's father. A low ceiling of clouds casts the breezeless summer day in a milky light. As Snow reads, his companions watch leaves and small branches collect in an eddy near his feet. Three empty bottles of Valentín Bianchi wine sit beside them.

The Argentines are recounting their dreams, something they do when the mood strikes. Luis, who dreams constantly about their work, describes his latest. He is sitting in a café in the Florida district with a beautiful woman beside him. He leans forward to kiss her. But just before their lips meet, she turns into a skeleton. Pato arches an eyebrow in Luis's direction. Still, she agrees that his dream tops his previous best, in which he sells all the bones.

Mimi goes next. She has had two dreams recently. One is recurring. A new military coup has toppled the civilian government and the police have captured the other members of the team and are holding them hostage. Only Mimi, who hasn't been found, can save them. Fighting her impulse to flee for her own life, she rushes through the streets of Buenos Aires searching frantically for her friends.

She then recounts her latest dream. It takes place at her sister's house. She is sleeping and is awakened by a noise from the closet. The closet door opens and a skeleton dressed in a woman's clothes walks out and dances around her bed. Mimi sits up, pulls her knees to her chest, and watches.

Pato draws a cigarette with her spidery fingers from an old fash-ioned metal box labeled "Sonny Boy." She lights it, inhales deeply, and describes her dream. A girlfiend needs an abortion and Pato gives her money. The girl calls Pato to the hospital. When she arrives, the doctor tells her that her friend needs blood, and that Pato is the only one who can give it. The doctor wraps a rubber cord around Pato's arm to raise the veins and turns to get a needle. Pato looks down and sees a baby's bones emerging from her arm.

The three Argentines fall silent and watch the eddies break the surface of the muddy stream as the rising tide pushes its waters up the bank.

"Clyde, do you ever dream?" Pato asks.

"Sure," Snow replies. "Just last night I dreamt I'd gone to hell but they threw me out."

Mimi smiles and translates for the others. "Why didn't they let you stay?" she asks Snow.

"Simple. My Visa card had expired."

The sun, as if cued by their laughter, breaks through the cloudy El Tigre sky. Shivering, Pato pulls her shawl over her shoulders.

"How can the sun make you cold?" Luis asks, wrapping his arm around her.

"Because it means we'll be digging again."

Snow looks up from his page. With a willow branch, he leans over the swirling knot of debris near his feet and pushes it free. They watch as it slowly floats downstream, out of sight, toward the sea.

NOTES

Chapter One

1. Texas Department of Highways and Public Transportation, *Texas Travel Handbook*, p. 63.

2. Clyde C. Snow, Herbert M. Reynolds, and Mackie A. Allgood, "Anthropometry of Airline Stewardesses," Office of Aviation Medicine, Federal Aviation Administration, AM 75-2, March 1975.

3. Clyde C. Snow, John Carroll, and Mackie Allgood, "Survival in Emergency Escape from Passenger Aircraft," Office of Aviation Medicine, Federal Aviation Administration, AM 70-16, October 1970.

4. Clyde C. Snow, "Forensic Anthropology," *Annual Review of Anthropology*, 1982; 11:97–131.

5. Clyde C. Snow and James L. Luke, "The Oklahoma City Child Disappearances of 1967: Forensic Anthropology in the Identification of Skeletal Remains," *Journal of Forensic Sciences*, 1970; 15(2):125–153.

6. John W. Forney, interview by the authors, March 1989.

Chapter Two

1. Jürgen Thornwald, *Century of the Detective* (New York: Harcourt, Brace & World, 1965), p. 201.

2. Orville T. Bailey, "Brahma, Parkman and Webster: Murder in Medical Boston," *Journal of the American Medical Association*, 1972; 220(1):70–74.

3. Hon. Robert Sullivan, "The Murder Trial of Dr. Webster, Boston, 1850," *Massachusetts Law Quarterly*, 1966; 51(4):367–396, and 1967; 52(1): 67–96.

4. Clyde C. Snow, "Forensic Anthropology," *Annual Review of Anthropology*, 1982; 11:97–131.

5. Ibid., p. 104.

6. T. W. Todd and D. W. Lyon, "Cranial Suture Closure: Its Progress and Age Relationship," Part IV, *American Journal of Physical Anthropology*,

1925; 8(2):149–168. Cited in Wilton M. Krogman, *The Human Skeleton in Forensic Medicine* (Springfield, Ill.: Charles C. Thomas, 1962), p. 76.

7. Robert Jay Lifton, *The Nazi Doctors: Medical Killing and the Psychology of Genocide* (New York: Basic Books, 1986), p. 17.

8. Krogman, *The Human Skeleton in Forensic Medicine*, p. 89.

9. Stephen Jay Gould, *The Mismeasure of Man* (New York: W. W. Norton & Company, 1981), pp. 122–143.

10. I. Taylor, P. Walton, and J. Young, *The New Criminology: For a Social Theory of Deviance* (London: Routlege and Kegan Paul, 1973), p. 41. Cited in Gould, *The Mismeasure of Man*, p. 124.

11. Cesar Lombroso, *Crime: Its Causes and Remedies* (Boston: Little, Brown, 1911), p. 437. Cited in Gould, *The Mismeasure of Man*, p. 139.

12. Henry T. F. Rhodes, *Alphonse Bertillon* (New York: Abelard-Schuman, 1956), p. 76.

13. Thornwald, *Century of the Detective*, p. 20.

14. Rhodes, *Alphonse Bertillon*, p. 146.

Chapter Three

1. T. Dale Stewart, "Forensic Anthropology," in *The Uses of Anthropology*, ed. Walter Goldschmidt (Washington, D.C.: American Anthropological Association, 1979, publication no. 10), pp. 169–183.

2. J. H. Wigmore, "The Luetgert Case," *American Law Review*, 1898; 32:187–207.

3. T. Dale Stewart, "George A. Dorsey's Role in the Luetgert Case: A Significant Episode in the History of Forensic Anthropology," *Journal of Forensic Sciences*, 1978; 23:786–791.

4. Clyde C. Snow, "Forensic Anthropology," *Annual Review of Anthropology*, 1982; 11:100.

5. Stewart, "Forensic Anthropology," p. 787.

6. Victor Cohn, *News and Numbers* (Ames, Iowa: Iowa State University Press, 1989), pp. 14–15.

7. T. Dale Stewart, ed., *Personal Identification in Mass Disasters* (Washington, D.C.: Smithsonian Institution, Museum of Natural History, 1970), p. 100 (report of a seminar).

8. Wilton M. Krogman, *The Human Skeleton in Forensic Medicine* (Springfield, Ill.: Charles C. Thomas, 1962), p. 162.

9. Ibid., p. 93.

10. Krogman, *The Human Skeleton in Forensic Medicine*. Cited by Curtis W. Wienker, "Sex Determination from Human Skeletal Remains: A Case of Mistaken Assumption," in *Human Identification — Case Studies in Forensic*

Anthropology, eds. Ted A. Rathbun and Jane E. Buikstra (Springfield, Ill.: Charles C. Thomas, 1984), pp. 229–243.

11. Eugene Giles, "Discriminant Function Sexing of the Human Skeleton," in *Personal Identification in Mass Disasters*, p. 100.

12. Stephen Jay Gould, *The Mismeasure of Man* (New York: W. W. Norton & Company, 1981), p. 50.

13. Krogman, *The Human Skeleton in Forensic Medicine*, p. 206.

14. David D. Thompson, "Forensic Anthropology," in *A History of American Physical Anthropology, 1930–1980*, ed. Frank Spenser (New York: Academic Press, Inc., 1982), pp. 358–359.

15. Stewart, "Forensic Anthropology," p. 175.

16. Mildred Trotter and Goldine Gleser, "A Reevaluation of Estimation of Stature Based on Measurements of Stature Taken During Life and of Long Bones After Death," *American Journal of Physical Anthropology*, 1958; 16(1):79–123.

17. Mildred Trotter, "Estimation of Stature from Intact Long Limb Bones," in *Personal Identification in Mass Disasters*, pp. 71–84.

18. Trotter and Gleser, "A Reevaluation of Estimation of Stature," pp. 79–123.

19. Thomas W. McKern, "Estimation of Skeletal Age from Combined Maturational Activity," *American Journal of Physical Anthropology*, 1957; 13:399–408.

20. Douglas Ubelaker, *Human Skeletal Remains: Excavation, Analysis, Interpretation* (Chicago: Aldine Publishing, 1978), p. 53.

21. T. Dale Stewart, "Medico-legal Aspects of the Skeleton," *American Journal of Physical Anthropology*, 1948; 6(3):315–322.

Chapter Four

1. Fred Jordan, interview by the authors, August 1988.

2. "American Airlines DC-10 Crashes After Takeoff at O'Hare," and related stories, *Chicago Tribune*, May 26, 1979, sec. N1, pp. 1–5.

3. Aircraft Accident Report, American Airlines, DC-10, N110AA, May 25, 1979, National Transportation Safety Board (NTSB-AAR-79-17).

4. Lowell J. Levine, "Forensic Odontology Today — A 'New' Forensic Science," *FBI Law Enforcement Bulletin*, August 1972, p. 7.

5. Elaine Markoutsas, "Grim Pursuit of Identities on Flight 191," *Chicago Tribune*, June 18, 1979, sec. 2, p. 1.

6. John J. Fitzpatrick, "Role of Radiology in Human Rights Abuse," *American Journal of Forensic Medicine and Pathology*, 1984; 5(4):321–325.

7. Douglas H. Ubelaker, "Positive Identification from the Radiographic Comparison of Frontal Sinus Patterns," in *Human Identification — Case Studies in Forensic Anthropology*, eds. Ted A. Rathbun and Jane E. Buikstra (Springfield, Ill.: Charles C. Thomas, 1984), pp. 399–411.

8. John J. Fitzpatrick, interview by the authors, January 1989.

9. Robert Kirschner, interview by the authors, January 1989.

Chapter Five

1. "Contractor Is Charged with Murder," and related stories, *Chicago Tribune*, December 23, 1978, sec. N1, p. 1.

2. "Few Parents of Missing Youths Contact Police in Mass Murder Case," *Chicago Tribune*, December 30, 1978, sec. N1, p. 5.

3. "Cook County Examiner Uses Facial Experts to Identify Murder Victims," *Chicago Tribune*, January 26, 1979, sec. N1, p. 1.

4. Clyde C. Snow, "Human Skeleton from Cook County, Illinois, 79–23, C.C.M.E. Case #1378 of December 1978, Body #17." Examination report to Cook County Medical Examiner, January 2, 1980.

5. John J. Fitzpatrick, interview by the authors, January 1989.

6. T. Dale Stewart, "Indications of Handedness," *Essentials of Forensic Anthropology* (Springfield, Ill.: Charles C. Thomas, 1979), pp. 239–244.

7. Stewart, *Essentials of Forensic Anthropology*, pp. 258–271.

8. Betty Pat Gatliff, interview by the authors, August 1988.

9. J. S. Rhine and H. R. Campbell, "Thickness of Facial Tissues in American Blacks," *Journal of Forensic Sciences*, 1980; 25(4):847–858.

10. M. F. A. Montagu, "A Study of Man Embracing Error," *Technical Review*, 1947; 49(6):345–347.

11. Wilton M. Krogman, "A Problem in Human Skeletal Remains," *FBI Law Enforcement Bulletin*, June 1948, pp. 7–12.

12. Clyde C. Snow, Betty P. Gatliff, and Kenneth R. McWilliams, "Reconstruction of Facial Features from the Skull: An Evaluation of its Usefulness in Forensic Anthropology," *American Journal of Physical Anthropology*, 1970; 33(2):221–227.

13. Clyde C. Snow, Betty P. Gatliff, and Frank Young, "Case History: Victim Identification through Facial Restoration," Civil Aeromedical Institute, FAA, January 1977 (Paper presented at the meeting of the American Academy of Forensic Sciences, San Diego, California, February 15–19, 1977), pp. 1–21.

14. E. N. Earley, "Murder Victim's Face No Longer Mystery," *Tulsa Tribune*, September 16, 1976, p. 1.

15. Gatliff interview, August 1988.

NOTES

Chapter Six

1. Clyde C. Snow, "The Life and Afterlife of Elmer J. McCurdy — A Melodrama in Two Acts," Special Supplement, Paleopathology Association, Detroit, Michigan, September 1977.

2. Joseph H. Choi, Forensic Laboratory Analysis Report C.C. NO. 76–14812, John Doe #255, FLC NO. 76–178, December 9, 1976.

3. Richard Campbell, "Sixty-five-Year 'Run' About to End in Rest," *Los Angeles Herald Examiner*, December 19, 1976, p. 17.

4. Snow, "The Life and Afterlife of Elmer J. McCurdy," p. 56.

5. "Amusement Park Dummy Found to Be Oklahoma Gunman Elmer McCurdy," *Los Angeles Times*, April 14, 1977, sec. 2, p. 1.

6. Judy Suchey, interview by the authors, September 1988.

7. Thomas D. Burrows and Donald N. Wood, *Television Production: Disciplines and Techniques* (Dubuque, Iowa: William C. Brown Publishers, 1978), pp. 149–170.

8. Arthur H. Lamb, *Tragedies of the Osage Hills* (Pawhuska, Okla.: Osage Printery, n.d.), pp. 193 et. seq. (In the Western history collection at the University of Oklahoma.)

9. "Tells of Taking Bandit M'Curdy," *Tulsa Daily World*, October 15, 1911, p. 10.

10. Lamb, *Tragedies of the Osage Hills*, p. 194.

11. "Desperado Body Finally Laid to Rest," *Lubbock* (Tex.) *Avalanche Journal*, April 23, 1977.

Chapter Seven

1. Robert M. Utley, *Custer Battlefield* (Washington, D.C.: Division of Publications, National Park Service, U.S. Department of the Interior, 1988, Handbook 132).

2. Douglas Scott, Melissa Connor, and Clyde C. Snow, "Nameless Faces of Custer Battlefield," *Greasy Grass, Annual for the Battlefield Dispatch* (Hardin, Mont.: Custer Battlefield Historical & Museum Association, May 1988), pp. 1–4.

3. Douglas Scott, interview by the authors, June 1989.

4. Clyde C. Snow and John J. Fitzpatrick, "Human Osteological Remains from the Battle of the Little Bighorn," in *Archaeological Perspectives on the Battle of the Little Bighorn*, eds. Douglas D. Scott, Richard A. Fox, Jr., Melissa A. Connor, and Dick Harmon (Norman, Okla.: University of Oklahoma Press, 1989), pp. 243–281.

5. Betty Pat Gatliff, interview by the authors, September 1988.

6. Snow and Fitzpatrick, p. 247.

NOTES

Chapter Eight

1. Alan Riding, "Key Man in Mengele Case: Romeu Tuma," *New York Times*, June 16, 1985, p. 3.

2. Ralph Blumenthal, interview by the authors, August 1988.

3. Mark Berkowitz, president, CANDLES (Children of Auschwitz Nazi Deadly Lab Experiment Survivors), prepared statement before the United States Senate, Subcommittee on Juvenile Justice, February 19, 1985.

4. Robert Jay Lifton, "What Made This Man? Mengele," *New York Times Magazine*, July 21, 1985, p. 21.

5. Robert Jay Lifton, *The Nazi Doctors: Medical Killing and the Psychology of Genocide* (New York: Basic Books, 1986), p. 22.

6. Arrest warrant and indictment issued in Frankfurt am Main on January 19, 1981, by the *Landgericht 22 Strafkammer* (State Court Number 22), file number (22)50/L Js340/68.

7. Gerald L. Posner and John Ware, *Mengele: The Complete Story* (New York: Dell Publishing Company, Inc., 1986), p. 62.

8. Richard Allan White, interview by the authors, December 1988.

9. Peggy C. Caldwell, report on photo comparison of possible Mengele suspects, February 3, 1985, in possession of the authors.

10. Ellis R. Kerley, report on photo comparison of possible Mengele suspects, February 3, 1985, in possession of the authors.

11. White interview, December 1988.

12. Neil Sher, quoted by Associated Press, April 22, 1985.

13. Hans Ebhard Klein, quoted by Posner and Ware, *Mengele: The Complete Story*, p. 334.

14. Posner and Ware, *Mengele: The Complete Story*, p. 336.

15. Morgan Hardiman, interview by the authors, November 1988.

16. Stephen S. Trott, Assistant Attorney General, Criminal Division, U.S. Department of Justice, prepared statement before the U.S. Senate, Subcommittee on Juvenile Justice, March 19, 1985.

17. Leslie Lukash, interview by the authors, August 1988.

18. Clyde C. Snow, interviewed by Charles Gibson for ABC-TV's *Nightline*, June 7, 1985.

19. Menachem Russek, quoted in Posner and Ware, *Mengele: The Complete Story*, p. 340.

20. Staff member of the U.S. Department of Justice, Office of Special Investigations, interview by the authors, November 1988.

21. Lowell J. Levine, interview by the authors, August 1988.

22. Blumenthal interview, August 1988.

23. David A. Crown, "Practical Aspects of the Mengele Handwriting Examination," *Journal of Forensic Science Society*, 1987; 27:5–11.

24. David A. Crown, "The Identification of the Handwriting of Josef Mengele," *Journal of Forensic Sciences*, 1987; 32:113–117.

25. Richard House, "U.S. Experts Identify Handwriting as Mengele's," *Washington Post*, June 15, 1985, p. A15.

26. One of the authors, Eric Stover, was present during the meeting at the Medico-Legal Institute in São Paulo on June 15, 1985, and for the duration of the scientific examination of the purported remains of Josef Mengele, which ended on June 21, 1985.

27. "Various Documents Concerning Josef Mengele's Genealogy and Racial Fitness" (*"Verschiedene Dokumente hinsichtlich der Genealogie und Rasentauglichkeit des Josef Mengele"*), 1938, Berlin Documentation Center archives, Berlin, in possession of authors.

28. Posner and Ware, *Mengele: The Complete Story*, p. 16.

29. David G. Marwell, memorandum to Mengele file, June 10, 1985, file number 146-2-47-145, Office of Special Investigations archives, Washington, D.C., in possession of the authors.

30. Donald J. Ortner and Walter G. J. Putschar, *Identification of Pathological Conditions in Human Skeletal Remains* (Washington, D.C.: Smithsonian Institution Press, 1981), pp. 105–129.

31. Ellis R. Kerley, "Osteomyelitis," unpublished report attached as "Exhibit K" in a report to the U.S. Attorney General, entitled "Examination of the Human Skeletal Remains Exhumed at Nossa Senhora do Rosario Cemetery, Embú, Brazil on 6 June 1985," by the forensic consultants representing the United States Marshals Service and Office of Special Investigations, the U.S. Department of Justice, and the Simon Wiesenthal Center, November 6, 1986, in possession of the authors.

Chapter Nine

1. Thomas Dwight, "The Size of the Articular Surface of the Long Bones As Characteristics of Sex: An Anthropological Study," *American Journal of Anthropology*, 1905; 4:19–32.

2. Stay of proceedings issued by SS and Police Court XV in Breslau (St. L.I7/43), dated September 28, 1943, in possession of the authors.

3. Lowell J. Levine, interview by authors, August 1988.

4. Ellis R. Kerley, "The Microscopic Determination of Age in Human Bone," *American Journal of Physical Anthropology*, 1965; 23:149–163; Ellis R. Kerley and Douglas H. Ubelaker, "Revisions in the Microscopic Method of Estimating Age at Death in Human Cortical Bone," *American Journal of Physical Anthropology*, 1978; 49:545–546.

5. Interview with Wolfram and Lisolette Bossert and Gitta Stammer at

the Medico-Legal Institute in São Paulo on June 18, 1985, by one of the authors, Eric Stover, and the forensic specialists sponsored by the Simon Wiesenthal Center and the governments of Brazil, the United States, and West Germany.

6. Richard Helmer, *Schadelidentifizierung durch elektronische Bildmischung: zugleich ein Beltrag zur Konstitutionsbiometrie und Dickenmessung der Gesichtsweichteile* (Heidelberg: Kriminalistik-Verlag, 1984).

7. One of the authors, Eric Stover, was present at the meeting of the American scientists at the U.S. Consulate in São Paulo, Brazil on June 20, 1985.

8. Leslie Lukash, interview by the authors, August 1988.

9. Telex from Rabbi Marvin Hier to Simon Wiesenthal delegation of forensic scientists, dated June 20, 1985, in possession of the authors.

10. The Federal Criminal Office of the Federal Republic of Germany, "Photo Analysis of an Unidentified Male," Case M-74 186 f.A., 7310.2–70/85, 1985, Frankfurt, in the possession of the authors.

11. "Examination of the Human Skeletal Remains Exhumed at Nossa Senhora do Rosario Cemetery, Embú, Brazil, on 6 June 1985: A Preliminary Report to Dr. Romeu Tuma, Superintendent, Federal Police in São Paulo, Brazil," submitted June 21, 1985, by the forensic science consultants sent by the Simon Wiesenthal Center and the United States Marshals Service, U.S. Department of Justice, on their studies carried out June 15–21, 1985, in the possession of the authors.

Chapter Ten

1. Lowell J. Levine, interview by the authors, August 1988.

2. "Israel Says It Reserves Judgment on Mengele," *New York Times*, June 24, 1985, sec. 1, p. 4.

3. "Meese Says U.S. Concurs on Mengele," *New York Times*, June 22, 1985, sec. 1, p. 8.

4. "Center '99 Percent' Sure," *New York Times*, June 22, 1985, sec. 1, p. 8.

5. David Marwell, "Evidence of Osteomyelitis," memorandum to Mengele file, Department of Justice, August 14, 1985, in possession of the authors.

6. Donald J. Ortner, "Observations on the Purported Skeleton of Josef Mengele, 14 January 1986–15 January 1986" (unpublished), in possession of the authors.

7. Donald J. Ortner, interview by the authors, October 1988.

8. David Marwell, "Medical Information from Mengele's Diaries and

Correspondence," memorandum to Mengele file, Department of Justice, August 14, 1985, in possession of the authors.

9. Idelle Davidson, "Shadowing the Angel of Death," *Pursuits*, Winter 1989, pp. 21–25.

10. Stephen Dachi, interview by the authors, July 1989.

Chapter Eleven

1. Federico García Lorca, *Selected Poems* (San Francisco: New Directions, 1952), p. 85.

2. Clyde C. Snow, "Forensic Anthropology in the Documentation of Human Rights Abuses" (Paper presented at the Annual Meeting of the American Association for the Advancement of Science, New York, May 27, 1984).

3. "Mrs. Perón Took Overthrow Calmly," *Buenos Aires Herald*, March 26, 1974, p. 1.

4. Marysa Navarro, "Evita and Peronism," in *Juan Perón and the Reshaping of Argentina*, eds. Frederick C. Turner and José Enrique Miquens (Pittsburgh: University of Pittsburgh Press, 1983), pp. 15–32.

5. The National Commission on the Disappeared, *Nunca Más* (London: Faber and Faber, 1986), pp. 51–208.

6. Marketa Freund, "The Law and Human Rights in Argentina," *Worldview*, May 1979, pp. 37–41.

7. The National Commission on the Disappeared, *Nunca Más*, pp. 29–31.

8. Ibid., p. 159.

9. Jacobo Timerman, *Prisoner Without a Name, Cell Without a Number* (New York: Alfred A. Knopf, Inc., 1981), p. 148.

10. The National Commission on the Disappeared, *Nunca Más*, pp. 121–131.

11. Ibid., p. 223.

12. Letter from Córdoba morgue workers to President Jorge Rafael Videla, June 30, 1980, file number 0126, National Commission on the Disappeared, Córdoba.

13. Francisco Rubén Bossio, deposition taken by the National Commission on the Disappeared, January 19, 1984, Córdoba, in possession of the authors.

14. Albano Jorge Harguindeguy, quoted in *"Disappearances": A Workbook* (New York: Amnesty International USA, 1981), pp. 11–12.

15. "Huge Crowds Celebrate Return to Democracy," *Buenos Aires Herald*, December 11, 1983, p. 1.

16. Lowell J. Levine, interview by the authors, August 1988.

17. Gustavo Angel R. Piccolo, deposition taken by the National Commission on the Disappeared, April 24, 1984, Villa Devoto, file number 3189.

18. Martin Andersen, "Letter from Argentina," *Boston Phoenix*, April 10, 1984, pp. 6–7.

19. Leslie Lukash, interview by the authors, August 1988.

20. Levine interview, August 1988.

21. Eric Stover, "The Disappeared of Argentina: Not Without Trace," *New Scientist*, November 15, 1984, pp. 14–15.

22. Hugo Rodolfo Ciarroca, deposition taken by the National Commission on the Disappeared, July 16, 1984, Rosario, file number 006527.

23. María Isabel "Chicha" Chorbik de Mariani, interview by the authors, April 1988.

24. Ana María Di Lonardo, Pierre Darlu, Max Baur, et al., "Human Genetics and Human Rights: Identifying the Families of Kidnapped Children," *American Journal of Forensic Medicine and Pathology*, 1984; 5: 339–347.

25. Rubén Lavallén, interviewed on "All Things Considered," National Public Radio, October, 1985.

26. Patricia Bernardi, interview by the authors, March 1988.

27. Morris Tidball Binz, interview by the authors, March 1988.

28. Mercedes Doretti, interview by the authors, March 1988.

Chapter Twelve

1. The National Commission on the Disappeared, *Nunca Más* (London: Faber and Faber, 1986), p. 289.

2. Testimonies of Ana María Martí and Sara Solarz de Osatinsky provided to the Abuelas de Plaza de Mayo in 1979, in possession of authors.

3. Hebe de Bonafini, "No Vamos a Claudicar," *Madres de Plaza de Mayo* newsletter, December 1984.

4. María Julia Bihurriet, interview by the authors, March 1988.

5. Mercedes Doretti, interview by the authors, March 1988.

6. Bihurriet interview, March 1988.

7. Luis Fondebrider, interview by the authors, March 1988.

8. Coche Pereyra, interview by the authors, March 1988.

9. See Néstor J. Montenegro, *Sera Justicia* (Buenos Aires: Editorial Distal, 1986), pp. 87–185.

10. Julio C. Strassera, quoted in Néstor J. Montenegro, *Sera Justicia*, p. 19.

11. Clyde C. Snow's videotaped testimony at the trial of the military juntas, April 24, 1985, is in the possession of the authors.

Chapter Thirteen

1. Clyde Snow and María Julia Bihurriet, "An Epidemiography of Homicide: *Ningun Nombre* Burials in the Province of Buenos Aires from 1970 to 1984," (unpublished, 1987).

2. "Fueron hallados 30 cadaveres en Pilar," *La Opinión*, August 8, 1976.

3. "La versión del comisario difiere de la del medico," *La Razón*, May 16, 1985, p. 13.

4. *La Opinión* (see n. 2.)

5. "Fueron identificados 3 cadaveres sepultados como N.N. en Derqui," *La Prensa*, September 28, 1983, p. 8.

6. Equipo Argentino de Antropología Forense, "The Fátima Case: A Brief Report," (unpublished, 1987), in possession of the authors.

7. Equipo Argentino de Antropología Forense, "A Forensic Anthropology Approach to Past Human Rights Violations in Argentina: The Spagnoli de Vera Case" (unpublished, June 22, 1987), in possession of the authors.

8. Clyde C. Snow, interview by the Argentine writer Mauricio Cohen, February 1, 1989; transcript in possession of the authors.

9. Richard P. Claude, Eric Stover, June P. Lopez, *Health Professionals and Human Rights in the Philippines* (Washington, D.C.: American Association for the Advancement of Science, 1987), pp. 49–52.

10. See "Truth and Partial Justice in Argentina," a report by America's Watch, New York, August 1987, pp. 64–68.

11. Ibid., pp. 68–72.

12. Alejandro Inchaurregui, interview by the authors, April 1988.

13. Horacio Verbitsky, "Falta compromiso con los derechos humanos," *El Periodista de Buenos Aires*, July 24–30, 1987, p. 10.

14. Inchaurregui interview, April 1988.

Chapter Fourteen

1. Rafael M. Perrota Bengolea, the son of Rafael Perrota, signed deposition before the National Commission on the Disappeared (CONADEP), January 24, 1984, in possession of the authors.

2. Mercedes Doretti, interview by the authors, March 1988.

3. Equipo Argentino de Antropología Forense, "Primera Etapa de la Planificación General Peritaje Antropológico Forense en el Cementerio de Avellaneda, Provincia de Buenos Aires," (unpublished, 1988), in possession of the authors.

4. Doretti interview, March 1988.

5. Avellaneda cemetery worker, interview by the authors, April 1988.

NOTES

6. Camille Peri, "Getting to Know the Lord of Life and Death," *Mother Jones*, September 1988, pp. 35–42.

7. Patricia Bernardi, interview by the authors, January 1989.

8. Eduardo Rabossi, letter to the editors, *Página 12*, July 22, 1988, p. 24.

9. Clyde C. Snow quoted in Mauricio Cohen, "La guerra sucia no debe ser tapada," *Página 12*, August 5, 1988, p. 12.

APPENDIXES

APPENDIX 1

HUMAN SKULL

1. Frontal
2. Greater wing, sphenoid
3. Lacrimal
4. Nasal
5. Zygomatic
6. Maxilla
7. Alveolar process
8. Incisor
9. Canine
10. Premolar
11. Molar
12. Mental foramen
13. Mandible
14. Coronoid process
15. Condylar process
16. Styloid process
17. External auditory meatus
18. Mastoid process
19. External occipital protuberance
20. Occipital
21. Temporal
22. Parietal
23. Superciliary ridge
24. Supraorbital margin
25. Optic canal
26. Infraorbital margin
27. Infraorbital foramen
28. Nasal septum
29. Mental protuberance
30. Superior orbital fissure
31. Inferior orbital fissure
32. Supraorbital foramen

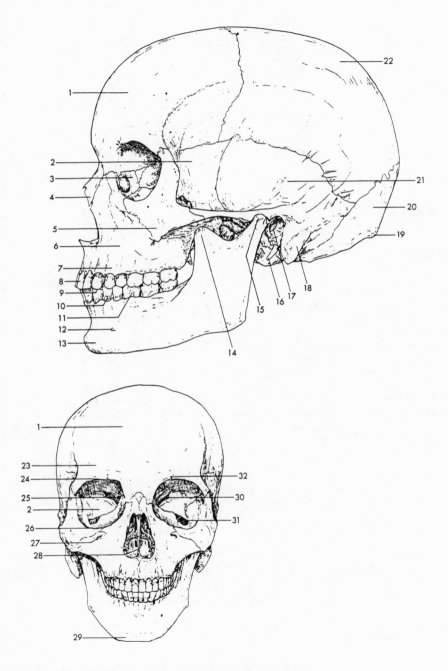

Illustration by Carolina Biological Supply Company, © 1991

321

APPENDIX 2

HUMAN SKELETON

1. Supraorbital for.
2. Optic for.
3. Sup. orbital fissure
4. Rotundum for.
5. Inf. orbital fissure
6. Ant. lacrimal ridge
7. Fossa for lacrimal sac
8. Infraorbital foramen and groove
9. Nasal cavity and inf. concha
10. Mandible
11. Condyle
12. Coronoid
13. Mandibular for. and lingula
14. Mental for.
15. Mylohyoid groove
16. Frontal sinus
17. Openings of maxillary sinus
18. Maxillary sinus
19. Pterygoid hamulus
20. Openings of post. ethmoid cells
21. Sphenopalatine for.
22. Sphenoid sinus and opening into nose
23. Sup. concha
24. Nasal bone
25. Middle concha and openings of nasofrontal duct and ant. ethmoid cells
26. Bulla ethmoidalis (openings of middle ethmoid cells)
27. Inf. concha and opening of nasolacrimal duct
28. Incisive for.
29. For. cecum
30. Crista galli and olfactory n. for.
31. Greater and lesser palatine for.
32. Zygomatic arch
33. Nasal septum
34. Ant. clinoid process
35. Pituitary fossa
36. For. ovale
37. Post. clinoid process
38. For. spinosum and groove for middle meningeal a.
39. For. lacerum
40. Orifice for Eustachian tube
41. For. carotid
42. Ext. auditory meatus
43. Styloid process
44. Jugular fossa
45. Occipital condyle and fossa
46. Mastoid process and stylomastoid for.
47. Petrous portion temporal bone and groove for sup. petrosal sinus
48. Int. auditory meatus
49. Hypoglossal canal
50. Jugular foramen
51. Foramen magnum
52. Mastoid foramen
53. Groove for occipital sinus
54. Groove for transverse sinus
55. Groove for sup. sagittal sinus
56. Orbit
57. Ant. and middle ethmoid cells
58. Middle concha

Anterior View

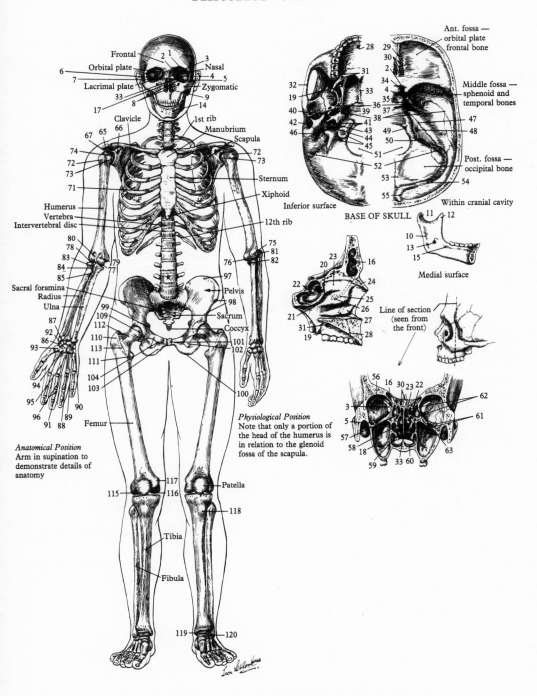

Anatomical Position
Arm in supination to
demonstrate details of
anatomy

Physiological Position
Note that only a portion of
the head of the humerus is
in relation to the glenoid
fossa of the scapula.

BASE OF SKULL
Inferior surface
Within cranial cavity
Medial surface
Line of section
(seen from
the front)

Schlossberg, Leon, and George D. Zuidema. *The Johns Hopkins Atlas of Human
Functional Anatomy*, 3rd ed. The Johns Hopkins University Press, Baltimore/London, 1986

59. Inf. concha
60. Nasal floor
61. Ant. ethmoid cells
62. Post. ethmoid cells
63. Lamina papyracea
64. Ext. occipital protuberance
65. Acromion
66. Coracoid process
67. Glenoid cavity
68. Spine
69. Inf. angle
70. Vert. and axillary borders
71. Costal cart.
72. Greater tubercle
73. Lesser tubercle
74. Head
75. Lat. epicondyle
76. Med. epicondyle
77. Trochlea
78. Capitulum
79. Coronoid fossa
80. Radial fossa
81. Olecranon
82. Coronoid process
83. Head
84. Neck
85. Radial tuberosity
86. Styloid processes
87. Navicular
88. Lunate
89. Triangular
90. Pisiform
91. Hamate
92. Capitate
93. Greater multangular
94. Lesser multangular
95. Metacarpal
96. Phalanges
97. Crest of ilium
98. Ant., sup., and inf. spines
99. Spine of ischium
100. Tuberosity of ischium

101. Symphysis pubis
102. Obturator foramen
103. Inf. ramus of pubis
104. Sub. ramus of pubis and pubic tubercle
105. Post., sup., and inf. spines
106. Greater sciatic notch
107. Sacral and coccygeal cornua
108. Sacral hiatus leading to caudal canal
109. Head of femur in acetabulum
110. Greater tronchanter
111. Lesser trochanter
112. Neck
113. Intertrochanteric line
114. Intertrochanteric crest
115. Lat. epicondyle
116. Med. epicondyle
117. Adductor tubercle
118. Tuberosity
119. Med. malleolus
120. Lat. malleolus
121. Talus
122. Calcaneus
123. Navicular
124. 1st cuneiform
125. 2nd cuneiform
126. 3rd cuneiform
127. Cuboid
128. Trans. process, pedicle, foramen, and groove for spinal n.
129. Vertebral foramen
130. Lamina
131. Spinous process
132. Sup. articular facet
133. Inf. articular facet
134. Odontoid process
135. Transverse process
136. Demi-facet for head of rib
137. Facet for articular part of tubercle of rib
138. Intervertebral foramen for spinal n.
139. Pedicle

Posterior and Lateral Views

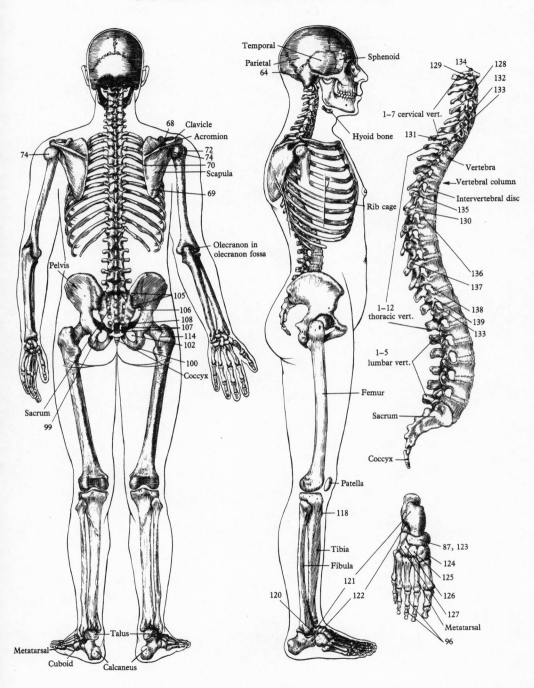

Schlossberg, Leon, and George D. Zuidema. *The Johns Hopkins Atlas of Human Functional Anatomy*, 3rd ed. The Johns Hopkins University Press, Baltimore/London, 1986

INDEX

INDEX

Bihurriet, María Julia, 255, 257–261, 270–271, 277
Binz, Morris Tidball. *See* Tidball, Morris
bite-mark identification, 96
blood, in forensic investigations, 71, 238–239
Blumenthal, Ralph (journalist), 150–151, 154–155, 157, 163–164, 201
blunt force trauma, 141
bones
  and determination of age, 34, 36, 53, 79, 86–88, 109, 119, 128, 141, 177–178, 183–184
  and disease, 78, 83
  and evolutionary changes, 24
  in forensic investigations, 3, 8, 33–38, 48–49, 71
  and determination of handedness, 111, 142, 178
  and determination of height, 35, 37, 53, 77–78, 84, 119, 141, 178
  identification of war dead, 83, 85
  and nutrition, 78, 83
  and pregnancy, evidence of, 275
  and determination of race, 53, 55, 80, 141–142, 178
  and racial destiny, 54
  and racial mixing, 78
  and determination of sex, 34–35, 53–54, 79, 89, 109, 177–178
  and signs of violence, 141
Bossert, Wolfram and Lisolette, 149–150, 158, 163–164, 178, 188–193
Boyer, Mitch, 140–144
brain size and criminality, 57
Brazil
  and Mengele, Josef, 149–150, 159

CAMI, 25–31, 91–92, 111, 116–117
Camps, General Ramón J., 269–270, 287, 290
Cantu, Antonio, 162
Caucasian, shape of skull, 80–81
Center for Social and Legal Studies
  Argentina, 232, 274
  Bolivia, 5
children, missing, 33–39. *See also* Abuelas
Choi, Dr. Joseph H. (medical examiner), 125–126
Civil Aeromedical Institute. *See* CAMI
computers
  in forensic investigations, 102–104, 270–274
CONADEP, 231–233, 236, 253–254, 273, 279, 289

coroners, 43–44
cranium. *See* skull
Crazy Horse, 137–139
criminal
  investigations, 3, 55, 69–75, 106–123
  photography, 67
criminal anthropology, 55–58
criminality
  and brain size, 57
  stigmata, physical, 55–58
Crown, David, 162–164
Custer, General George Armstrong, 135–146
Custer's Last Stand, 135–138

Dachi, Stephen (oral pathologist), 205–209
dactylography. *See* fingerprints
d'Amato, Senator Alphonse, 159–160, 162–163
death
  causes, 44–45, 125
  and decomposition, 38, 48
  manner, 44–45
death squads in Argentina, 220–225
decomposition and time of death, 38, 48
de Mello, Dr. José, 168, 170–171
dentistry. *See* teeth
deoxyribonucleic acid. *See* DNA
discriminant function analysis, 81, 109
disease and bones, 78, 83
DNA, 238
  and forensic investigations, 209–211
Doretti, Mercedes. *See* Mimi
Dorsey, George, 69, 71, 73–74
Dreyfus, Captain Alfred, 67
Dwight, Thomas (anatomist), 53–54, 69

Ecumenical Movement for Human Rights.
  See MEDH
El Diario del Juicio, 263
embalming and arsenic, 129
Endris, Rolf (odontologist), 163, 195
engineering and air safety, 27
Epstein, Gideon, 162–164
Equipo Argentino de Antropología Forense.
  See Argentine Forensic Anthropology Team
eugenics and Mengele, Josef, 152–153
evidence
  accuracy of, 74
  circumstantial, 71
  improper admission, 51
  and probability, 76
evolution and stigmata of criminality, 56

328

INDEX

INDEX

Vera, Marita, 255, 257–261
Videla, General Jorge Rafael, 221–227, 263
video superimposition, 143, 145, 163, 204
  by Helmer, Richard (forensic anthropologist), 193–196
Vietnam, 278
Viola, General Roberto Eduardo, 227, 263

Wagner, Gustav Franz (war criminal), 168
Weathermen, 96
Webster, John White, 45–52
Webster-Parkman case. *See* Parkman case
White, Richard, 155–157

Wiesenthal, Simon, 154, 157–158
work camps, 3–4
  closure, 8–9
  Granja de Espejos, 4–9
  treatment of inmates, 5–7
Wyman, Dr. Jeffries (anatomist), 48–49, 52–53

X rays
  use of antemortem, 100, 102–103, 181
  in forensic investigations, 83, 96, 99–103, 181–182, 204, 208, 235–236